# DIGESTIVE TRACT TUMORS

## GANN Monograph on Cancer Research

The "GANN Monograph on Cancer Research" series is promoted by the Japanese Cancer Association. This semiannual series of monographs was initiated in 1966 by the late Dr. Tomizo Yoshida (1903–1973) and is now published jointly by Japan Scientific Societies Press, Tokyo and Plenum Press, New York and London. Each volume consists of collected contributions on current topics in cancer problems and allied research fields. The publication of these monographs owes much to the financial support given by the late Professor Kazushige Higuchi, the Jikei University School of Medicine.

The planning for each volume is done by the Board of Executive Directors of the Japanese Cancer Association, with the final approval of the Board of Directors. It is hoped that the series will serve as an important source of information in the field of cancer research.

Japanese Cancer Association

JAPANESE CANCER ASSOCIATION
**GANN** Monograph on Cancer Research No.31

# DIGESTIVE TRACT TUMORS

FUNDAMENTAL AND CLINICAL ASPECTS

Edited by

KIYOSHI INOKUCHI
G. P. MURPHY
HARUO SUGANO
TAKASHI SUGIMURA
U. VERONESI

JAPAN SCIENTIFIC SOCIETIES PRESS, Tokyo
PLENUM PRESS, New York and London

ISBN 978-1-4684-5151-1          ISBN 978-1-4684-5149-8 (eBook)
DOI 10.1007/978-1-4684-5149-8
© JAPAN SCIENTIFIC SOCIETIES PRESS, 1986
Softcover reprint of the hardcover 1st edition 1986

January 1986

Published jointly by
JAPAN SCIENTIFIC SOCIETIES PRESS
2-10 Hongo, 6-chome, Bunkyo-ku, Tokyo 113, Japan
ISBN  978-1-4684-5151-1
        and
PLENUM PRESS
233 Spring Street, New York, NY 10013, USA
ISBN 978-1-4684-5151-1

Distributed in all areas outside Japan and Asia between Pakistan and Korea by PLENUM PRESS, New York and London.

# PREFACE

The problem of digestive tract tumors presents multifaceted aspects which involve epidemiology, pathogenesis, histopathology, surgery and adjuvant multidisciplinary modality. Time trends in cancer mortality vary in the individual cancers. Mortality from stomach cancer shows a decreasing tendency in most countries, although Japan still has the highest incidence in the world. Intestinal other than rectum and pancreatic cancers have shown an increase in most countries, while mortality due to liver cell and gallbladder cancer vary greatly by locality. Since most cancers are considered to be related to environmental and lifestyle exposures, such as diet, smoking or excessive drinking, there is hope that action on these factors may serve to substantially reduce occurrence of the disease.

Recent progress in early diagnosis has made it feasible to detect small and minute cancers, and these have proven possible to cure with relatively favorable results. The most important advancement has come from a multidisciplinary approach to cancer treatment, utilizing a balanced application of surgery, radiation therapy and chemotherapy. A considerable increase in the five-year survival rate has been realized in stomach cancer.

While progress is being made in the practical treatment of this disease, it remains far better to prevent than to cure. For the first time immunization offers a unique opportunity to prevent liver cell cancer.

The UICC Fukuoka Symposium held in the fall of 1984 in Japan centered on Fundamental and Clinical Aspects of Digestive Tract Tumors. It offered the most comprehensive and newest information on this type of cancer from scientists around the world. The selections in this book were authored by experts who participated in that meeting.

We hope that by virtue of the in-depth and contemporary reports it contains, this volume can play a role in advancing the work being done in cancer research.

*December 1985*

K. INOKUCHI
G. P. MURPHY
H. SUGANO
T. SUGIMURA
U. VERONESI

# CONTENTS

viii

IV.  LONG-TERM SURVIVAL AND COMBINED MODALITY
BY DIGESTIVE TRACT CANCER

V.  RISK OF CARCINOMA AFTER PARTIAL GASTRECTOMY

VI.  MULTIDISCIPLINARY APPROACH TO CANCER PREVENTION

# CARCINOGENESIS

# MORTALITY OF CANCER OF THE DIGESTIVE ORGANS: THE PAST, PRESENT, AND FUTURE

Minoru Kurihara[*1] and Kunio Aoki[*2]

*Department of Epidemiology and Social Medicine, Research Institute for Nuclear Medicine and Biology, Hiroshima University[*1] and Department of Preventive Medicine, Nagoya University School of Medicine[*2]*

The purpose of this study was to suggest the common causal factors of cancer related to place, time, and individual by reviewing the frequency-distribution and trends in cancer mortality of the digestive organs in various countries of the world. Age-adjusted death rates from 1950–51 to 1978–79 in 24 countries and those in 1978–79 in 15 other countries were compiled. The estimated mortality rates for the period of 1980 to 2000 were computed for seven countries, based on the mortality rates by sex, age, and birth cohort before 1980. By reviewing these basic data, the authors attempted to point out not only the considerable variations but also the strikingly similar patterns of cancer mortality in time and space.

The target organs of the digestive system presented in this report are the esophagus, stomach, intestine except rectum, rectum, liver, gallbladder and bile ducts, and pancreas.

Cancer is one of the leading causes of death in most countries of the world, accounting for more than four million deaths each year. Mortality statistics are an important indicator in cancer epidemiology because of the homogeneous data available for many years in various countries of the world and the high fatality rate of many types of cancer.

By compiling and reviewing the past and present frequency-distribution of cancer of the digestive organs in different countries, and also by estimating future mortalities by site, the authors have attempted to point out not only the considerable variations but also the strikingly similar patterns in time and space and to ascertain some epidemiological factors relating to cancer incidence.

*Calculation of Age-adjusted Rate and Simulation for Trends in Death Rates in the Past and Near Future*

Age-adjusted death rates of cancer by site in 39 countries in 1978–79 were computed using the mortality statistics obtained from the WHO data base through the courtesy of Dr. Hansluwka of WHO. The age-adjusted death rates of cancer in 24 countries for the period between 1950 and 1967 were published earlier by Segi and Kurihara (4) and those between 1968 and 1977 were computed biennially by the authors. Segi's "world population" (4) was used as the standard for calculating age-adjusted rates, and the age-adjusted death rate was employed for calculating the sex ratio of death rates (male

[*1] Kasumi 1-chome, Minami-ku, Hiroshima 734, Japan (栗原　登).

[*2] Tsurumai-cho, Showa-ku, Nagoya 466, Japan (青木国雄).

to female). The annual rates of increase or decrease in age-adjusted death rates in the period between 1954–55 and 1976–77 in 24 countries were calculated based on a log-linear regression line fitted to the trend curve related to such rates for these two decades.

The future trend in cancer mortality for the period between 1980 and 2000 was predicted by using the following regression models based on the age-specific death rates by birth cohort.

It was assumed that the number of deaths due to cancer for each age group in each birth cohort has a Poisson distribution and the following two types of regression models were prepared for description of the age-specific cancer mortality rate $R(k, i)$ for $i$-th age group in $k$-th cohort.

1.   Model I:     $R(k, i) = (a + bi)^{k-1} c_i,$
2.   Model II:    $R(k, i) = (ab^i)^{k-1} c_i,$

where $a$ and $b$ are constants which are independent of $i$ and of $k$, and $c_i$ is a constant depending only on $i$.

In these models, it should be noted that the ratio $r$ between the expectation of the mortality of the $i$-th age group in $(k+1)$-th cohort and that in $k$-th cohort can be expressed in terms of $a$ and $b$ as $r = a + bi$ in Model I, $r = ab^i$ in Model II, respectively.

The unknown parameters $a$, $b$ and $c_i$'s in Model I or II could be estimated by the maximum likelihood method.

The above regression models were compared by the Akaike minimum-AIC method (1) to obtain the best fitted model.

Future mortality values were calculated by this best fitted model in varying $k$ in the future direction. However, in those cases (stomach cancer in Japan, etc.) when a decreasing tendency followed an increasing tendency in the older cohorts, the regression models were calculated excluding the data of old cohorts in the increasing tendency.

The predicted age-adjusted death rates were calculated for each calendar year from these values, using Doll-Segi's "world population" (2) as a standard. The prediction could be made for seven countries.

The target organs of the digestive system studied in the report are the esophagus, stomach, intestine except rectum, rectum, liver, gallbladder and bile ducts, and pancreas.


*International Variation and Similarity of Cancer Incidence*

*1.  Esophagus*

The highest age-adjusted death rate of esophageal cancer for males in 1978–79 was observed in Uruguay with more than 11 per 100,000 population followed by France, Hong Kong, Singapore, and U.S. nonwhite, and that for females was seen in Chile with more than 4 per 100,000 followed by Ireland, Uruguay, and Scotland, but most countries showed less than 2 per 100,000. Lower rates were seen in Guatemala, Balkan countries, and Israel for both sexes.

The mortality rate was always higher in males than in females, and the countries with high mortality in males differed from those with high mortality in females.

A marked intercountry difference in sex ratio of age-adjusted death rates was observed. For instance, the highest sex ratio was 12:1 in France, while the lowest was only 1.6:1 in Finland (Table I).

Trends in age-adjusted death rates in males in some countries between 1950–51 and 1978–79 are shown in Fig. 1. An increasing trend was observed after 1950–51 in

TABLE I. Sex Ratios (%) (Male to Female) of Age-Adjusted Death Rates for Cancers of
Esophagus, Stomach, Intestine except Rectum, Rectum, and Gallbladder and
Bile Ducts, in 39 Countries in 1978–79

| Country | Esophagus | Stomach | Intestine except rectum | Rectum | Gallbladder and bile ducts |
|---|---|---|---|---|---|
| Argentina | 334 | 209 | 109[a] | 154 | —[c] |
| Australia | 235 | 210 | 119 | 171 | — |
| Austria | 620 | 202 | 138 | 178 | — |
| Belgium[a] | 403 | 195 | 114 | 150 | 69[a] |
| Bulgaria | 263 | 164 | 117 | 144 | 70 |
| Canada | 290 | 231 | 112 | 167 | 76[b] |
| Chile | 213 | 224 | 89 | 117 | — |
| Costa Rica | 220 | 186 | 105 | 73 | — |
| Cuba[a] | 253 | 178 | 77 | 118 | — |
| Denmark | 285 | 189 | 108 | 179 | 65 |
| England and Wales | 195 | 217 | 110 | 176 | 95 |
| Finland | 157 | 193 | 109 | 150 | 52 |
| France | 1,222 | 223 | 140 | 191 | 72 |
| Germany, Fed. Rep. | 527 | 190 | 115 | 164 | 55 |
| Greece | 306 | 182 | 102 | 151 | 59 |
| Guatemala | 186 | 98 | 132[a] | 54 | — |
| Hong Kong | 479 | 210 | 115 | 170 | 113 |
| Hungary | 613 | 217 | 116 | 161 | 43 |
| Ireland[a] | 180 | 154 | 109 | 162 | 61 |
| Israel | 170 | 158 | 120 | 125 | 55 |
| Italy[a] | 535 | 206 | 125 | 157 | 62 |
| Japan | 490 | 197 | 119 | 157 | 93 |
| Netherlands | 262 | 230 | 111 | 160 | 57 |
| New Zealand | 179 | 228 | 100 | 144 | 80 |
| Northern Ireland | 212 | 195 | 92 | 164 | 98 |
| Norway | 376 | 201 | 99 | 162 | 72 |
| Paraguay | 577 | 139 | 105[a] | 289 | — |
| Poland | 453 | 257 | 117 | 141 | — |
| Portugal | 353 | 201 | 109 | 181 | — |
| Romania[a] | 323 | 228 | 110 | 121 | — |
| Scotland | 217 | 206 | 105 | 176 | 78 |
| Singapore | 417 | 245 | 120 | 145 | 124 |
| Spain | 569 | 193 | 109 | 145 | 51 |
| Sweden | 320 | 190 | 111 | 187 | 50 |
| Switzerland | 807 | 205 | 133 | 178 | 61[a] |
| United States, white[a] | 355 | 203 | 125 | 175 | 80 |
| United States, nonwhite[a] | 390 | 211 | 108 | 158 | 75 |
| Uruguay[a] | 400 | 198 | 115 | 171 | — |
| Venezuela[a] | 246 | 165 | 71 | 74 | 55 |
| Yugoslavia | 464 | 202 | 124 | 149 | 47 |

Segi's "world population" figures were used as standard for age-adjusted death rates.

[a] 1978 only.

[b] 1979 only.

[c] — not available.

England and Wales and in U.S. nonwhite, while a marked decreasing trend was seen in
Switzerland, Finland, Federal Republic of Germany, Poland, and Norway for both
sexes. In Japan, the mortality rate in males slightly increased until 1970, but thereafter

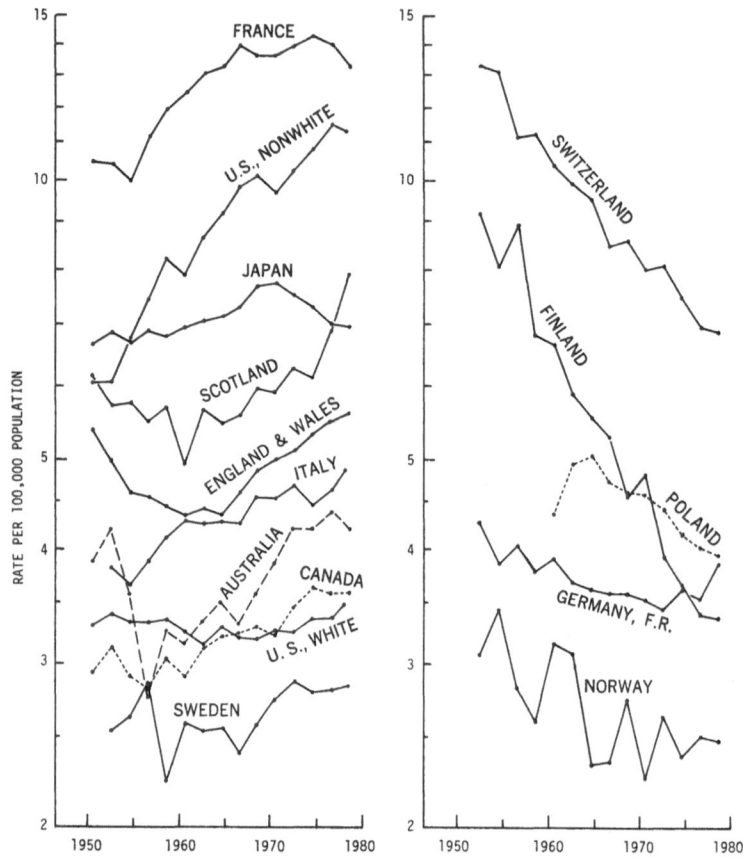

Fig. 1.   Trends in age-adjusted death rates for cancer of esophagus in males in
selected countries, from 1950–51 to 1978–79.

it decreased, while that in females showed a markedly decreasing trend after 1970.

The rates of increase or decrease per year in age-adjusted death rates of esophageal cancer between 1954–55 and 1976–77 by log-linear regression were noted in 24 countries. When the rate of increase is 5% per year, for example, the death rate doubles in about 15 years, and the doubling time is about 70 years if the rate is 1% per year.

In males, as shown in Fig. 2, an increasing trend was noted in 16 countries, while for females, an increasing trend was observed in only seven countries. A sex discrepancy in the trend, that is, increase in males and decrease in females, was seen in eight countries including France, Italy and Japan.

Figure 3 shows the trends in estimated age-adjusted death rates for esophageal cancer until 2000. A remarkably high mortality in U.S. nonwhite of both sexes is expected until 2000, but such increasing trend may be levelling off, because the rate of increase in age-specific death rates by birth cohort became smaller among the cohorts born after 1930. Some countries show slightly increasing trends for both sexes, and Denmark, Poland, and Federal Republic of Germany indicate a definite declining trend for females.

Considering the marked difference in mortality, sex discrepancy in the death rate, and the variety of trends by country or ethnic group, deaths due to esophageal cancer might be affected by multiple causative factors which may differ by sex.

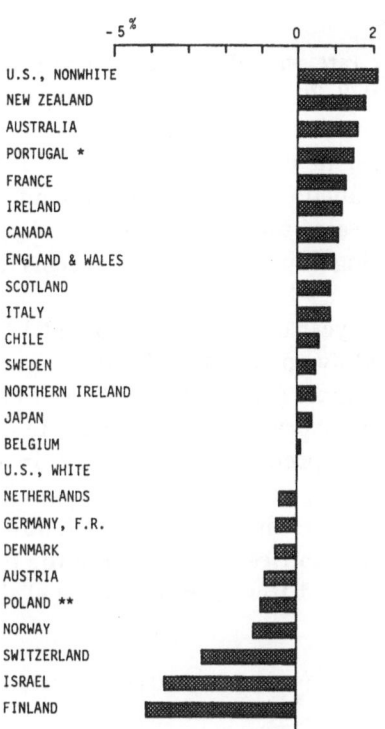

FIG. 2. Rates of change per year in age-adjusted death rates for cancer of esophagus in males in 24 countries, from 1954–55 to 1976–77.
* From 1956–57 to 1976–77,   ** from 1960–61 to 1976–77.

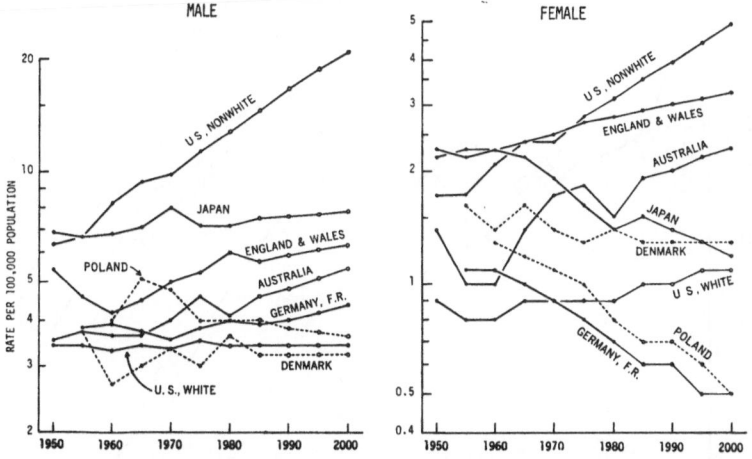

FIG. 3. Estimated age-adjusted death rates for cancer of esophagus in seven countries until 2000.
● observed;  ○ estimated.

## 2. *Stomach*

The highest mortality rate was observed in Japan for both sexes among these 39 countries of the world in 1978–79, followed by Chile and Costa Rica. U.S. white showed the lowest rates, being about 1/8 that in Japan.

Figure 4 shows a constant declining trend since 1950 in most of the countries. Among them, a marked reduction was seen in Finland, U.S. white and Norway. In Portugal, the death rate increased until 1970. Poland and Japan began to show a decrease around 1965, and the declining slope in recent years seems to be as steep as that in western countries.

The reduction rates per year between 1954–55 and 1976–77 range 1 to 5% for both sexes among 23 countries. Only one country, Portugal, presented a tendency to increase in males. A marked reduction rate greater than 3.5% was observed in Finland, Denmark, U.S. white, Switzerland, and Norway. A reduction rate of 3.5% per year implies that a reduction of about 50% is expected within 20 years. In Japan, the reduction rate was about 1.2% in males and 1.4% in females, but it was 2.7% and 3.3%, respectively, during the last decade. It appears that Japan might follow a similar declining course in mortality which the western countries experienced in the past.

The observed and estimated trends in age-adjusted death rates between 1950 and

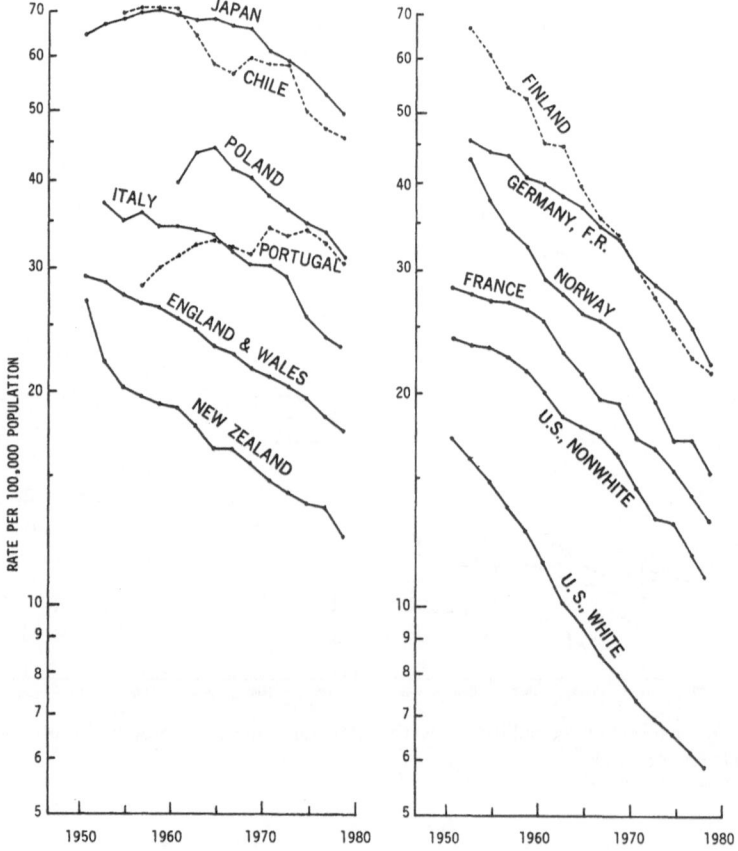

FIG. 4. Trends in age-adjusted death rates for cancer of stomach in males in selected countries, from 1950–51 to 1978–79.

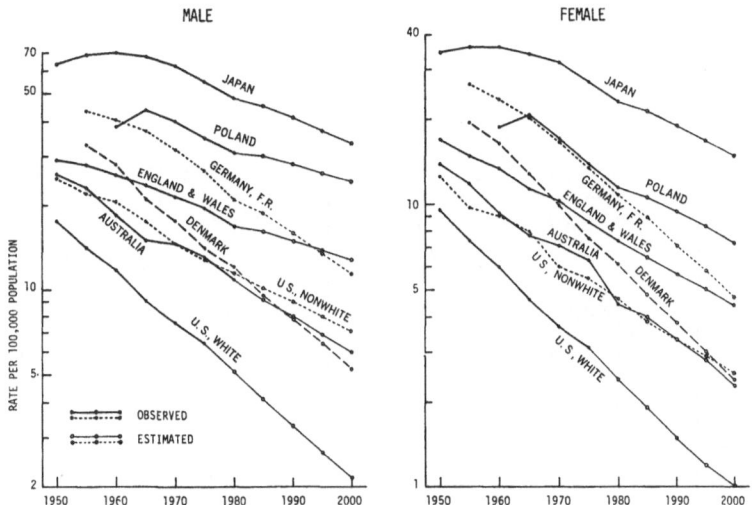

FIG. 5. Estimated age-adjusted death rates for cancer of stomach in seven countries until 2000.

● observed; ○ estimated.

2000 are shown in Fig. 5. The declining trends in the past are expected to linearly continue for the next two decades. In the U.S. white in particular, stomach cancer will become a rare disease by 2000, the estimated deaths being 2 per 100,000 population for males and 1 for females, but in Japan, stomach cancer will continue to be a prevalent disease even in 2000.

The remarkable reduction in mortality of stomach cancer in the developed countries is attributable to various factors. The improvement of treatment is one of them, but reduction in morbidity undoubtedly contributes to this declining trend, as the morbidity rate of stomach cancer has gradually been declining in many areas where cancer registry has been established.

It is assumed that common causal factors are involved in the reduced mortality of stomach cancer in view of the fact that many countries show a similar decreasing trend in mortality. The modernization of dietary pattern observed all over the world during this century is considered one of the major common causal factors. In examining the reduction rate in stomach cancer mortality by prefecture in Japan (3), the prefecture with more urban factors shows a higher reduction rate than that with less urban factors, and westernization of dietary pattern is more prevalent in cities than in rural areas.

## 3. Intestine except rectum

In 1978–79, the countries in Western Europe and North America showed high age-adjusted mortality rates with little difference in frequency. No significant difference was observed among the countries of Central and South America, Eastern Europe and Japan, these countries showing death rates as low as 5–7 per 100,000 population. It is noted that the death rate in Guatemala was exceptionally low.

One of the particular characteristics of this cancer is that the sex ratio of the death rates was approximately 100% in all 39 countries, which is in great contrast to the sex ratio of esophageal cancer. The highest sex ratio of 140% was observed in France and the

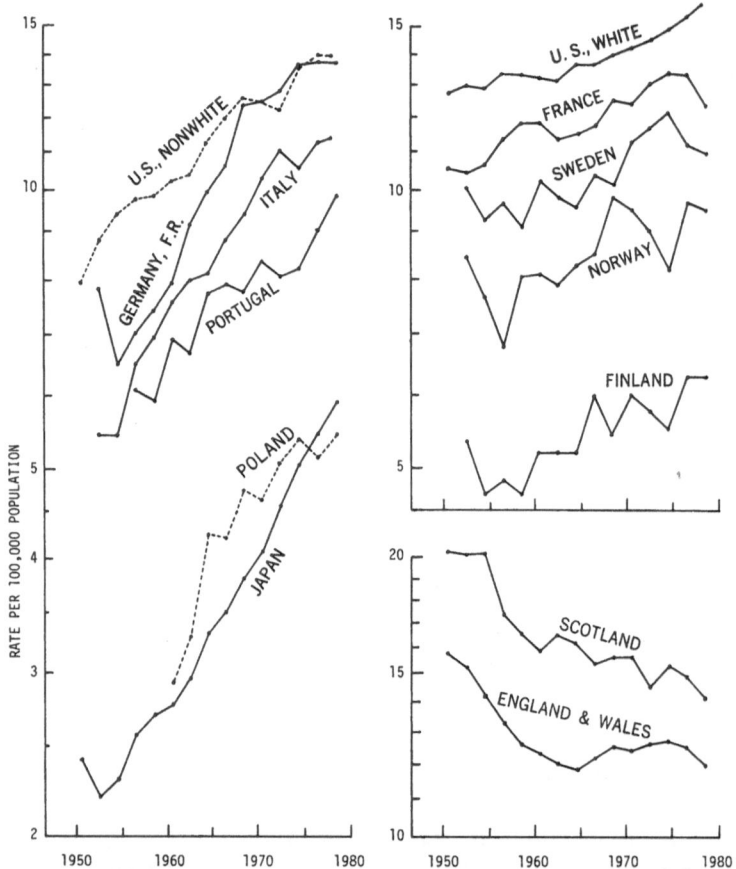

FIG. 6.  Trends in age-adjusted death rates for cancer of intestine except rectum in males in selected countries, from 1950–51 to 1978–79.

lowest of 71% in Venezuela, and in most countries the males exceeded the females (Table I).

Trends in mortality in some countries for males since 1950 are shown in Fig. 6. An abrupt increasing trend was observed in Japan, U.S. nonwhite, Federal Republic of Germany, and Poland, while some countries such as England and Wales and Scotland showed a decreasing trend.

The rates of increase per year between 1954–55 and 1976–77 were large in Japan, Federal Republic of Germany, Poland, and Italy for both sexes. The increase rate was smaller in females than in males. A decrease rate was seen in England and Wales, Scotland, and Denmark in both sexes.

Prediction of future age-adjusted death rates was made only for colon cancer (Fig. 7). An increasing trend is expected in Japan, Federal Republic of Germany, and U.S. white for both sexes, while a decreasing trend is predicted in England and Wales. Japan may exceed England and Wales by 2000.

It is considered that modernization of dietary pattern might bring about an increase in colon cancer, a phenomenon contrary to the case of stomach cancer. Although improvement in treatment of colon cancer might affect the fatality rate, it is natural to

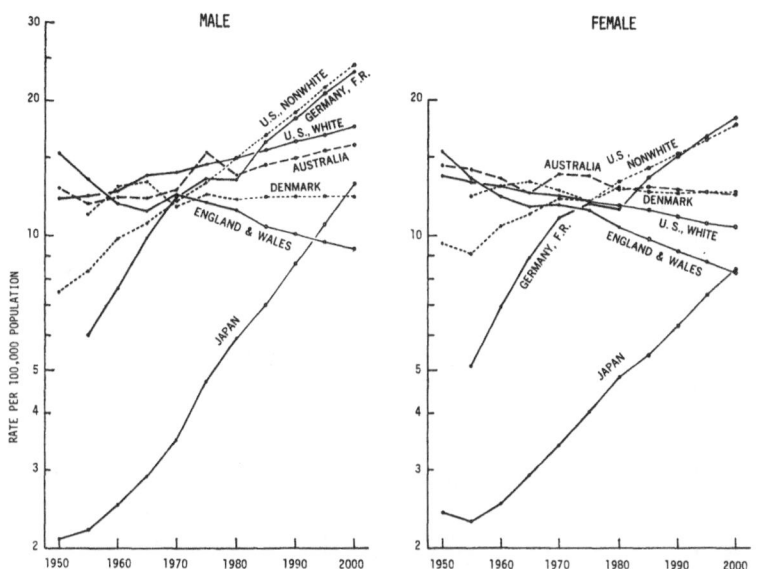

FIG. 7. Estimated age-adjusted death rates for cancer of colon in six countries until 2000.

● observed; ○ estimated.

assume that causal factors have not increased in recent years in these countries with a decreasing trend. Females as well as males might be equally exposed to such causal factors, since sex difference in mortality is very small.

### 4. Rectum

A high death rate was observed in Denmark, Hungary, Austria, and New Zealand, and a low rate was seen in Guatemala, Greece, Paraguay, and both white and nonwhite in the U.S. in 1978–79.

The sex ratio in mortality exceeded 150% in most of the countries, the highest being 280% in Paraguay. These values differ from those of cancer of the intestine except rectum (Table I).

As shown in Fig. 8, Poland showed a steep increasing trend, while Austria, Federal Republic of Germany, Italy, and Japan have tended to level off in recent years after a marked increase until 1970. Several countries showed a steadily declining trend, and a remarkable decrease was observed in U.S. white and nonwhite.

The rates of change in mortality between 1954–55 and 1976–77 showed a decreasing trend in about half of the countries. The highest increase rate of more than 5% per year was observed in Poland, while the highest decrease rate of more than 2% was seen in U.S. white for both sexes.

The trends in age-adjusted death rates in the past and until 2000 are shown in Fig. 9. An extraordinarily steep increasing trend is observed in Poand, while Japan and Federal Republic of Germany show a moderately increasing trend. In other countries, decreasing trends are shown until 2000, although Australia maintains a stable level for both sexes. It is therefore expected that the order of the death rate among countries will be changed by 2000. However, the increasing trend in Poland may level off before 2000, considering the trends of other types of cancer and other biological conditions,

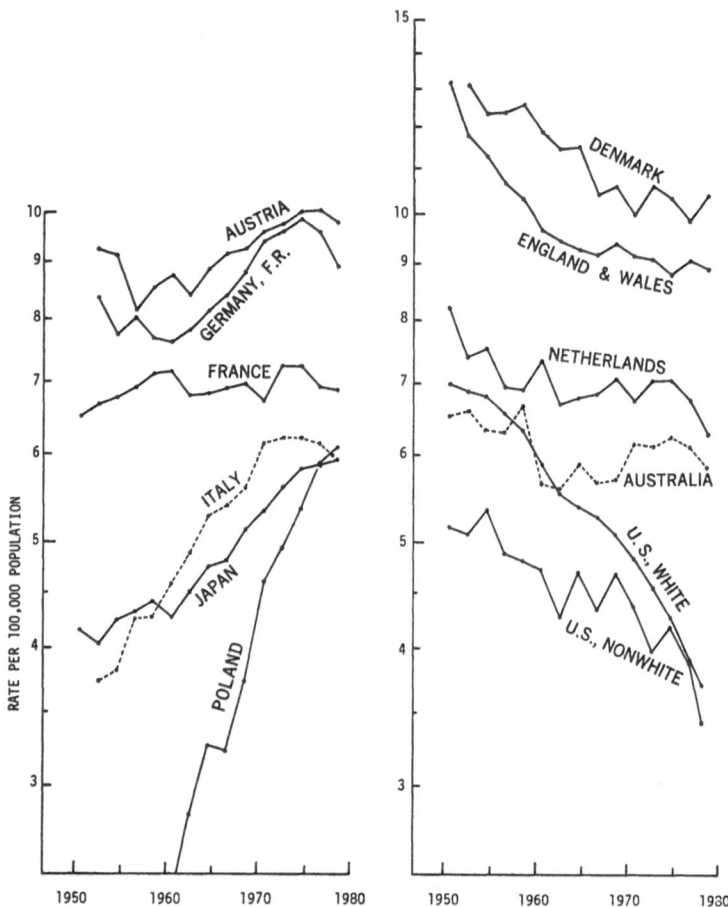

FIG. 8.   Trends in age-adjusted death rates for cancer of rectum in males in selected countries, from 1950–51 to 1978–79.

The foregoing frequency-distribution of rectal cancer suggests that it is very difficult to speculate on common epidemiological factors of this disease and that causal factors might be quite specific in each area.

### 5.   Liver

Primary liver cancer is relatively uncommon in Western countries but the incidence has been observed in developing countries in Asia and Africa.

Descriptive epidemiology has faced obstacles with the changes made in the International Classification of Diseases in recent decades and in different diagnostic levels between countries, especially the divergent usage of the primary and secondary liver cancer. Cancer of the liver includes both primary liver cancer and liver cancer not specified as primary or secondary, but not secondary liver cancer, in this study.

Figure 10 shows a large difference in mortality between countries. Singapore males have an exceedingly high rate, followed by Greece, Japan, Spain, and Italy, while the countries in Northern and Western Europe, North America, and Oceania show low rates. In females, the similar tendency was observed.

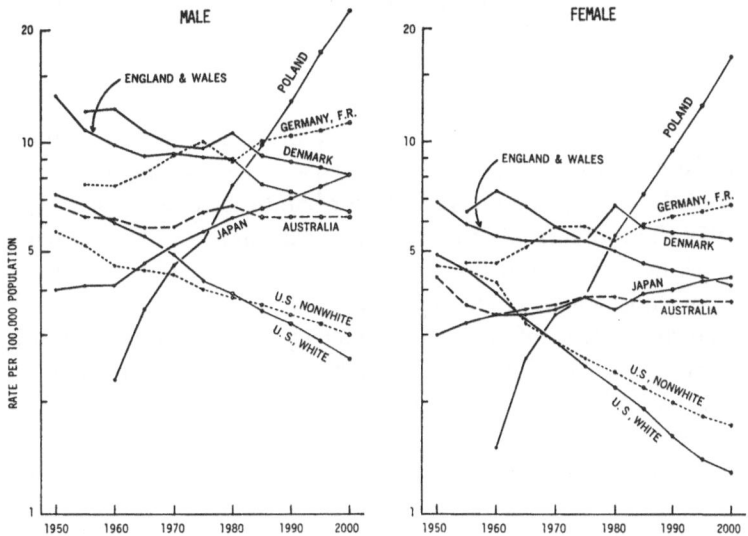

FIG. 9. Estimated age-adjusted death rates for cancer of rectum in seven countries until 2000.

● observed; ○ estimated.

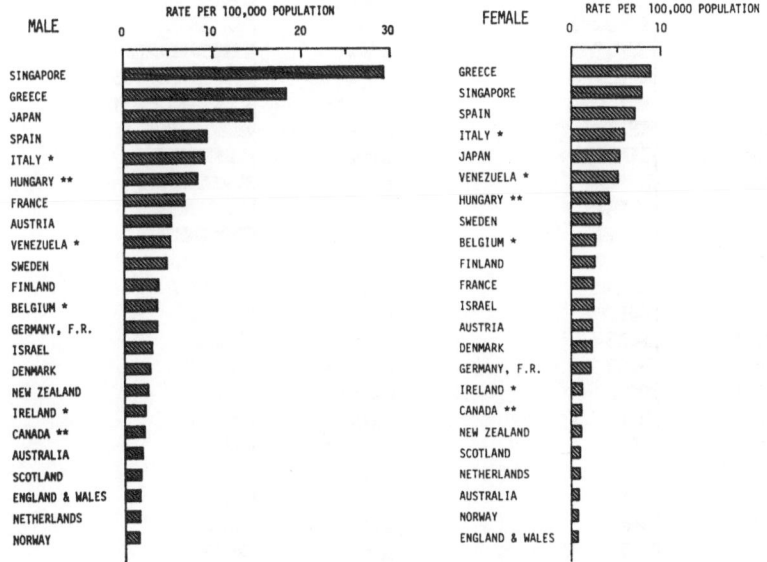

FIG. 10. Age-adjusted death rates for cancer of liver in 23 countries in 1978–79.
* 1978 only, ** 1979 only.

The trends in age-adjusted death rates could be observed in 12 countries since 1958–59. A downward trend in mortality was observed in European countries except Sweden and Finland, especially in females. Japanese males have shown an increasing trend since 1975, but a continuously decreasing trend was seen in females.

As mentioned previously, there are some obstacles in understanding the descriptive epidemiology of liver cancer. However, it is noteworthy that the remarkable decreasing trend in mortality for females in developed countries may suggest a reduction in common etiological factors.

## 6. *Gallbladder and bile ducts*

The biliary tract is an inaccessible organ by ordinary medical techniques and the inability of the International Classification of Diseases to distinguish between cancers of the liver and of the biliary system was a major handicap in descriptive epidemiological study before 1958. The diversity of diagnostic level might hinder the comparability of mortality statistics between countries. However, recent developments in diagnosis may overcome the above obstacle in epidemiological study.

Age-adjusted death rates of the biliary tract in 1978–79 which could be calculated in 29 countries are shown in Fig. 11. The highest rate was observed in Hungarian females, and Japan, Austria, and Federal Republic of Germany show relatively high frequency for both sexes.

In most countries, females exceed males except Singapore and Hong Kong. The

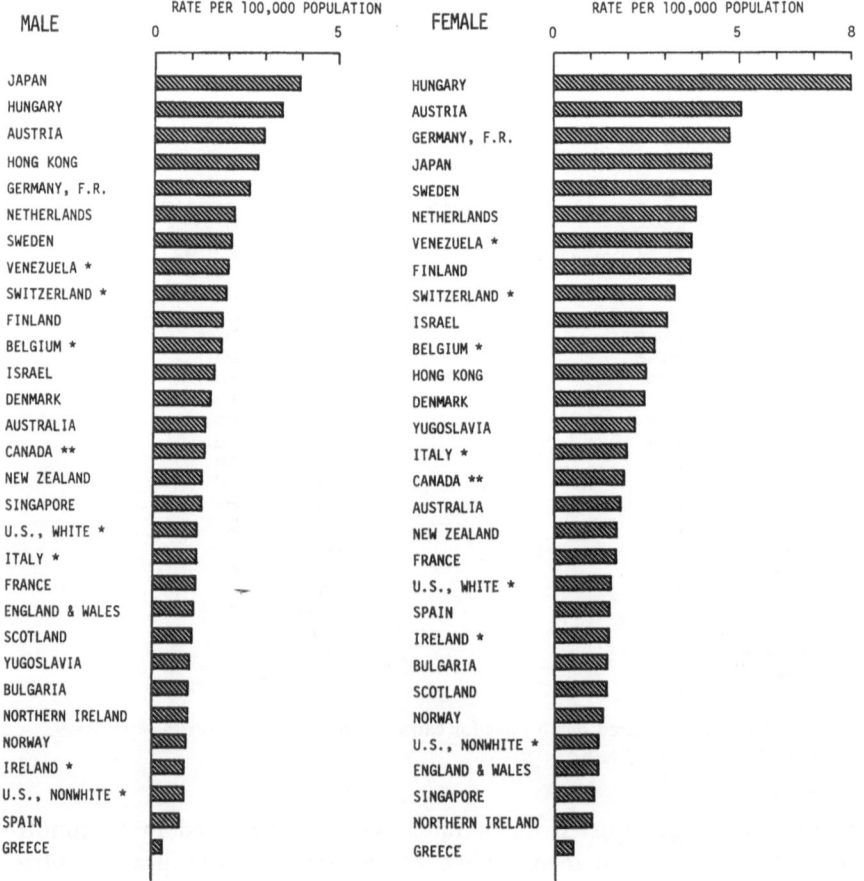

FIG. 11.  Age-adjusted death rates for cancer of gallbladder and bile ducts in 29 countries in 1978–79.
* 1978 only, ** 1979 only.

death rates for females in Hungary, Yugoslavia, and Sweden were more than twice those for males.

Trends in age-adjusted death rates between 1958–59 and 1978–79 were observed in 11 countries. Marked increase trends were seen in Japan, Sweden, and Finland, while U.S. white and nonwhite, Australia, Canada, Federal Republic of Germany, and England and Wales show declining trends.

Geographic variations in this cancer cannot suggest any epidemiological factors, because of divergent diagnostic levels, different medicare systems and poor etiological studies in the past. However, some differences in mortality, different trends in Western countries and also excessive female mortality may serve as clues in future studies.

### 7. *Pancreas*

Reliability of the mortality rate of such a well-hidden organ as the pancreas might *per se* depend on the diagnostic level and medicare system in each area, and these have been changing with time. Therefore the descriptive epidemiology of this disease should be carefully evaluated, although the authors have reviewed it in the same manner as that of other cancers.

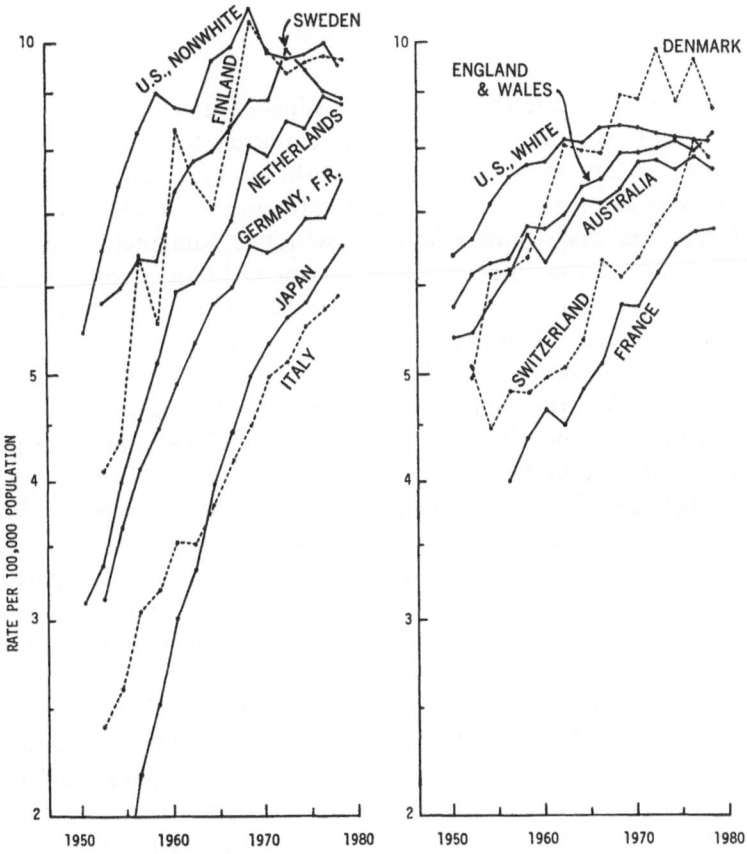

FIG. 12. Trends in age-adjusted death rates for cancer of pancreas in males in selected countries, from 1950–51 to 1978–79.

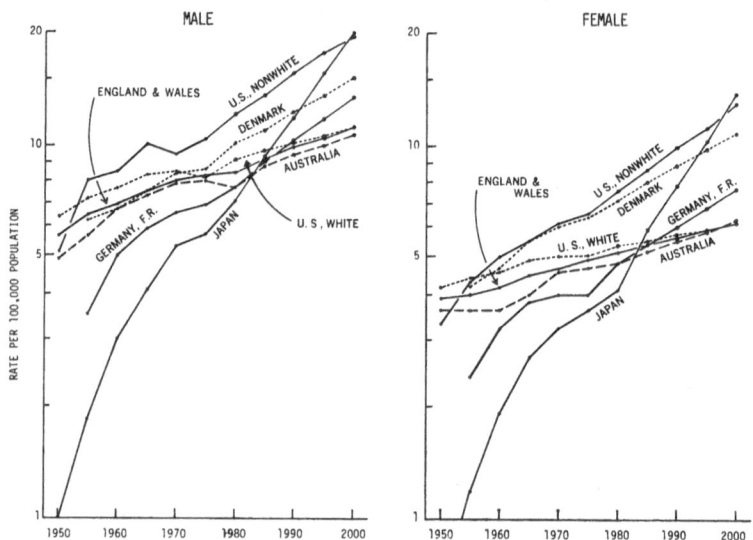

Fig. 13. Estimated age-adjusted death rates for cancer of pancreas in six countries until 2000.
● observed; ○ estimated.

There is only a little difference in the age-adjusted death rates for 1978–79 among 20 countries with a high rate for males and 15 countries for females. Also, a little difference was observed among seven countries with low rates, although some difference was evident between countries with high death rates and those with low rates. Countries in Eastern Europe and Asia show relatively low rates. Nonetheless, an accurate comparison is difficult due to the difference in diagnostic techniques employed in each area.

The mortality rates have been increasing markedly since 1950 in most countries, but recently have levelled off in several. In general, the increasing slope in mortality was steeper in males than in females (Fig. 12).

Among 21 countries, the highest rate of increase between 1954–55 and 1976–77 was observed in Japan, being 5.3% per year in males and 4.4% in females, followed by Belgium, Italy and the Netherlands.

The estimated age-adjusted death rates in the future are shown in Fig. 13. Japan shows the steepest increasing trend until 2000. Such a trend might be attributable in part to improved diagnostic techniques during the last decade and in part to change in dietary pattern, but it is still difficult to explain this steep trend. Some other factors might exist in the estimation method, that is, the increasing trend might level off before 2000, as the basic data for the last decade seem inadequate to estimate mortality rate more than 10 years in the future. Other countries show mild or moderately increasing trends and thus the death rates in Japan might level off and not exceed those of western countries.

The little difference in mortality among the western countries and the slight difference between developed and developing countries suggest that causal factors of pancreas cancer are related to the increasing uniformity of dietary pattern in many countries of the world; also, the gradual increasing trends in mortality in many developed countries may indicate improvement in both diet and diagnostic level.

*Implication of Cancer Mortality Statistics*

Recent advances in cancer therapy and in preventive strategies, especially secondary prevention through screening programs, have gradually been changing the role of mortality statistics in cancer epidemiology. However, such data are still useful in identifying variations in cancer frequency over time and among different populations or areas, because the availability of morbidity incidence data is limited in the world.

The purpose of this study was to provide cancer mortality statistics for the past three decades, the present situation of cancer mortality in countries of the world and also to estimate cancer mortality in the near future. Through a review of the above data, some epidemiological factors related to cancer were discussed.

The quality of mortality data depends on diagnostic level, reporting system, classification and medicare system, *etc.* in a community. Good quality data have continuously been available in the 24 countries, but the comparability of data for cancers of the liver, biliary tracts, and pancreas seems to be weaker than that of other digestive organs. Therefore, interpretation of this data should be carefully done by the readers.

Some epidemiological factors related to cancer incidence were ascertained through review of the above sources, but most of them have been presented before. These data will be immensely useful for examining hypotheses derived from clinical and experimental studies and for evaluating the preventive cancer measures carried out in the previous period.

Lastly, the authors would like to recommend a birth cohort study using such data over a long period, which might more clearly reflect the effect of changes in lifestyle habits and environmental factors.

## REFERENCES

1. Akaike, H. Information theory and an extension of the maximum likelihood principle. *In* "2nd International Symposium on Information Theory," ed. B. N. Petrov and F. Csáki, pp. 267–281 (1973). Akadémiai Kiado, Budapest.
2. Doll, R. and Cook, P. Summarizing indices for comparison of cancer incidence data. *Int. J. Cancer*, **2**, 269–279 (1976).
3. Kurihara, M. Geographical pathology on stomach cancer (in Japanese). *Igan to Shudan Kenshin*, No. 52, 38–47 (1981).
4. Segi, M. and Kurihara, M. "Cancer Mortality for Selected Sites in 24 Countries No. 6 (1966–1967)" (1972). Japan Cancer Society, Tokyo.

# PRECANCEROUS LESIONS OF THE STOMACH

Jeremy R. Jass

*ICRF Colorectal Cancer Unit, St. Mark's Hospital**

The term precancerous lesion is defined and the following examples
are presented in relation to human stomach—chronic gastritis, intestinal
metaplasia, dysplasia, and adenoma. Particular emphasis is placed on the
histopathology of these lesions and the variants of intestinal metaplasia
are considered in detail. Reference is also made to Menetrier's disease
and non-adenomatous polyps. The relevance of precancerous lesions to
cancer prevention programmes is briefly summarised.

A precancerous lesion may be defined as a histopathological abnormality in which
cancer is more likely to occur than in its normal counterpart (*14, 15*). The term precancerous does not imply that the development of malignancy is inevitable, but rather
that the probability of such an event is increased. The most important precancerous
lesions of the stomach include chronic gastritis, intestinal metaplasia, dysplasia, and
adenoma.

## Chronic Gastritis and Intestinal Metaplasia

Chronic gastritis occurs as an autoimmune disease (in association with pernicious
anaemia), in acid hypersecretors and in patients from high risk countries for gastric
cancer (" envrionmental " chronic gastritis) (*1*). The precise pathogenesis of "hypersecretory " and " environmental " chronic gastritis is not known. Autoimmune gastritis
mainly involves body mucosa, hypersecretory gastritis the antrum, and environmental
gastritis commences patchily within the intermediate zone (*1*). Only the first and last
are associated with gastric cancer (*1*). Chronic gastritis is recognised histologically by
the presence of mucosal inflammation, fibrosis of lamina propria, glandular atrophy,
pyloric metaplasia, intestinal metaplasia (IM), and rarely dysplasia. Some authors recognise a relationship between chronic cystic gastritis and gastric carcinoma (*14*). IM
has been regarded for many years not only as the end-point in the spectrum of changes
associated with chronic gastritis, but also as the lesion which statistically most predis-
poses to malignancy (excluding dysplasia).

Gastric carcinomas fall into two principal groups. One type is well differentiated
with an expanding pattern of growth (intestinal type) and the other is poorly differentiated with a diffusely infiltrating growth pattern (*11*). Intestinal type carcinoma more
often arises in or is associated with IM than the diffuse type (*11, 17, 20*). Both intestinal
type carcinoma (*16*) and IM (*4*) are more common in patients from high risk countries
for gastric cancer. However, not only have exceptions to these findings been recorded,

---

* City Road, London EC1V 2PS, U.K.

but it is widely acknowledged that IM arises too frequently in clinical practice to be a valuable marker of increased cancer risk.

### Intestinal Metaplasia Variants

Two main types of IM have been described (6). Complete or type I IM closely resembles normal intestinal epithelium (usually small intestine) but lacks well-developed villi and presents within a thin, atrophic mucosa. The crypts are generally simple, un-branched tubules and are lined by goblet cells secreting acid mucins (mainly sialomucin) and brightly eosinophilic columnar cells with a well-developed brush border (Photo 1). The columnar cells stain intensely for IgA and secretory component (5). Paneth cells positive for lysozyme (5) and immature columnar cells secreting small amounts of mucus are present in the crypt base. Small intestinal brush border enzymes are fully repre-sented (12) and carcinoembryonic antigen is detected as a fine delineation of the brush border (9).

Incomplete or type II IM may be divided into two groups. In the first (type IIA) goblet cells secreting acid mucins are scattered amongst apparently normal gastric foveolar cells secreting neutral mucins and sometimes small amounts of sialomucin (6). This probably represents early IM and may be termed goblet cell metaplasia. In the second (type IIB IM) goblet cells are bordered by immature mucous cells showing ambiguous differentiation and secreting neutral and acid mucins in varying combinations, but often with sulphomucins predominating (6) (Photo 2). The crypts of type IIB IM are often hyperplastic (elongated, tortuous, sometimes with papillary infolding) (Photo 3). Nuclei are typically vesicular with a prominent nucleolus and slightly enlarged. The goblet cells and columnar mucous cells are taller than their normal counterparts within type I IM (6). Staining for carcinoembryonic antigen is increased with a positive cytoplasm in some cases (9) whereas IgA and secretory component staining are limited to the crypt base columnar cells (9). Paneth cells are usually absent. However, absence of Paneth cells should *not* be used as the only criterion for diagnosing incomplete IM. Brush border enzymes are reduced or absent (12) and the brush border is correspondingly poorly developed.

The evidence linking type IIB IM with gastric cancer is as follows. a) Type IIB IM shows a more selective association with gastric cancer than the other IM variants (6, 18, 19). b) Most gastric adenomas arise in type IIB IM (8). c) Careful studies of microcarcinomas of intestinal type indicate their usual origin within incomplete IM (3, 12). d) Histological and histochemical transitions through dysplasia to carcinoma (intestinal type) can be demonstrated (7).

### Gastric Dysplasia

Dysplasia (intraepithelial neoplasia) is regarded as the most selective precancerous marker (2, 7, 14, 15) but is uncommon. It presents either as a patchy or diffuse change in flat gastric mucosa, or as a discrete, circumscribed, and usually raised lesion (ade-noma). The latter is typically sessile rather than pedunculated and shows either a tubular (borderline lesion), villous, or tubulovillous configuration. Tubular adenomas are more common in Japan than elsewhere and this may be related to the relatively low incidence of malignant change in Japanese adenomas or borderline lesions (13). Some adenomas may be flat or even depressed, but all show an abrupt transition with the adjacent non-neoplastic mucosa.

Dysplasia is recognised histologically by a combination of architectural changes, cytological atypia, and a failure of differentiation. Various types of dysplasia have been recognised. Adenomatous (2) or type I (7) dysplasia shows elongated, pseudostratified, hyperchromatic nuclei and a dark amphophilic cytoplasm (Photo 4). In hyperplastic (2) or type II (7) dysplasia the nuclei are basally sited, enlarged, ovid, and vesicular with a coarse nuclear membrane and prominent nucleolus. Cytoplasm is eosinophilic and often pale. These contrasting types of dysplasia probably reflect different levels and directions of differentiation of the constituent cells. Type II dysplasia arises in flat gastritic mucosa (usually incomplete IM), is often difficult to recognise and grade, but gives rise to the more poorly differentiated carcinomas of intestinal type (Photo 5) (7).

Dysplasia is graded according to the severity of the change (14, 15). For example, low grade dysplasia deviates minimally from normal whereas high grade dysplasia approximates to intramucosal carcinoma. Problems in interpretation include the distinction between regenerative change and dysplasia (especially type II) and separating high grade dysplasia and intramucosal carcinoma. Tumour markers offer no help with these diagnostic difficulties as yet, but *in situ* hybridisation techniques and monoclonal antibody developments may lead to future breakthroughs. Dysplastic cells often secrete small amounts of sulphomucin, suggesting a histogenetic link with type IIB IM (7).

### Gastric Polyps

Gastric polyps have been split into three principal subgroups 1) adenomatous (neoplastic), 2) hyperplastic (regenerative), and 3) hamartomatous (including fundic gland cyst, juvenile, and Peutz-Jeghers polyps) (13).

Adenomas have a lobulated surface and tend to be sessile, solitary, and located in the antrum. The incidence of malignant change ranges from 6–75% in reported series (13). The histology has been described under gastric dysplasia.

Hyperplastic polyps are the commonest type, but rarely undergo malignant change (1–2% incidence in reported series) (13). Co-existent cancers occurred in about 1/3 of all stomachs harbouring hyperplastic polyps (21) but this figure is biased by case selection. One follow-up study has shown that a small proportion of hyperplastic polyps gradually increase in size, show dysplastic change and even malignant transformation (10). Hyperplastic polyps are usually less than 1.5 cm in diameter, show a smooth surface (except when ulcerated) and are either sessile or pedunculated. They are multiple in about 1/3 of cases and often occupy the intermediate zone between antrum and body. They are composed of gastric type epithelium showing mild architectural disorder. Goblet cell metaplasia (type IIA IM; see above) is sometimes seen (14).

Fundic gland cyst polyps are most commonly observed in patients with familial adenomatosis (14). They are not premalignant. Peutz-Jeghers and juvenile polyposis are associated with a slightly increased risk of gastrointestinal malignancy (14).

### Menetrier's Disease

This condition is probably precancerous but the risk is unknown and the mode of histogenesis is not understood (14).

## CONCLUSION

When precancerous lesions are fully typed and characterised, it should be possible to ascertain their natural history by means of prospective studies. Such programmes might be carried out in high risk countries or in patients with precancerous conditions such as gastric stumps, pernicious anaemia or Menetrier's disease. It is vital that such studies publish representative photomicrographs of the precancerous lesions; dysplasia is often overdiagnosed and this will result in rapid disenchantment with the term. Until the natural history of the various precancerous lesions is ascertained, firm guidelines for the management of individual patients cannot be given.

## REFERENCES

1.  Correa, P. The epidemiology and pathogenesis of chronic gastritis. Three aetiological entities. *In* "Frontiers of Gastrointestinal Research," ed. L. van der Reis, pp. 98–108 (1980). Karger, Basel.
2.  Cuello, C., Correa, P., Zarama, G., Lopez, J., Murray, J., and Gordillo, G. Histopathology of gastric dysplasias. *Am. J. Surg. Pathol.*, **3**, 491–500 (1979).
3.  Iida, F. and Kusama, J. Gastric carcinoma and intestinal metaplasia. *Cancer*, **50**, 2854–2858 (1982).
4.  Imai, T., Kubo, T., and Watanabe, H. Chronic gastritis in Japanese with reference to the high incidence of gastric carcinoma. *J. Natl. Cancer Inst.*, **47**, 179–195 (1971).
5.  Isaacson, P. Immunoperoxidase study of the secretory immunoglobulin system and lysozyme in normal and diseased gastric mucosa. *Gut*, **23**, 578–588 (1982).
6.  Jass, J. R. Role of intestinal metaplasia in the histogenesis of gastric carcinoma. *J. Clin. Pathol.*, **33**, 801–810 (1980).
7.  Jass, J. R. A classification of gastric dysplasia. *Histopathology*, **7**, 181–193 (1983).
8.  Jass, J. R. and Filipe, M. I. Sulphomucins and precancerous lesions of the human stomach. *Histopathology*, **3**, 191–199 (1980).
9.  Jass, J. R. and Strudley, I. Immunohistochemical demonstration of carcinoembryonic antigen-like material, secretory component and epithelial IgA within complete and incomplete intestinal metaplasia. *IRCS Med. Sci.*, **11**, 1117–1118 (1983).
10. Kamiya, T., Morishita, T., Asakura, H., Miura, S., Munakata, Y., and Tsuchiya, M. Histoclinical long-standing follow-up study of hyperplastic polyps of the stomach. *Am. J. Gastroenterol.*, **75**, 275–281 (1981).
11. Lauren, P. The two main types of gastric carcinoma; diffuse and so-called intestinal type carcinoma. *Acta Pathol. Microbiol. Scand.*, **64**, 31–49 (1965).
12. Matsukura, N., Suzuki, K., Kawachi, T. Aoyagi, M., Sugimura, T., Kitaoka, H., Numajiri, H., Shirota, A., Itabashi, H., and Hirota, T. Distribution of marker enzymes and mucin in intestinal metaplasia in human stomachs and relation of complete and incomplete types of intestinal metaplasia in minute gastric carcinomas. *J. Natl. Cancer Inst.*, **65**, 231–240 (1980).
13. Ming, S. C. The classification and significance of gastric polyps. *In* "The Gastrointestinal Tract," ed. J. H. Yardley, B. C. Morson, and M. R. Abell, pp. 149–175 (1979). Williams and Wilkins, Co., Baltimore.
14. Morson, B. C., Jass, J. R., and Sobin, L. H. Precancerous lesions of the gastrointestinal tract. A histological classification (1984). Bailliere Tindall, London-Philadelphia-Toronto.
15. Morson, B. C., Sobin, L. H., Grundmann, E., Johansen, A., Nagayo, T., and Serck-Hansen, A. Precancerous conditions and epithelial dysplasia in the stomach. *J.Clin.Pathol.*, **33**, 711–721 (1980).

16.  Munoz, N., Correa, P., Cuello, C., and Duque, E. Histologic types of gastric carcinoma in high and low risk areas. *Int. J. Cancer*, **3**, 809–818 (1968).
17.  Nakamura, K., Sugano, H., and Takagi, K. Carcinoma of the stomach in incipient phase; its histogenesis and histological appearances. *Gann*, **59**, 251–258 (1968).
18.  Segura, D. I. and Montero, C. Histochemical characterization of different types of intestinal metaplasia in gastric carcinoma. *Cancer*, **52**, 498–503 (1983).
19.  Sipponen, P. Intestinal metaplasia and gastric carcinoma. *Ann. Clin. Res.*, **13**, 139–143 (1981).
20.  Sipponen, P., Kekki, M., and Siurala, M. Atrophic gastritis and intestinal metaplasia in gastric carcinoma. *Cancer*, **52**, 1062–1068 (1983).
21.  Tomasulo, J. Gastric polyps. Histologic types and their relationship to gastric carcinoma. *Cancer*, **27**, 1346–1355 (1971).

## EXPLANATIONS OF PHOTOS

PHOTO 1.   Complete or type I intestinal metaplasia of gastric mucosa. The metaplastic crypts are lined by goblet cells and columnar cells with a well-developed brush border. A small focus of incomplete IM is included (arrow). Haematoxylin-Eosin stain (H-E). ×150.

PHOTO 2.   Incomplete IM type IIB. Goblet cells (arrows) stain grey (blue in colour) and the intervening columnar mucous cells stain black (brown/black in colour). High iron diamine-Alcian blue stain. ×150.

PHOTO 3.   Incomplete IM. Goblet cells are scattered inconspicuously amongst tall columnar mucous cells. The mucosa is thickened and the hyperplastic crypts show a serrated configuration. Superficial inspection may result in a missed diagnosis. H-E. ×150.

PHOTO 4.   Adenomatous or type I dysplasia. The nuclei are enlarged, hyperchromatic, and pseudostratified with loss of polarity. The cytoplasm is dark and amphophilic. H-E. ×300.

PHOTO 5.   Hyperplastic or type II dysplasia. The nuclei are enlarged, vesicular, and basally sited. The nuclear membrane is coarse and there is nucleolar prominence. Cytoplasm is pale and eosinophilic. Photos 4 and 5 both show high grade dysplasia, but the appearances are quite different. H-E. ×300.

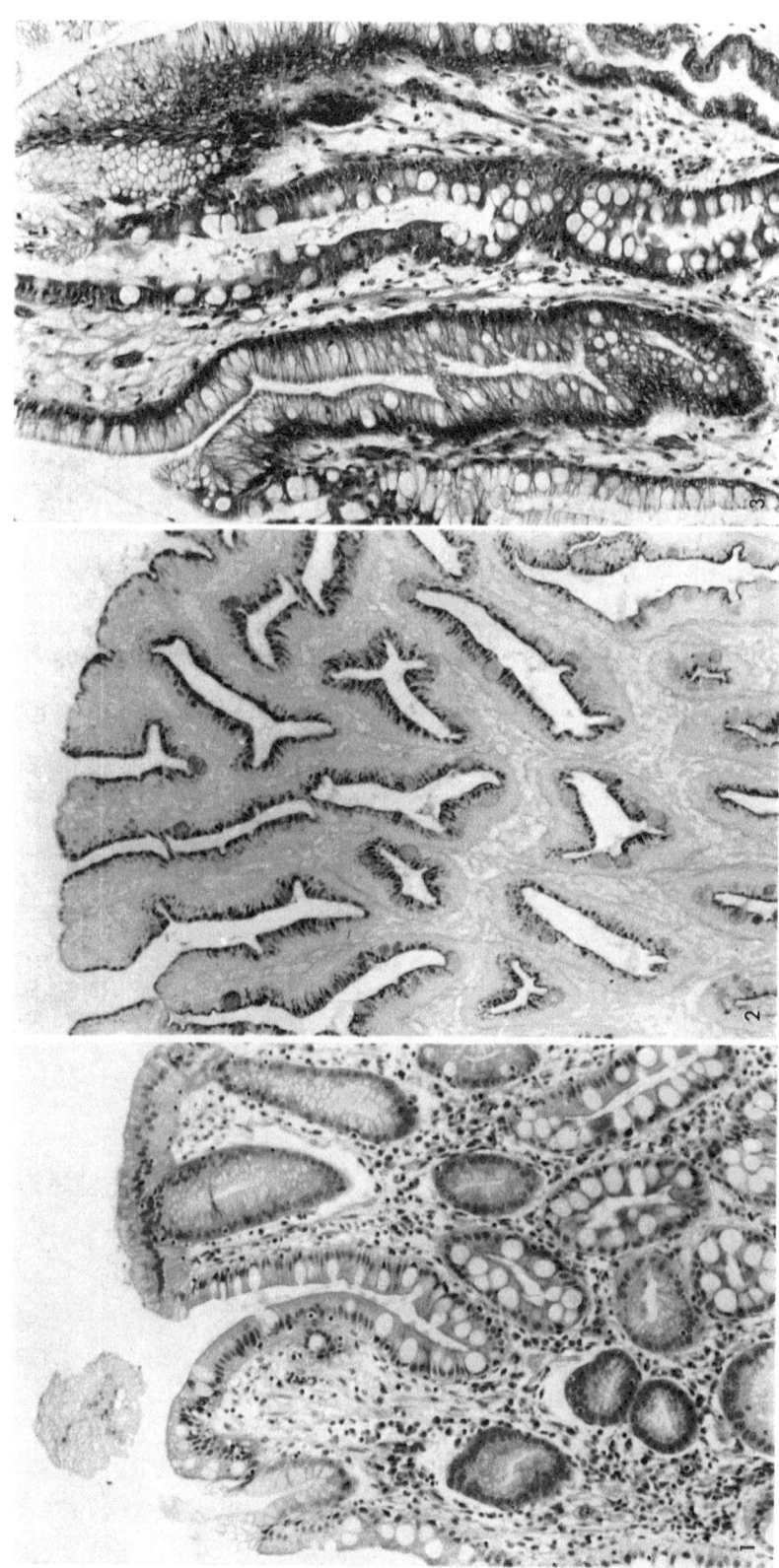

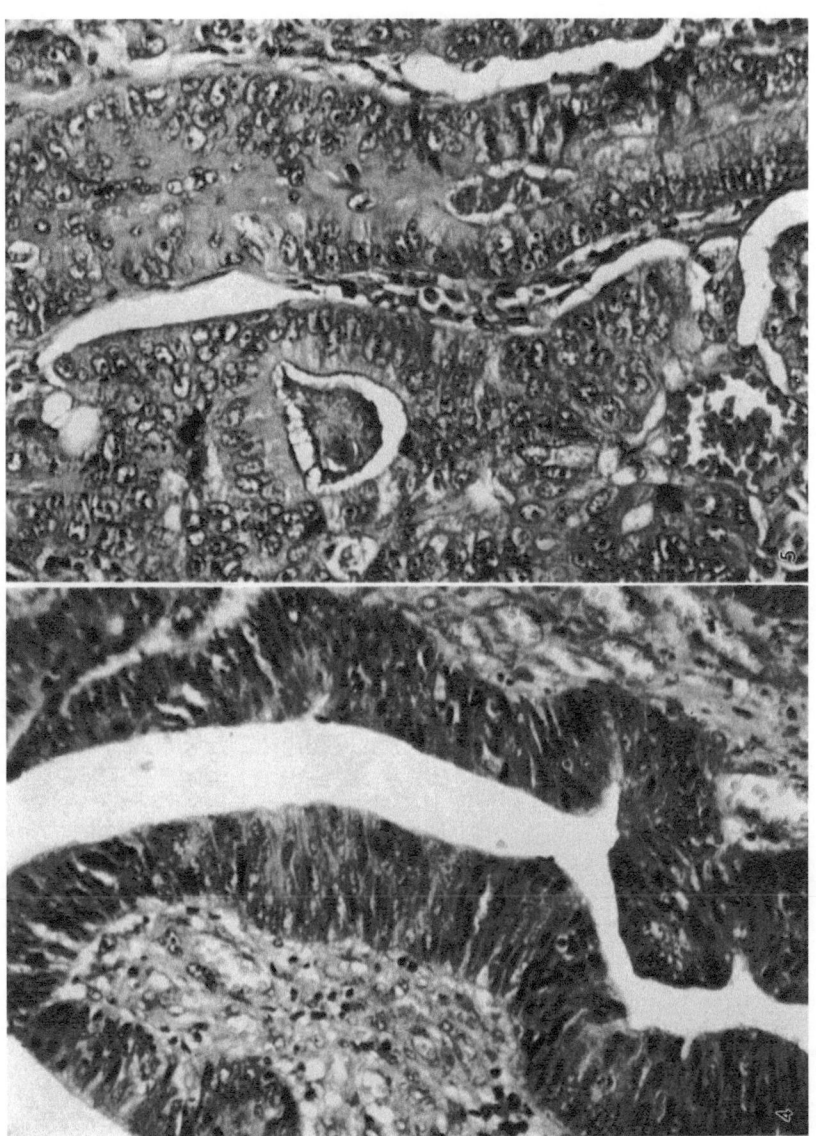

# PRECANCEROUS LESIONS OF THE OESOPHAGUS AND THEIR RISK FACTORS

Nubia Muñoz[*1] and Massimo Crespi[*2]

*International Agency for Research on Cancer[*1] and Istituti Regina Elena[*2]*

Precursor lesions of oesophageal cancer have been described for the first time in two high-risk populations in Iran and China (Linxian) (*2, 10*) and in a low-risk population in China (Jiaoxian). These lesions were identified in three endoscopic surveys which included 430, 527, and 252 individuals, respectively. These precursor lesions include a chronic oesophagitis accompanied in some cases by atrophy of the epithelium and later on by dysplasia. That these lesions are in fact precancerous is suggested by:

1. The higher prevalence of these lesions in high-risk populations as compared to low-risk populations for oesophageal cancer;
2. The similar location of these lesions and of oesophageal cancer: both involve mainly the middle and lower thirds of the oesophagus;
3. The results of a limited follow-up study in China, which showed that in 8 out of 20 individuals, re-examined one year after the first endoscopic examination, the lesions had progressed to more advanced lesions. In 4 of them, a progression from mild oesophagitis with atrophy or dysplasia was observed and in the remaining 4, oesophagitis with atrophy or dysplasia had progressed to cancer.

Alcohol and tobacco, which account for over 70% of the risk in populations of Europe and America, appear to play a minor role in the development of oesophageal cancer in Iran and China. Biochemical analyses showed that riboflavin deficiency was widespread in both populations, but it was more severe in Linxian, the high-risk population. No clear difference between the two populations was observed in relation to the level of $\beta$-carotene, retinol, and zinc. To clarify the role of this vitamin deficiency in the development of precancerous lesions of the oesophagus an intervention study is in progress as a blind randomized trial in which one group receives treatment with riboflavin, retinol, and zinc, and the other group receives a placebo, once a week for one year. Should this trial be positive, its impact on the primary prevention of oesophageal cancer will be enormous.

Identification of precancerous lesions of the oesophagus and their risk factors may have a significant impact on the primary prevention of oesophageal cancer as it might be easier to induce regression of very early lesions than those more advanced. Knowledge of precancerous lesions of the oesophagus in man is scarce. The available information is

[*1] 150 cours Albert Thomas, 69372 Lyon, France.

[*2] Viale Regina Elena 291, 00161 Rome, Italy.

derived from a limited number of postmortem studies on subjects dying from diseases other than oesophageal cancer. In this way dysplasia has been proposed as a precancerous lesion, but up to now no information was available on the lesions preceding the dysplasia (8, 9, 12, 15). In a high-risk population in Central Asia, submucosal fibrosis has been incriminated as a precancerous condition (6). To gather information on these lesions that will enable us to construct the natural history of this disease, epidemiological and endoscopic surveys have been carried out in two high-risk populations in northern Iran and northern China and in a low-risk population on the northeast coast of China.

## Methodology of Analysis

In the Islamic Republic of Iran a total of 430 subjects (218 males and 212 females) from the northern Turkoman villages of Khoran, Hottan, and Ghappan, were included in this study. Initially, persons with gastro-intestinal symptoms and those with close relatives who had had cancer of the oesophagus were encouraged to attend. Later in the study symptom-free individuals and individuals with no family history of oesophageal cancer were also included. In northern China 527 individuals (292 males and 235 females) from the Chen Guam commune of Linxian were included in the study. Results of these surveys have been published elsewhere (2, 10, 11).

In Jiaoxian, a low-lying county in Shandong province, situated on the northeast coast of China with a low-risk for oesophageal cancer, 301 subjects were randomly selected, and in 252 individuals (152 males and 100 females) endoscopic examination was performed. The detailed results are reported elsewhere (3).

The following procedure was followed with each of the subjects examined:
1. A questionnaire containing information on basic demographic data and information on smoking and drinking habits and cancer family history was completed together with a clinical form recording personal medical history and symptoms of upper gastrointestinal disease. In addition, in the Iranian village of Ghappan, questions on opium smoking or eating of opium pyrolysates were asked and in northern China information on dietary habits was also obtained.
2. A physical examination including evaluation of general health and signs of specific vitamin deficiencies was performed.
3. Specimens of blood and hair were collected in a sample of 111 of the subjects from Linxian and 120 from Jiaoxian for analysis of vitamin A, riboflavin, and zinc.
4. An endoscopic examination was performed in all subjects and guided cytology and at least two biopsies were taken from each individual.
5. The histological slides were read without knowledge of clinical data.

The criteria previously described were used to evaluate the endoscopical and histological findings (2, 3, 10). Briefly, oesophagitis was classified endoscopically as: *mild*, mucosa with slightly irregular surface, mild hyperaemia with or without slight scattered leukoplasia; *moderate*, irregular rough mucosa with pronounced hyperaemia and scattered or confluent leukoplasia, friable mucosa, bleeding easily at the touch of the oesophagoscope, and readily tearing at biopsy; or *severe*, irregular swollen mucosa, pronounced hyperaemia, and multiple leukoplasia, ridged mucosa consisting of white folds separated by hyperaemic areas. Biopsy specimens were fixed in 10% formalin and stained with haematoxylin and eosin. Slides were read without knowledge of clinical data. Because chronic oesophagitis was noted in many cases, the following criteria were used to grade this lesion: *mild*, characterized by slight lymphoplasmacytic infiltration, slight oedema of the submucosa, vascular proliferation and dilatation, and slight papillomatosis; *severe*, when the inflammatory infiltrate oedema and papillomatosis were more pronounced; and *moderate*, when the changes were between the two above extremes.

Riboflavin, vitamin A, and zinc status were measured using the same techniques as previously described (*12, 14*). Briefly, riboflavin was measured by the erythrocyte glutathion reductase activity test, retinol and β-carotene by a colorimetric method, and zinc by atomic absorption spectrophotometry.

## Precursor Lesions in High- and Low-risk Populations

### 1. Endoscopical findings

The results of the endoscopical findings are summarized in Table I. Oesophagitis was found in 85.3 and 88.4% of the males from the high-risk areas of Iran and Linxian and in 50.6% of the males in Jiaoxian, the low-risk area. The corresponding figures for females were 87.7 and 70.2% in Iran and Linxian respectively and 28.0% in Jiaoxian. Most of the oesophagitis was classified as mild or moderate and the severe type was found much more frequently in the high-risk populations than in the low-risk population, and in the former it was more frequent among males than among females. The oesophagitis was located mainly in the medium and lower thirds of the oesophagus. The involvement of the lower third was not accompanied by disease in the precardial region or signs of gastric reflux.

Inconspicuous oesophageal varices and incompetent cardia were found more frequently among the high-risk populations than among the low-risk one. Hiatal hernia was very rare in all populations.

The higher prevalence of oesophagitis, varices, and incompetent cardia in the high-risk populations than in the low-risk population of Jiaoxian, especially among women, is remarkable.

### 2. Histological findings

Table II summarizes the results of the histological evaluation. It shows that most of the oesophagitis diagnosed endoscopically was confirmed histologically. Its prevalence

TABLE I. Precursor Lesions of Oesophageal Cancer in High- and Low-risk Populations (Endoscopical Findings)

|  |  | Male | | | Female | | |
|  |  | High-risk | | Low-risk | High-risk | | Low-risk |
|  |  | Iran Turkoman | China Linxian | China Jiaoxian | Iran Turkoman | China Linxian | China Jiaoxian |
|---|---|---|---|---|---|---|---|
| Number of subjects |  | 218 | 292 | 152 | 212 | 235 | 100 |
|  | Mild | 37.6% | 41.1% | 32.2% | 59.9% | 53.6% | 17.0% |
| Oesophagitis | Moderate | 36.7 | 38.4 | 17.1 | 23.1 | 14.9 | 11.0 |
|  | Severe | 11.0 | 8.9 | 1.9 | 4.7 | 1.7 | 0.0 |
|  | Total | 85.3 | 88.4 | 50.6 | 87.7 | 70.2 | 28.0 |
| Varices |  | 13.2 | 7.2 | 1.3 | 18.4 | 9.4 | 2.0 |
| Incompetent cardia |  | 7.3 | 9.2 | 2.0 | 8.5 | 9.8 | 0.0 |
| Hiatal hernia |  | 0.9 | 0.7 | 0.7 | 0.9 | 0.0 | 1.0 |

TABLE II.  Precursor Lesions of Oesophageal Cancer in High- and Low-risk
Populations (Histological Findings)

| | | Male | | | Female | |
| | | High-risk | | Low-risk | High-risk | | Low-risk |
| | | Iran Turkoman | China Linxian | China Jiaoxian | Iran Turkoman | China Linxian | China Jiaoxian |
|---|---|---|---|---|---|---|---|
| Number of subjects | | 213 | 292 | 152 | 205 | 235 | 100 |
| | Mild | 58.7% | 55.8% | 33.5% | 57.6% | 56.2% | 18.0% |
| Oesophagitis | Moderate | 21.6 | 7.5 | 0.7 | 17.6 | 6.4 | 0.0 |
| | Severe | 2.8 | 1.7 | 0.0 | 1.0 | 0.9 | 0.0 |
| | Total | 83.1 | 65.0 | 34.2 | 76.2 | 63.5 | 18.0 |
| Clear cell acanthosis | | 66.2 | 80.8 | 82.9 | 64.9 | 72.4 | 85.0 |
| Atrophy | | 12.7 | 11.6 | 0.7 | 8.3 | 9.8 | 0.0 |
| Dysplasia | | 4.7 | 7.9 | 0.0 | 2.9 | 8.1 | 0.0 |

was higher in the high-risk populations than in the low-risk population. In males, it was 83.1% in Iran, 65.0% in Linxian, and 34.2% in Jiaoxian. In females, the prevalence of oesophagitis was 76.2% in Iran, 63.5% in Linxian, and 18.0% in Jiaoxian. The absence of the most advanced types in Jiaoxian is noteworthy. The second most common lesion was clear cell acanthosis characterized by a squamous epithelium thickened by swollen clear cells which, in most instances, were periodic acid / Schiff (PAS) negative. This lesion was unrelated to oesophagitis and its prevalence was similar in the high- and low-risk populations. Epithelial atrophy was diagnosed in 8–13% of the subjects from the high-risk populations and in 0.7% of the males in the low-risk area, and no case was diagnosed among the females. Epithelial dysplasia was diagnosed in 5 and 8% of the males from Iran and Linxian respectively, and 3 and 8% of the females, but no case was found in the low-risk area. In the high-risk populations the prevalence of oesophagitis was equally high in all age groups, even in those subjects under 20 years of age, but there was a tendency for the more severe types, especially those accompanied by dysplasia, to be higher in the older age groups.

## 3.  Risk factors

Table III shows the prevalence of the suspected risk factors in the two Chinese populations. The data for Iran are not shown as the questionnaire used there was different from the one used in China. The higher prevalence of a positive family history for oesophageal cancer in the high-risk population than in the low-risk population is remarkable

TABLE III.  Prevalence of Risk Factors in High- and Low-risk
Populations for Oesophageal Cancer in China

| | High-risk Linxian | Low-risk Jiaoxian |
|---|---|---|
| Family history of oesophageal cancer | 61.0% | 1.2% |
| Cigarette smokers | 45.0 | 64.0 |
| Alcohol drinkers | 17.0 | 64.0 |
| Angular stomatitis | 6.0 | 2.0 |
| Riboflavin status (mean A.C. and S.D.) | 1.69 (0.23) | 1.48 (0.19) |
| Oral leukoplasia | 20.0 | 2.0 |

as well as lack of correlation with smoking and drinking habits. The higher prevalence of angular stomatitis, one of the signs of riboflavin deficiency in Linxian than in Jiaoxian is in line with the more severe biochemical deficiency observed in Linxian. The higher prevalence of oral leukoplasia in the high-risk population deserves further study.

In Ghappan, one of the Turkoman villages, the subjects were asked whether they used opium. Of the 142 subjects, 35 (25%) admitted to using opium regularly (smoked or eaten), 70% of these had chronic oesophagitis compared with 77% of the 107 non-users. However, oesophageal cancer was found in 2 (5.7%) of the users and in 2 (1.8%) of the non-users.

## Aetiological Consideration

The oesophagitis firstly described by us in the high-risk populations of Iran and China, differs from that reported from low-risk populations in Europe and America. In Iran and China oesophagitis is characterized endoscopically by an irregular friable mucosa with varying degrees of oedema, hyperaemia, and leukoplasia but without erosions or ulceration and it usually involves the middle and lower thirds of the oesophagus, leaving the precardial region free. On the other hand, in the low-risk populations in Europe, oesophagitis is characterized by erosions and ulcerations, which usually involve the precardial region, as it is in general due to reflux.

The difference in the prevalence of chronic oesophagitis, diagnosed either endoscopically or histologically, between populations at high and low risk for oesophageal cancer is exceptional. The much lower prevalence of atrophy in the low-risk population and the absence of severe oesophagitis, dysplasia, and oesophageal cancer are also remarkable. These findings further support the model for the natural history of oesophageal cancer that was suggested by us previously,

i.e., Chronic oesophagitis $\longrightarrow$ Atrophy $\longrightarrow$ Dysplasia $\longrightarrow$ Cancer

That these lesions are in fact precancerous is suggested by:

a. The higher prevalence of these lesions in high-risk populations as compared to low-risk populations for oesophageal cancer;
b. The similar location of these lesions and of the oesophageal cancer: both involve mainly the middle and lower thirds of the oesophagus;
c. The results of a limited follow-up study in Linxian, which showed that in 8 out of 20 individuals examined endoscopically in May 1980 and May 1981, the lesions had progressed to a more advanced stage. In 4 of these, progression from mild oesophagitis to oesophagitis with atrophy and dysplasia was observed; and in the remaining 4, oesophagitis with atrophy or dysplasia had progressed to cancer. Details of this follow-up study are described elsewhere (10).

With regard to chronic oesophagitis, it should be pointed out that its presence, location, and severity are not correlated with any of the symptoms considered to be specific for oesophageal disease, such as dysphagia and retrosternal pain. This finding suggests that these symptoms are of no value for the selection of high-risk individuals.

The higher frequency of a positive family history for oesophageal cancer in Linxian (61.0%) than in Jiaoxian (1.2%) is remarkable. Although appropriate genetic studies have not been undertaken in Linxian, it has been assumed that this family clustering probably reflects a common exposure to environmental risk factors. Alcohol and tobacco, which account for about 70% of the oesophageal cancer in western societies, appear to play a less important role in the high-risk areas of Iran and China (4). The lower prevalence of smokers and drinkers in Linxian than in Jiaoxian supports this observation.

The search for aetiological factors associated with these precancerous lesions has been oriented to nutritional deficiencies. The vitamin analysis carried out in Linxian and Jiaoxian showed that riboflavin deficiency was widespread in both populations but it was more severe in Linxian. In order to clarify the role of these vitamin deficiencies in the development of precancerous lesions of the oesophagus, a blind, randomized trial having as its end-point an assessment of the precancerous lesions we have described is now underway in Huixian, China. One group receives a capsule containing riboflavin, retinol, and zinc, and the other, a placebo once a week for one year. The effects of the vitamin treatment will be evaluated by endoscopy, with cytology and histology, and the prevalence of the precancerous lesions will be compared in the two groups. Should the results of this trial be positive, the implication for primary prevention will be enormous.

Other factors suspected of being associated with the precancerous lesions of the oesophagus are thermal injury caused by drinking very hot beverages and physical injury due to eating very coarse food (10). The specific carcinogens responsible for the high incidence of oeosphageal cancer in Iran and China remain to be identified, but there is evidence suggesting that opium may be the main carcinogen in Iran (5), and N-nitroso compounds in China (1, 7).

## REFERENCES

1. Bartsch, H., Ohshima, H., Muñoz, N., Crespi, M., and Lu, S. H. Measurement of endogenous nitrosation in humans: potential applications of a new method and initial results. In "Human Carcinogenesis," ed. C. C. Harris and H. N. Alltrup, pp. 833–855 (1983). Academic Press, New York.

2. Crespi, M., Muñoz, N., Grassi, A., Aramesh, B., Amiri, G., and Mojtabai, A. Oesophageal lesions in northern Iran: a premalignant condition? *Lancet*, ii, 217–221 (1979).

3. Crespi, M., Muñoz, N., Grassi, A., Shen Qiong, Wang Kuo Jing, and Lin Jing Jien. Precursor lesions of oesophageal cancer in a low-risk population in China: comparison with high-risk populations. *Int. J. Cancer*, 34, 599–602 (1984).

4. Day, N. E. and Muñoz, N. Esophagus. In " Cancer Epidemiology and Prevention," ed. D. Schottenfeld and J. F. Fraumeni, pp. 596–623 (1982). W. B. Saunders & Co., Philadelphia.

5. Day, N. E., Malaveille, C., Friesen, M., and Bartsch, H. The possible role of opium and tobacco pyrolysates in esophageal cancer. In "Carcinogens and Mutagens in the Environment," Vol. II, " Naturally Occurring Compounds," ed. H. F. Stich, pp. 59–72 (1983). CRC Press, Boca Raton.

6. Kolysheva, V. J. Data on the epidemiology and morphology of precancerous changes and of cancer of the oesophagus in Kazakhstan, USSR. Thesis, Alma Ata (1974).

7. Lu, S. H., Bartsch, H., and Ohshima, H. Recent studies on nitrosamine and oesophageal cancer. In "N-Nitroso Compounds: Occurrence, Biological Effects and Relevance to Human Cancer," ed. I. K. O'Neill, R. C. von Borstel, J. E. Long, C. T. Miller, and H. Bartsch, IARC Scientific Publication No. 57, Lyon (1984), in press.

8. Mandard, A. M., Chasle, J., and Marnay, J. Autopsy findings in 111 cases of esophageal cancer. *Cancer*, 48, 329–335 (1981).

9. Mukuda, T., Sato, E., and Sasano, N. Comparative studies on dysplasia of esophageal

epithelium in four prefectures of Japan (Miyagi, Nara, Wakayama and Aomori) with reference to risk of carcinoma. *Tohoku J. Exp. Med.*, **119**, 51–63 (1976).

10. Muñoz, N., Crespi, M., Grassi, A., Wang Guo Qing, Shen Qiong, and Li Zhang Cai. Precursor lesions of oesophageal cancer in high-risk populations in Iran and China, *Lancet*, **i**, 876–879 (1982).

11. Muñoz, N. and Crespi, M. High-risk condition and precancerous lesions of the oesophagus. *In* "Precancerous Lesions of the Gastro-intestinal Tract," ed. P. Sherlock, B. C. Morson, L. Barbara, and U. Veronesi, pp. 53–63 (1983). Raven Press, New York.

12. Postelthwait, R. W. and Wendell Musser, A. Changes in the esophagus in 1,000 autopsy specimens. *J. Thorac. Cardiovasc. Surg.*, **68**, 953–956 (1974).

13. Thurnham, D. I., Rathakette, P., Hambidge, K. M., Muñoz, N., and Crespi, M. Riboflavin, vitamin A, and zinc status in Chinese subjects in a high-risk area for oesophageal cancer in China. *Hum. Nutr.: Clin. Nutr.*, **36C**, 337–349 (1982).

14. Thurnham, D. I., Zheng, S. F., Muñoz, N., Crespi, M., Grassi, A., Hambidge, K. M., and Chai, T. F. Comparison of riboflavin, vitamin A, and zinc status in high and low-risk regions for oesophageal cancer in China. Submitted to *Nutr. Cancer* (1985).

15. Ushigome, S., Spjut, H. J., and Noon, G. P. Extensive dysplasia and carcinoma *in situ* of esophageal epithelium. *Cancer*, **20**, 1023–1034 (1967).

# EXPERIMENTAL GASTRIC CARCINOGENESIS

Michihito TAKAHASHI

*Department of Pathology, National Institute of Hygienic Sciences\**

Utilizing a two-step carcinogenesis model with $N$-methyl-$N'$-nitro-$N$-nitrosoguanidine (MNNG) plus high salt diet as the initiator, we examined the promoting effect of sodium chloride in gastric carcinogenesis and compared the results with the actions of other chemicals.

In the first experiment, male outbred Wistar rats were given MNNG in the drinking water (100 mg/liter) for 8 weeks, and during this period they were fed on diet supplemented with 10% sodium chloride. Thereafter, they were divided into 5 groups and fed on the basal diet or one of various diets supplemented with 10% sodium chloride, 5% sodium saccharin, a known bladder promoter, 0.05% phenobarbital, a hepatic promoter, or 1% aspirin, a muscosal damaging agent until the end of the experiment. The incidence of adenocarcinoma was increased in the group given sodium chloride following the initiation treatment as compared with the basal diet group, though not significantly. However, the incidence of preneoplastic hyperplasia was significantly increased in this group. Phenobarbital and aspirin did not enhance tumor development, and aspirin, in fact, rather showing a tendency to decrease tumor incidence.

We further examined the promoting potential of ethanol in gastric carcinogenesis and compared with the other mucosal damaging agents. Rats were simultaneously given MNNG and sodium chloride for initiation, as in the first experiment. Thereafter, they received drinking water alone or drinking water supplemented with 10% ethanol, 1% potassium metabisulfite, 0.5% formalin (formaldehyde), or 1% hydrogen peroxide until the end of the experiment. The incidence of adenocarcinoma was increased in the groups given potassium metabisulfite and formaldehyde. However, neither ethanol nor hydrogen peroxide showed any modification of tumor development.

These results strongly suggest that sodium chloride, in addition to possessing co-initiator action, may also exert a promoting influence on gastric carcinogenesis. In contrast, ethanol does not appear active in this respect.

Cancer of the stomach is still the commonest cause of cancer death in Japan. Although the etiology of gastric cancer is unknown, a number of epidemiological studies have suggested that environmental factors such as dietary salt levels could explain, for example, the higher incidence in northern than in southern areas of this country. However, these studies of human population groups provide very little information about the evaluation and pathogenesis of gastric cancer. In recent years the discovery of $N$-methyl-$N'$-nitro-$N$-nitrosoguanidine (MNNG) has provided investigators with a specific

---

\* Kamiyoga 1-18-1, Setagaya-ku, Tokyo 158, Japan (高橋道人).

tool for elucidation of aspects of human gastric cancer. This compound when administered to rodents induces benign and malignant neoplasms of the stomach which are strikingly similar in most respects to gastric tumors in man, thus providing an opportunity to study, under controlled laboratory conditions, the effects of diet (25, 26), exogenous chemicals (23), and pathologic conditions in the stomach such as ulcer (27, 28), partial gastrectomy (2), genetic (11), and other factors (4) on tumor production.

## MNNG-Induced Gastric Cancer

Although gastric cancers have been induced in animals by various means, MNNG has been found to be a very advantageous gastric carcinogen when given in drinking water to rats and dogs (17). The method is simple, avoids stress associated with administration by gavage or injection, and is reproducible, yielding a high incidence of stomach tumors. This model was first established by Sugimura and Fujimura in 1967, who demonstrated a selective induction of high yields of gastric neoplasms after oral administration of MNNG at a dose of 83 $\mu$g/ml to Wistar rats (15).

Although randomly bred Wistar rats have been used most frequently, Donryu, Sprague-Dawley, ACI, Wistar / kob, BD IX, and BN rats also develop gastric tumors at a high frequency in response to MNNG treatment (11). However, Bralow et al. (1) found that rats of the Buffalo strain were not susceptible to induction of stomach cancer by MNNG and recently, Ohgaki et al. (11) reported on the role of genetic control. By studying the induction of gastric tumors by MNNG in susceptible ACI rats, resistant Buffalo rats, and their $F_1$ and $F_2$ offsprings, these authors showed that the gene controlling resistance to MNNG was autosomal in the Buffalo strain and was inherited dominantly by the $F_1$ and $F_2$ offsprings.

MNNG-induced gastric adenocarcinomas in rats usually develop in the pyloric region with rare neoplastic changes in the fundic region. A few tumors are also produced in the duodenum.

The histopathological features of MNNG-induced gastric neoplasms in rats and dogs have been described in detail by several investigators (8, 16). A histological classification of different types of experimental gastric adenocarcinoma is shown in Table I. Most MNNG-induced carcinomas demonstrate a highly differentiated glandular morphological pattern although diffuse and signet-ring cell carcinomas have also occasionally been reported (18). Electron microscopic and histochemical studies have revealed that most tumors are composed predominantly of undifferentiated cells originating from the gastric pyloric mucosa (9, 20). Pepsinogen isozyme studies have indicated that the pattern of

TABLE I.   Histological Types of Experimental Gastric Adenocarcinoma

Common type
  Papillary adenocarcinoma
  Tubular adenocarcinoma
    Well differentiated
    Moderately differentiated
    Poorly differentiated
  Mucinous adenocarcinoma
  Signet-ring cell carcinoma
Specific type

pepsinogen isozymes evident in gastric adenocarcinomas of rats is similar to that of normal pyloric mucosa, suggesting a histogenesis from pyloric mucosal cells (7, 21).

Macroscopically, early adenocarcinomas are usually characterized by small elevations of the mucosa. However, several other lesions may present the same appearance, making microscopic examination necessary for accurate diagnosis. Thus, in addition to early MNNG-induced adenocarcinomas (Photo 1), the possibilities include preneoplastic hyperplasias which are mostly early manifestations of adenocarcinoma (Photo 2), submucosal lymphoid hyperplasias (Photo 3), early mesenchymal tumors such as leiomyomas or leiomyosarcomas (Photo 4) and pyloric metaplasias of the fundus.

Sequential morphological investigations in the rat showed that the earliest gastric lesions observed during MNNG treatment consisted of mucosal erosion and atrophy followed first by regenerative hyperplasia and then by adenomatous hyperplasia (so-called adenoma), leading finally to invasive cancer. Although a number of authors have suggested that intestinal metaplasias may be precursor lesions for gastric carcinogenesis, the intestinal phenotype is most often observed within regions of advanced cancer. Such observations would suggest that the intestinal type of cell arises usually by a process of changed differentiation of gastric cancer cells rather than originating by metaplasia.

## Modulation of Experimental Gastric Carcinogenesis

Our earlier experiments on modulation of carcinogenesis were designed to survey the effects of various conditions on gastric carcinogenesis (5, 23). For example, it was demonstrated that concomitant administration of several surfactants with MNNG enhances the incidence of the more malignant and poorly differentiated type of adenocarcinoma. The presence of the surfactant may be effective in facilitating absorption of the carcinogen and thus enhancing the direct effects of the carcinogen on the target cells. Furthermore, it was shown that after the induction of chronic ulcers by administration of iodoacetamide (28), by freezing (27) or by intramural injections of formalin (13), subsequent ingestion of MNNG produces cancers at the ulcer site. The role of changes in gastric acidity has also been investigated by hormonal manipulation. Thus, lowering of pH by gastrin given during MNNG treatment led to enhancement of tumor yield together with a shift toward the carcinoid type of morphology (19). However, when gastrin was administered after removal of carcinogenic insult a reduction in the incidence of induced tumors resulted (29). Vagotomy carried out prior to MNNG administration gives rise to an increase in the yield of gastric tumors in the dog, presumably by increasing the duration of exposure to carcinogen (3).

## Effect of Salt as a Co-Initiator on Gastric Carcinogenesis

Our earlier study (22) demonstrated experimentally in rats that excess intake of sodium chloride concomitant to carcinogen treatment increased tumor incidences in the forestomach induced by 4-nitroquinoline 1-oxide (4-NQO) and in the glandular stomach induced by MNNG. More recently, we confirmed the effect of sodium chloride as a co-initiator in experimental gastric carcinogenesis (25).

Male outbred Wistar rats were simultaneously administered sodium chloride in the diet (10%) and MNNG in drinking water (100 mg/liter) for 20 weeks. Sacrifice at week 40 revealed a clear increase in both the incidence and size of tumors induced. On the other hand, administration of sodium chloride during the second 20 week period, after removal of the carcinogen, did not result in any enhancement of tumor development.

These data indicate that excess intake of sodium chloride enhances carcinogenesis only at the initiation stage, thus clarifying the results gained from our initial experiments (22) where no separation of the stages of carcinogenesis was made.

## Effect of Salt as a Promoter of Two-Step Carcinogenesis in an Experimental Gastric Cancer Model

It is widely accepted that carcinogenesis is a multistep process with each step probably representing one of a number of unknown discontinuous rare events. Experimentally, at least two and possibly more stages can be separated, namely, initiation and promotion. Two-step carcinogenesis was originally demonstrated in skin and subsequently was shown to occur in several other tissues.

While previous works (14, 25) failed to demonstrate the promoting potential of sodium chloride in gastric carcinogenesis after MNNG initiation, the possibility was raised that this was an inappropriate experimental design (26).

Therefore, utilizing a two-step carcinogenesis model with MNNG plus high salt diet as the initiator, we examined the promoting effects of sodium chloride in gastric carcinogenesis and compared the results with the actions of saccharin, a known bladder

TABLE II. Promoting Effects of Various Chemicals on Gastroduodenal Carcinogenesis Initiated by MNNG and NaCl in Male Wistar Rats (24, 26)

| Group No. | Chemical | Total No. of rats | No. of tumor bearing animals (%) | Forestomach | Glandular stomach | | | | Duodenum | |
|---|---|---|---|---|---|---|---|---|---|---|
| | | | | | Fundus | | Pylorus | | | |
| | | | | Papilloma | Adeno-carcinoma | Hyper-plasia | Adeno-carcinoma | Preneo-plastic hyper-plasia | Adeno-carcinoma | Others |
| Experiment I | | | | | | | | | | |
| 1 | None | 39 | 6(15.4) | 0 | 0 | 0 | 3( 7.7) | 5(12.8) | 3 | 0 |
| 2 | NaCl | 20 | 7(35.0) | 0 | 0 | 0 | 4(20.0) | 8(40.0)* | 3(15.0) | 0 |
| 3 | Saccharin | 20 | 5(25.0) | 0 | 0 | 0 | 3(15.0) | 5(25.0) | 1( 5.0) | 2(10.0)a |
| 4 | Pheno-barbital | 19 | 2(10.5) | 0 | 0 | 0 | 1( 5.3) | 4(21.1) | 1( 5.3) | 1( 5.3)b |
| 5 | Aspirin | 20 | 1( 5.0) | 0 | 0 | 0 | 0 | 2(10.0) | 1( 5.0) | 0 |
| Experiment II | | | | | | | | | | |
| 1 | None | 30 | 4(13.3) | 0 | 0 | 0 | 1( 3.3) | 7(23.3) | 3(10.0) | 0 |
| 2 | Ethanol | 21 | 2( 9.5) | 0 | 0 | 1( 4.8) | 0 | 1( 4.8) | 2( 9.5) | 0 |
| 3 | Potassium metabisulfite | 19 | 6(31.6) | 2(10.5) | 0 | 1( 5.3) | 5(26.3)* | 4(21.1) | 1( 5.3) | 0 |
| 4 | Form-aldehyde | 17 | 5(29.4) | 15(88.2)** | 0 | 15(88.2)** | 4(23.5)* | 7(41.2) | 1( 5.9) | 0 |
| 5 | Hydrogen peroxide | 21 | 2( 9.5) | 21(100)** | 0 | 8(38.1)** | 2( 9.5) | 6(28.6) | 0 | 0 |

Data for groups 6–10 in both experiments are omitted.

a One fibrosarcoma and one hemangiosarcoma.

b Hepatocellular carcinoma.

* $p < 0.05$, ** $p < 0.001$.

promoter, phenobarbital, a hepatic promoter, and aspirin, a mucosal damaging agent (26) (Experiment I). Male outbred Wistar rats were given MNNG in the drinking water (100 mg/liter) for 8 weeks, and during this period were fed on diet supplemented with 10% sodium chloride. Thereafter, they were divided into 5 groups and fed on a basal diet or one of various diets supplemented with 10% sodium chloride, 5% sodium saccharin, 0.05% phenobarbital, or 1% aspirin until the end of the experiment. All animals were killed at the 40th experimental week for necropsy and histological examination. The incidence of adenocarcinoma (Table II) was increased in the group given sodium chloride following initiation by MNNG and sodium chloride as compared with the respective control group given MNNG and sodium chloride initiation only, but not significantly. However, the incidence of preneoplastic hyperplasia was significantly increased in this group. Saccharin also enhanced the development of adenocarcinomas of the glandular stomach. The results indicated a tendency for dietary administration of sodium chloride or saccharin to promote tumor development. Phenobarbital and aspirin, on the other hand, did not enhance tumor development, and aspirin, in fact, rather showing a tendency to decrease tumor incidence.

In a further experiment (Experiment II) we examined the promoting potential of ethanol in gastric carcinogenesis and compared the results with the actions of potassium metabisulfite, formaldehyde and hydrogen peroxide (24). Rats were given MNNG as initiator in the drinking water for 8 weeks and during this period they were fed on diet supplemented with 10% sodium chloride, similarly as in Experiment I. Thereafter, they were divided into 5 groups, receiving drinking water alone or drinking water supplemented with 10% ethanol, 1% potassium metabisulfite, 0.5% formalin (formaldehyde), or 1% hydrogen peroxide until the end of the experiment. All animals were killed at the 40th experimental week for necropsy and histological examination. The incidence of adenocarcinoma was increased in the groups given potassium metabisulfite and formaldehyde. Neither ethanol nor hydrogen peroxide showed any enhancement of tumor development. Papillomas in the forestomach were observed in formaldehyde- and hydrogen peroxide-treated rats, but the incidence of these lesions did not differ between the groups with and without initiation treatment.

These results strongly suggest that sodium chloride, in addition to possessing co-initiator action, may also exert a promoting influence on gastric carcinogenesis. In contrast, ethanol does not appear active in this respect.

Recently Salmon et al. (12) and Kobori et al. (10) reported a significant enhancement of MNNG-induced gastric tumorigenesis respectively by taurocholic acid or sodium taurocholate mixed with diet, indicating that bile salts could also be gastric promoters.

## CONCLUSION

Although progress in experimental gastric carcinogenesis has recently been made with the utilization of different animal models, the results have not yet to be translated into effective means for controlling the human disease. The availability of experimental models permits evaluation of risk factors such as high salt consumption and, furthermore, allows such risk factors to be investigated with regard to their relative importance in the initiation and promotion stages of multi-step carcinogenesis.

While the results of the present study provide suggestive evidence for the promotional role of dietary sodium chloride in gastric carcinogenesis, the mechanism remains unclear. One possibility is that high doses of sodium chloride have hyperplasiogenic potential: this study revealed that the enhancement of tumor induction with sodium chloride and saccharin was associated with diffuse proliferative changes in the superficial epithelium or generative zone of the glandular stomach (Photo 5). In contrast, the non-enhancers phenobarbital and aspirin caused neither effect. Although erosive lesions could be seen in the aspirin treated groups, these were focal in nature and no diffuse hyperplasia was apparent. Recently, Furihata *et al.* (*6*) reported an induction of ornithine decarboxylase (ODC) activity and DNA synthesis in the glandular stomach mucosa of rats by sodium chloride as well as by MNNG. This phenomenon is reminiscent of the changes in ODC and DNA synthesis observed after 12-O-tetradecanoylphorbol-13-acetate (TPA) or mezerein treatment of skin, although much higher concentrations of sodium chloride were required for significant induction.

## REFERENCES

1. Bralow, S. P., Gruenstein, M., and Meranze, D. R. Strain resistance to gastric adeno-carcinoma in rats ingesting NG. *Proc. Am. Assoc. Cancer Res.*, **12**, 3 (1971).
2. Dahm, K. and Werner, B. Susceptibility of the resected stomach to experimental carcino-genesis. *Z. Krebsforsch.*, **85**, 219–229 (1976).
3. Fujita, M., Takami, M., Usugane, M., Nampei, S., and Taguchi, T. Enhancement of gastric carcinogenesis in dogs given N-methyl-N'-nitro-N-nitrosoguanidine following vagotomy. *Cancer Res.*, **39**, 811–816 (1979).
4. Fukushima, S., Hananouchi, M., Shirai, T. Tatematsu, M., Hirose, M., Yoshida, S., and Takahashi, M. Effect of plastic bead on gastric carcinogenesis in rats treated with N-methyl-N'-nitro-N-nitrosoguanidine. *Gann*, **67**, 197–205 (1976).
5. Fukushima, S., Tatematsu, M., and Takahashi, M. Combined effect of various surfactants on gastric carcinogenesis in rats treated with N-methyl-N'-nitro-N-nitrosoguanidine. *Gann*, **65**, 371–376 (1974).
6. Furihata, C., Sato, Y., Hosaka, M., Matsushima, T., Furukawa, F., and Takahashi, M. NaCl induced ornithine decarboxylase and DNA synthesis in rat stomach mucosa. *Biochem. Biophys. Res. Commun.*, **121**, 1027–1032 (1984).
7. Furihata, C., Tatematsu, M., Shirai, T., Yokochi, K., Takahashi, M., and Sugimura, T. Pepsinogens and stomach cancer. *In* "Pathophysiology of Carcinogenesis in Digestive Organs," ed. E. Farber *et al.*, pp. 49–63 (1977). Japan Sci. Soc. Press, Tokyo/Univ. Park Press, Baltimore.
8. Kobori, O. Analytical study of precancerous lesions in rat stomach mucosa induced by N-methyl-N'-nitro-N-nitrosoguanidine. *GANN Monogr. Cancer Res.*, **25**, 141–150 (1980).
9. Kobori, O., Gedigk, P., and Totović, V. Adenomatous changes and adenocarcionoma of glandular stomach in Wistar rats induced by N-methyl-N'-nitro-N-nitrosoguanidine. An electron microscopic and histochemical study. *Virchows Arch. A (Pathol. Anat.)*, **373**, 37–54 (1977).
10. Kobori, O., Watanabe, J., Shimizu, T., Shoji, M., and Morioka, Y. Enhancing effect of sodium taurocholate on N-methyl-N'-nitro-N-nitrosoguanidine-induced stomach tumorigenesis in rats. *Gann*, **75**, 651–654 (1984).
11. Ohgaki, H., Kawachi, T., Matsukura, N., Morino, K., Miyamoto, M., and Sugimura, T. Genetic control of susceptibility of rats to gastric carcinoma. *Cancer Res.*, **43**, 3663–3667 (1983).
12. Salmon, R. J., Laurene, M., and Thierry, J. P. Effect of taurocholic acid feeding on methyl-nitro-N-nitrosoguanidine induced gastric tumors. *Cancer Lett.*, **22**, 315–320 (1984).

13. Saito, T., Sasaki, O., Matsukuchi, T., Iwamatsu, M., and Inokuchi, K. Experimental gastric cancer: pathogenesis and clinicohistopathologic correlation. *In* "Gastric Cancer," eds. Ch. Herfarth and P. Schlag, pp. 22–31 (1979). Springer-Verlag, Berlin.

14. Shirai, T., Imaida, K., Fukushima, S., Hasegawa, R., Tatematsu, M., and Ito, N. Effects of NaCl, Tween 60 and a low dose of *N*-ethyl-*N'*-nitro-*N*-nitrosoguanidine on gastric carcinogenesis of rat given a single dose of *N*-methyl-*N'*-nitro-*N*-nitrosoguanidine. *Carcinogenesis*, **3**, 1419–1422 (1982).

15. Sugimura, T. and Fujimura, S. Tumour production in glandular stomach of rats by *N*-methyl-*N'*-nitro-*N*-nitrosoguanidine. *Nature*, **216**, 943–944 (1967).

16. Sugimura, T. and Kawachi, T. Experimental stomach carcinogenesis. *In* "Gastrointestinal Tract Cancer," ed. M. Lipkin and R. A. Good, pp. 327–341 (1978). Plenum Publ. Co., New York.

17. Sugimura, T., Fujimura, S., Kogure, K. Baba, T., Saito, T., Nagao, M., Hosoi, H., Shimosato, Y., and Yokoshima, T. Production of adenocarcinomas in the glandular stomach of experimental animals by *N*-methyl-*N'*-nitro-*N*-nitrosoguanidine. *GANN Monogr.*, **8**, 157–196 (1969).

18. Tahara, E. and Haizuka, S. Effect of gastro-entero-pancreatic endocrine hormones on the histogenesis of gastric cancer in rats induced by *N*-methyl-*N'*-nitro-*N*-nitrosoguanidine; with special reference to development of scirrhous gastric cancer. *Gann*, **66**, 421–426 (1975).

19. Tahara, E., Shimamoto, F., Taniyama, K., Ito, H., Kosako, Y., and Sumiyoshi, H. Enhanced effect of gastrin on rat stomach carcinogenesis induced by *N*-methyl-*N'*-nitro-*N*-nitrosoguanidine. *Cancer Res.*, **42**, 1781–1787 (1982).

20. Tatematsu, M., Katsuyama, T., Fukushima, S. Takahashi, M., Shirai, T., Ito, N., and Nasu, T. Mucin histochemistry by paradoxical concanavalin A staining in experimental gastric cancers induced in Wistar rats by *N*-methyl-*N'*-nitro-*N*-nitrosoguanidine or 4-nitroquinoline 1-oxide. *J. Natl. Cancer Inst.*, **64**, 835–843 (1980).

21. Tatematsu, M., Saito, D., Furihata, C., Miyata, Y., Nakatsuka, T., Ito, N., and Sugimura, T. Initial DNA damage and heritable permanent change in pepsinogen isoenzyme pattern in the pyloric mucosae of rats after short-term administration of *N*-methyl-*N'*-nitro-*N*-nitrosoguanidine. *J. Natl. Cancer Inst.*, **64**, 775–781 (1980).

22. Tatematsu, M., Takahashi, M., Fukushima, S., Hananouchi, M., and Shirai, T. Effects in rats of sodium chloride on experimental gastric cancers induced by *N*-methyl-*N'*-nitro-*N*-nitrosoguanidine or 4-nitroquinoline-1-oxide. *J. Natl. Cancer Inst.*, **55**, 101–106 (1975).

23. Takahashi, M., Fukushima, S., and Sato, H. Carcinogenic effect of *N*-methyl-*N'*-nitro-*N*-nitrosoguanidine with various kinds of surfactant in the glandular stomach of rats. *Gann*, **64**, 211–218 (1973).

24. Takahashi, M., Hasegawa, R., Furukawa, F., Toyoda, K., Sato, H., and Hayashi, Y. Effects of ethanol, potassium metabisulfite, formaldehyde and hydrogen peroxide on gastric carcinogenesis in rats after initiation with *N*-methyl-*N'*-nitro-*N*-nitrosoguanidine. *Gann*, **77**, in press (1986).

25. Takahashi, M., Kokubo, T., Furukawa, F., Kurokawa, Y., Tatematsu, M., and Hayashi, Y. Effect of high salt diet on rat gastric carcinogenesis induced by *N*-methyl-*N'*-nitro-*N*-nitrosoguanidine. *Gann*, **74**, 28–34 (1983).

26. Takahashi, M., Kokubo, T., Furukawa, F., Kurokawa, Y., and Hayashi, Y. Effects of sodium chloride, saccharin, phenobarbital and aspirin on gastric carcinogenesis in rats after initiation with *N*-methyl-*N'*-nitro-*N*-nitrosoguanidine. *Gann*, **75**, 494–501 (1984).

27. Takahashi, M., Shirai, T., Fukushima, S., Ito, N., Kokubo, T., and Kurata, Y. Ulcer formation and associated tumor production in multiple sites within stomach and duodenum of rats treated with *N*-methyl-*N'*-nitro-*N*-nitrosoguanidine. *J. Natl. Cancer Inst.*, **67**, 473–479 (1981).

28. Takahashi, M., Shirai, T., Fukushima, S., Hananouchi, M., Hirose, M., and Ito, N. Effect of fundic ulcers induced by iodoacetamide on development of gastric tumors in rats treated with $N$-methyl-$N'$-nitro-$N$-nitrosoguanidine. *Gann*, **67**, 47–54 (1976).
29. Tatsuta, M., Itoh, T., Okuda, S., Taniguchi, H., and Tamura, H. Effect of prolonged administration of gastrin on experimental carcinogenesis in rat stomach induced by $N$-methyl-$N'$-nitro-$N$-nitrosoguanidine. *Cancer Res.*, **37**, 1808–1810 (1977).

## EXPLANATION OF PHOTOS

PHOTO 1.   A small elevation of the mucosa showing underlying adenocarcinoma. Hematoxylin-Eosin stain (H-E). ×40.

PHOTO 2.   A small elevation of the mucosa showing preneoplastic hyperplasia. H-E. ×40.

PHOTO 3.   A small elevation of the mucosa showing submucosal lymphoid hyperplasia. H-E. ×40.

PHOTO 4.   A small elevation of the mucosa showing leiomyoma. H-E. ×40.

PHOTO 5.   Histological appearance of the glandular stomach in a control rat (A), in a sodium chloride-treated rat showing deep gastric pits with a markedly increased number of mucous neck cells (B), and in a saccharin-treated rat showing increased number of dark cells in the generative zone (C). H-E. ×200.

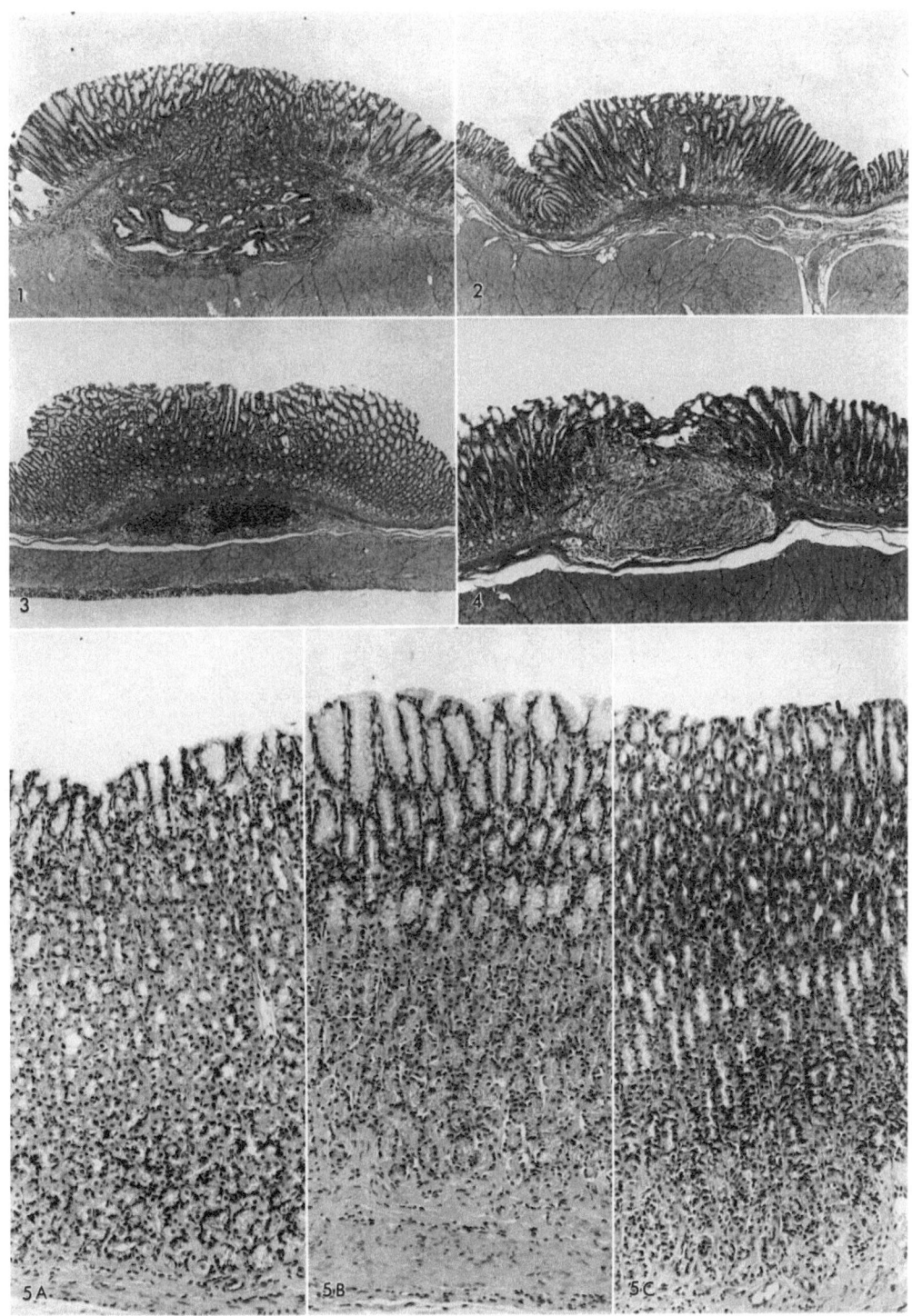

# MORPHOLOGICAL CHANGES OF THE ILEAL EPITHELIUM TRANSPOSED INTO THE COLON, AND ITS EFFECTS ON THE DMH CARCINOGENESIS OF RATS

Masayuki Yasutomi, Taiji Matsuda, Masaaki Ogawa, Zenji Iwasa, Jiro Maruyama, Ikuhiro Sakata, Kazuyoshi Kurooka, and Yasuhiro Katsura

*Department of Surgery, Kinki University Faculty of Medicine\**

It is well-known that dimethylhydrazine (DMH)-induced cancer of the rat has a specificity for the colon and a histological resemblance to human cancer of the intestine. In order to elucidate this organ specificity of the colon, DMH (10 mg/kg weekly×16) was administered after surgery transposing an ileal segment into the colon. DMH administration was begun at two different times, the early administration started 2 weeks after the surgery and the late administration 16 weeks afterwards. Cancer developed in the ileal segment transposed into the colon in both groups 30 weeks after DMH administration, but did not develop at all in the ileum of a sham operation or of non-operated control animals. To clarify the cause for such an increase in tumor incidence changes in the stalked interposed ileum were studied without the administration of DMH. After 6 weeks, the number of cells composing the crypt of the transposed ileal epithelium had increased 1.4-fold, and microautoradiography by $^3$H-thymidine showed an increase of labelling index of the crypt and an upward expansion of the germinal zone. Histochemistry of an HID-AB stain showed a change in mucin composition in the epithelial cells with sialomucin predominant. Bacterial flora of the transposed ileum, both aerobes and anaerobes, increased more than $10^2$ times. It was suspected that in the early administration mechanical injury of the intestinal mucosa by the operation promoted carcinogenesis, while in the late administration carcinogenesis was due to a change in the transposed ileal epithelium.

In the modelling of human cancer of the large intestine, there have recently been many reports on experimental carcinogenesis with dimethylhydrazine (DMH) and the related compound azoxymethane (AOM). Cancer induced by these carcinogens develops in the colon at a high incidence, like human cancer of the intestine, but rarely develops in the small intestine or other organs. In order to elucidate this organ specificity, Gennaro *et al.* (1973) (*3*) and Celik *et al.* (1981) (*1*) performed a transposition of the small intestine into the colon and of the colon into the small intestine, and then administered either AOM or DMH. Since cancer did not develop in the small intestine transposed into the colon, both groups concluded that the mucosa of the small intestine itself resists carcinogens, while the colonic mucosa is sensitive. Yamada *et al.* (*9*) and Ogawa *et al.* (*7*), who administered DMH after practically the same operation, however, reported that cancer

---

\* Sayamacho, Minamikawachi-gun, Osaka 589, Japan (安富正幸, 松田泰治, 小川雅昭, 岩佐善二, 丸山次郎, 坂田育弘, 黒岡一仁, 桂　康博)

also developed in the small intestine transposed into the colon, as it did in the colon, their conclusions thus contradicting those reached by Gennaro *et al.* and Celik *et al.* Surgical operations of the intestinal tract, such as resection, anastomosis, *etc.*, influence carcinogenesis in different ways. Therefore carcinogens must be administered after sufficient time has elapsed after surgery. Further, after a long period the epithelium of the small intestine may change and become sensitive to the carcinogens as does the colon. To test this theory, after surgical transposition of an ileal segment into the colon, DMH was administered after a short time in one group of animals and after a longer time in another.

*Transposition of the Intestine and Experimental Carcinogenesis*

Male Sprague-Dawley rats, each weighing 200–250 g, were used and were raised with CE-2 rat feed (Nippon-Clea Co., Ltd.). After 24 hr of fasting, the rats were subjected to the following surgery under ether anesthesia:
1. Transposition of the ileal segment into the colon: a stalked ileal segment, about 5 cm long and 20 cm from the terminal ileum, was transposed into the proximal colon.
2. Transposition of the colonic segment into the ileum: a 5 cm colonic segment was transposed into the ileum 20 cm from the terminal ileum.
3. Transection and anastomosis of the ileum: as a sham operation, the ileum 20 cm from the terminal ileum was divided into lengths of about 5 cm, and then anastomosed again at the same site.
4. No operation: 1,2-DMH dihydrochloride (Aldrich) was administered once a week for 16 weeks at a dose of 10 mg/kg. Gennaro *et al.* (*3*) performed transpositions between the jejunum and the distal colon, but in our experiment the transposition was between the ileum and the proximal colon. Further, they used AOM as the carcinogen, whereas we used DMH at a lower dose of 10 mg/kg. According to the literature, when DMH at 20 mg/kg is administered for 16 weeks, cancer develops in more than 80% of rats, but at the dose of 10 mg/kg × 16 the incidence of tumors is as low as 30–40%. DMH administration was begun at two times: in the early administration group it was at an average period of 2 weeks, while in the late administration group it averaged 16 weeks after surgery. At 2 weeks, as reported by Celik *et al.* (*1*), Williamson *et al.* (*8*), Yamada *et al.* (*9*) and others, the influence of surgery is still present. One hundred twenty-seven rats were sacrificed 30 weeks after DMH administration, and their intestinal carcinogenesis was examined by macroscopical and microscopical methods. Cancer was defined as a tumor which had invaded histologically. Noninvasive mucosal cancer was defined as adenoma, since discrimination from adenoma was often difficult.

*1. DMH early administration group*

The incidence of intestinal cancer with early administration was 26.6%, and that of tumor, including adenoma and cancer, was 60.9%. The incidence of cancer and tumor in the two experimental groups was as high as 57.1 and 95.2% in the transposition group, compared with 7.7 and 23.1% in the control (Table I). The tumor distribution of the intestine was most frequent at the anastomosis site of the colon to the ileum 23.8%, followed by the colon 19.0% and the transposed ileum 9.5%, as shown in Table II-A. The area of the anastomosis site included 1 cm on both the oral and anal sides of the

TABLE I. DMH-Induced Intestinal Tumor

A. Early administration group: DMH started 2 weeks after operation

| Operation performed | Total No. of rats | No. of rats | |
|---|---|---|---|
| | | With cancer | With cancer and/or adenoma |
| Transposition of ileal segment into the colon | 21 | 12 (57.1%) | 20 (95.2%) |
| Sham operation (transection and anastomosis of the ileum) | 30 | 15 (50.0%) | 18 (60.0%) |
| Control (no operation) | 13 | 1 ( 7.7%) | 3 (23.1%) |
| Total | 64 | 17 (26.6%) | 39 (60.9%) |

B. Late administration group: DMH started 16 weeks after surgery

| Operation performed | Total No. of rats | No. of rats | |
|---|---|---|---|
| | | With cancer | With cancer and/or adenoma |
| Transposition of ileal segment into the colon | 31 | 9 (29.0%) | 16 (51.6%) |
| Sham operation (transection and anastomosis of the ileum) | 17 | 8 (47.2%) | 8 (47.1%) |
| Control (no operation) | 15 | 2 (13.3%) | 10 (66.7%) |
| Total | 63 | 19 (30.1%) | 34 (54.0%) |

suture line, and a tumor developing there was regarded as a tumor developing at the anastomosis site. No neoplasmas were found in the ileum or other organs.

## 2. DMH late administration group

DMH administration was started about 16 weeks after the operation. As shown in Table I-B, the incidence of cancer on the whole was 30.1%, and that of cancer and adenoma was 54.0%. The incidence of cancer and of tumor including cancer and adenoma were 29.0 and 51.6% in the ileal transposition, while 13.3 and 66.7% in control. The intestinal tumor distribution is shown in Table II-B. Tumors were frequently observed at the anastomosis site of transposition and in the colon of all groups, however, this was true in fewer cases than in the early administration group except for the control. Also, cancer and adenoma were noted in the ileal segment transposed into the colon while no cancers were found in the ileum between anastomoses in the sham operation or in the normal ileum in all groups. Taking the incidence of cancer per mucosal area of the ileum transposed into the colon as 100, the incidence in the large intestine was 64 in the early administration group, and 29 in the late administration group. The incidence per unit mucosal area was higher in the transposed ileum than in the large intestine. The transposed ileum is small in area and cancer seems to be rare.

Since the reports of Gennaro et al. (3) and Celik et al. (1), it has been generally accepted that the mucosa of the small intestine itself is resistant to carcinogens. However, this study has shown that adenoma and cancer develop in the ileum transposed into the colon. When DMH administration was started 2 weeks after the operation, tumors developed simultaneously at a high incidence on the suture line; this is due to the fact that carcinogenesis is promoted by mucosal injury during the operation. Concerning the reason for the development of tumors at the site of intestinal anastomosis, Williamson et al. (8) state that here mucosal defects and repairs are repeated, and the synthesis of

TABLE II.   Distribution of DMH-Induced Intestinal Tumor

A.   Early administration (2 weeks after 10 mg/kg × 16)

| | No. of rats | |
| --- | --- | --- |
| | With cancer (%) | With cancer (%) and/or adenoma (%) |
| Transposition of ileum into the colon (21 rats) | | |
| Jejunum | 3 (14.3) | 3 (14.3) |
| Ileum | 0 | 0 |
| Transposed ileal segment | 2 ( 9.5) | 3 (14.3) |
| Anastomosis (colon to ileum) | 5 (23.8) | 7 (33.3) |
| Anastomosis (ileum to ileum) | 2 ( 9.5) | 2 ( 9.5) |
| Colon | 4 (19.0) | 4 (19.0) |
| Sham operation (transection and anastomosis of the ileum) (10 rats) | | |
| Jejunum | 0 | 0 |
| Ileum | 0 | 0 |
| Transectioned ileal segment | 1 ( 3.3) | 1 ( 3.3) |
| Anastomoses (ileum to ileum) | 15 (50.0) | 18 (60.0) |
| Colon | 6 (20.0) | 8 (26.6) |
| No operation (13 rats) | | |
| Jejunum | 0 | 0 |
| Ileum | 0 | 0 |
| Colon | 1 ( 7.7) | 2 (15.4) |

B.   Late administration (16 weeks after 10 mg/kg × 16)

| | No. of rats | |
| --- | --- | --- |
| | With cancer (%) | With cancer (%) and/or adenoma (%) |
| Transposition of ileum into the colon (31 rats) | | |
| Jejunum | 1 ( 3.2) | 1 ( 3.2) |
| Ileum | 0 | 0 |
| Transposed ileal segment | 2 ( 6.4) | 3 ( 9.7) |
| Anastomosis (ileum to colon) | 5 (16.1) | 7 (22.6) |
| Anastomosis (ileum to ileum) | 1 ( 3.2) | 4 (12.9) |
| Colon | 2 ( 6.4) | 7 (22.6) |
| Sham operation (transection and anastomosis of the ileum) (17 rats) | | |
| Jejunum | 0 | 1 ( 5.9) |
| Ileum | 0 | 0 |
| Transectioned ileal segment | 0 | 0 |
| Anastomosis (ileum to ileum) | 1 ( 5.9) | 8 (47.1) |
| Colon | 7 (41.2) | 7 (41.2) |
| No operation (18 rats) | | |
| Jejunum | 0 | 0 |
| Ileum | 0 | 1 ( 5.6) |
| Colon | 2 (11.1) | 9 (50.0) |

DNA is accelerated, which has a promoting effect on carcinogenesis. Hagihara (4) reported that acute colitis caused by acetic acid promoted carcinogenesis with DMH. The acceleration of carcinogenesis at the anastomosed site in this study may have the same mechanism.

Gennaro *et al.* (3) stated that cancer did not develop in the small intestine transposed into the colon, but he used only 9 rats in each group. Celik *et al.* (*1*) also started DMH 10–12 days after the operation and did not exclude the effect of the operation on carcinogenesis. In order to exclude the effect of the surgery, DMH was administered 16 weeks after the operation in the late administration group. The incidence of tumor decreased notably at the site of anastomosis; however, in the transposed ileum both cancer and adenoma developed.

In order to elucidate the causes for such an increase in tumor incidence in the interposed ileum, changes in the stalked interposed ileum were studied without the administration of DMH.

### Changes of Ileal Mucosal Epithelium Transposed into Colon

It was believed that changes occurred in the ileal epithelium transposed into the colon, which accelerated carcinogenesis. Three separate types of operation were carried out: 1) transposition of the ileum into the colon (21 rats), 2) sham operation (20 rats), and 3) no operation (10 rats), and successive changes in the ileal mucosal epithelium were followed after 6, 12, and 18 weeks without administration of a carcinogen.

a. Changes in the number of epithelial cells composing villi and crypts of the ileal mucosa: the number of epithelial cells composing villi of the normal ileum was 46±3.1, and there was no difference between the no-operation group and the sham operation group after 6, 12, and 18 weeks. By contrast, in the ileal epithelium interposed into the colon, the number increased to 66±7.9 after 6 weeks, and again significantly after 12 and 18 weeks. The number of cells composing the crypts also increased markedly, 1.4-fold, in the ileum interposed into the colon group, compared with that of the control group.

b. Cell population kinetics of the epithelium of the crypt: a labelling index of the epithelium of the crypt was studied by microautoradiography with $^3$H-thymidine. It was 19.1% in the control, whereas it increased to 27.6–30.8% in the transposed ileum. Further, the germinal zone was noted to expand to the upper segment of the crypt, though normally it is in the lower half. This increase in the labelling index of the crypt column, and the expansion of the germinal zone are changes indicating histological hyperplasia with high risk of tumor genesis, corresponding to Lipkin's phase I change of carcinogenesis (*6*).

c. Mucin histochemical studies of the epithelial cells were performed by HID-AB stain; staining was positive in the normal and control while in the ileum interposed into the colon Alcian blue staining became positive. The change in mucin composition from sulfomucin to sialomucin is one seen in the transitional mucosa of Fillipe (*2*), which he indicates as a precancerous lesion.

d. Such changes in the transposed ileal mucosa, promoting carcinogenesis, may be due to changes in the bacterial flora of the intestine, and this was studied next. In the transposed ileum the bacterial count increased more than $10^2$ times, in both aerobes and anaerobes, compared with the normal ileum or the ileum of the sham operation. The change in the bacterial flora of the intestine is believed to change the cell cycle of the ileal epithelium, causing a state of hyperplasia, and simultaneously also to change the properties of mucus and act to enhance carcinogenesis.

## REFERENCES

1. Celik, C., Mittelman, A., Paolini, N. S., Jr., Lewis, D., and Evans, J. T. Effects of 1,2-symmetrical dimethylhydrazine on jejunocolic transposition in Sprague-Dawley rats. *Cancer Res.*, **41**, 2908–2911 (1981).
2. Fillipe, M. I. Mucous secretion in rat colonic mucosa during carcinogenesis induced by dimethylhydrazine. A morphological and histochemical study. *Br. J. Cancer*, **32**, 60–77 (1975).
3. Gennaro, A. R., Villanueva, R., Sukonthaman, Y., Vathanophas, V., and Rosemond, G. P. Chemical carcinogenesis in transposed intestinal segments. *Cancer Res.*, **33**, 536–541 (1973).
4. Hagihara, P. F. Experimental colitis as a promoter in large-bowel tumorigenesis. *Arch. Surg.*, **117**, 1304–1307 (1982).
5. Katsura, Y. and Yasutomi, M. Histochemical and cytokinetic studies on promoting effect of DMH carcinogenesis of the transposed ileal epithelia into the colon *Jpn. J. Gastroenterol.*, **18** (9), 2049–2056 (1985).
6. Lipkin, M. Proliferative changes in the colon. *Dig. Dis.*, **19** (11), 1029–1032 (1974).
7. Ogawa, M., Katsura, Y., Maruyama, J., Matsuda, T., Sakata, I., and Yasutomi, M. Studies on effect of intestinal microflora on DMH-induced cancer (in Japanese). *Med. J. Kinki Univ.*, **8** (1), 23–38 (1983).
8. Williamson, R.C.N., Bauer, F.L.R., and Terpstra, O. T. Contrasting effects of subtotal enteric bypass, enterectomy, and colectomy on azoxymethane-induced intestinal carcinogenesis. *Cancer Res.*, **40**, 538–543 (1980).
9. Yamada, Y., Hosoda, S., and Nagayo, T. The effects of DMH carcinogenesis on the jejunal segment interposed into the colon (in Japanese). *Proc. Meet. Jpn. Cancer Soc.*, **40**, 65 (1981).

# TUMOR CHARACTERISTICS

# HISTOPATHOLOGY OF GI TRACT TUMOR

Haruo SUGANO,*¹ Yo KATO*¹, and Kyoichi NAKAMURA*²

*Department of Pathology, Cancer Institute*¹ *and Department
of Pathology, Tsukuba University*²

From histopathologic and histogenetic viewpoints, gastric carcinoma can be classified into two subtypes: poorly differentiated (diffuse) (PCA) and differentiated (intestinal) (DCA). The former arises from the non-intestinalized ordinary epithelium and often occurs in young persons, especially in females. The latter originates from the intestinalized epithelium and frequently occurs in older persons, especially in males. The time trend data indicates that in both sexes the incidence of DCA has decreased, but that of PCA is steady.

Based on the natural history of cancer and environmental carcinogenesis, we proposed the concept of basic cancer and variable cancer. Basic cancer is a proper cancer of a certain organ and less changeable in its incidence, while the variable one is a cancer whose incidence is modified by environmental conditions. In the stomach, PCA is a basic cancer group which is less affected by dietary change, whereas, DCA is a variable one which is clearly decreasing in incidence.

Colonic cancer histologically is a type of differentiated adenocarcinoma and no significant difference is observed in the histology of types in the colon and rectum. The increase in its incidence, however, is more rapid and higher in the colon than in the rectum. Such increase occurs in older age suggesting that it is an environmental cancer.

It is presumed that the basic cancer tends to be genetic or familial in nature, while the variable one is environmental. The variable should therefore be preventable, but the basic one is harder to avoid.

Gastric cancer is one of the most common cancers in the world. Although its mortality rate has decreased in most countries, it is still a leading carcinoma in many others. In Japan, it is at the very top in the list of cancer deaths, 52.89 per 100,000 population in males and 27.04 in females in 1976–1977. Colonic cancer is another important cancer and is known to have a high incidence in industrialized countries, but in other countries, including Japan, its incidence increased. In this paper, histopathology and time trend data on gastric cancer and colonic cancer will be discussed in relation to environmental carcinogenesis.

## Two Different Carcinomas of the Stomach

### Histologic subtype and clinicopathological behavior

Gastric cancer can be classified into two subtypes, poorly differentiated carcinoma

---

*¹ Kami-Ikebukuro, Toshima-ku, Tokyo 170, Japan (菅野晴夫, 加藤　洋)

*² Ibaraki 305, Japan (中村恭一)

(PCA) and differentiated carcinoma (DCA). PCA includes signet ring cell carcinoma and scirrhous-anaplastic adenocarcinoma whose cells spread individually and/or show a cord-like arrangement. DCA consists of tubular and papillotubular adenocarcinoma in which cancer cells form distinct tubuli with or without papillary projections (8–11, 15). These two types generally respectively correspond to a diffuse type carcinoma and an intestinal type, by Lauren's classification (5).

The clinicopathological differences between these two types are distinct (8, 13, 16). Macroscopic appearance, growth pattern, and spread of the carcinoma differ by histologic subtype. Consequently, the prognosis of patients is different: both sexes with DCA have better prognosis than those with PCA. The prognosis of the two types differs by tumor depth: DCA shows a tendency to metastasize to the liver *via* the portal vein, and PCA shows a tendency to give rise to peritoneal carcinomatosis.

*Microcarcinoma and morphogenesis of the two subtypes*

We observed that in cases of early cancer DCA was often surrounded by the intestinalized epithelium, whereas PCA was surrounded by the non-intestinalized one. We therefore postulated that DCA may originate from the intestinalized epithelium and PCA from the non-intestinalized normal epithelium. In order to prove this postulation, we examined very small carcinomas, called microcarcinomas, which were measured less than 5 mm in the diameter and were found incidentally by detailed histologic examination using the serial step sections of the resected stomach for gastric cancer, ulcer and other diseases (8–11, 15). Microcarcinoma or smaller carcinoma is the incipient phase of gastric carcinoma and its neighboring mucosa is presumed to preserve relatively well the nature of the mucosa when the cancer developed. The results supported our postulation: most DCA are surrounded by the intestinalized mucosa, while most PCA are surrounded by the non-metaplastic ordinary mucosa (Fig. 1).

Furthermore, studies using advanced gastric cancers showed that the ratio of PCA to DCA decreases with age. In other words, the frequency of PCA decreases, but that of DCA increases with increasing age. The frequency of the intestinalized mucosa of the stomach in the control group also increased with age. There was a clear parallel relation between intestinal metaplasia and DCA on one side and non-intestinal metaplasia and PCA on another. Further, ultra-structural and histochemical examinations of cancer cells and gastric epithelia supported these relations (8, 11, 13, 15, 16).

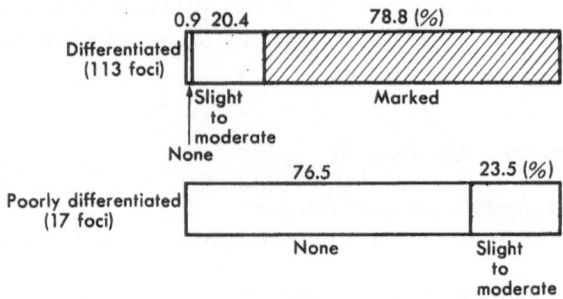

FIG. 1.  Relationship between histologic subtype of gastric carcinoma and the grade of intestinal metaplasia of its surrounding mucosa.
Analysis of 130 foci of microcarcinoma less than 5 mm in diameter.

From these observations, we concluded that the PCA arises from the ordinary mucosa of the stomach, whereas DCA arises from or is closely related to the intestinalized mucosa of the stomach.

## The Incidence of the Two Subtypes

Statistics show that PCA is more common in younger persons, especially females, and DCA in older people, especially males. The incidence of gastric cancer by sex is revealing (13, 15): when the number of cases is divided by subtypes, the number of PCA is roughly the same in both sexes, while there are many more cases of DCA in males (Fig. 2). Therefore, we can postulate that a basic carcinogenic burden which can sufficiently produce PCA is almost the same in both sexes, while additional carcinogenic factors which induce both DCA and intestinalization of the gastric mucosa act much more on males than on females.

To determine the histomorphological state of gastric cancer which corresponds to its decreased incidence in Japan, the change in histologic subtype was investigated (3, 13). The ratio of DCA to PCA (DPR) was calculated for the decades 1955–64 and 1965–74. The DPR decreased from 1.28 to 1.18 in males and from 0.67 to 0.50 in females during the 20-year period (Fig. 3), indicating that a relative decrease in DCA among Japanese is now taking place.

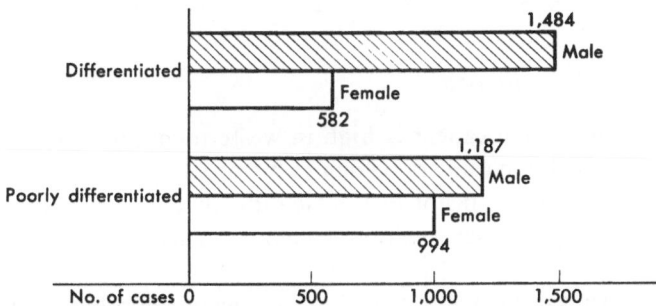

FIG. 2. The frequency of two histologic subtypes of gastric carcinoma in males and females.

Classification of 4,247 cases surgically removed at the Cancer Institute Hospital (CIH) during 1955–1979.

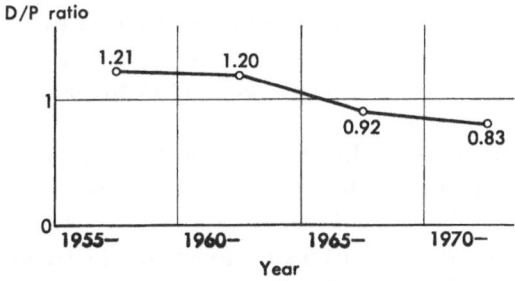

FIG. 3. Chronological change in the DPR (ratio of DCA to PCA) of gastric carcinoma in both sexes.

Total of 3,966 cases during 1955–1975.

Recent patho-epidemiological studies revealed that when there is decrease in the incidence of gastric cancer, the rate of decrease in DCA is more rapid than that in PCA (6, 7, 12). Hanai et al. (2) found the same result in the Osaka area.

## The Concept of Basic and Variable Cancer

It is now obvious that PCA and DCA are different in various aspects. PCA of the stomach arises from ordinary mucosa and shows characters resembling those of normal gastric epithelia. Its incidence is not greatly different in the two sexes and shows little chronological change. DCA of the stomach, on the other hand, is closely related to the intestinalized mucosa in its development and shows characters similar to the intestinalized epithelia. Its incidence is different in the sexes, but has decreased in both.

We proposed previously the concept of basic cancer and variable cancer (13, 15). Basic cancer is a proper cancer of a certain organ and often occurs in younger people. It is stable or less influenced in incidence by environmental conditions, while variable cancer frequently occurs in older people and is one whose incidence is modified by environmental changes. From the viewpoint of carcinogenesis, the two cancer types are caused by a different mode of action. Presumably the basic cancer relates to the exposure to strong or excess carcinogens in the early life of patients and/or to a susceptibility to carcinogens of host cells which are genetically unstable. Variable cancer, on the other hand, is a result of long and continuous involvement with carcinogens and promoters. In the stomach, therefore, PCA is thought to be a basic cancer and DCA a variable one.

## Carcinoma of the Colon and Rectum

The incidence of colonic cancer is high in western countries and low in Japan and other countries. Most colonic cancers belong to histopathologically differentiated adenocarcinoma and there is no significant histologic difference in carcinoma of the colon and rectum (4, 14). Here, the present status of colonic cancer in Japan will be discussed briefly.

The age-standardized incidence rate of carcinoma of the colon in Okayama, Japan is 5.0 per 100,000 population in males and 4.7 in females, while it is 30.1 and 26.1, respectively, in Connecticut in the U.S.A. In Okayama, the rate of rectal carcinoma is 7.0 in males and 5.5 in females and in Connecticut respectively 18.2 and 11.1 (1). The incidence of carcinoma of the colon and rectum is low and almost the same in both sexes in Japan, while in the U.S.A. it is high and the colon carcinoma incidence is much higher than rectal carcinoma. Comparing the incidence of colonic cancer by age in the two countries reveals that it is distributed in more older Americans than in Japanese. These findings indicate that colonic cancer tends to more common in the colon and in aged people in western countries.

In Japan, carcinoma of the colon and rectum has increased, with the former increasing more rapidly (Fig. 4). Further, the age distribution shifted slightly to an older age during the periods 1955–64 and 1975–77 (Fig. 5) (13). These findings suggest that carcinoma of the colon and rectum in Japan is following the trend in the West.

Colonic cancer among Hawaiian Japanese may be an example of colonic cancer in Japan in the future. The incidence of carcinoma of the colon is 22.4 in males and 18.8 in females and carcinoma of the rectum is 16.3 in males and 10.1 in females (1). These

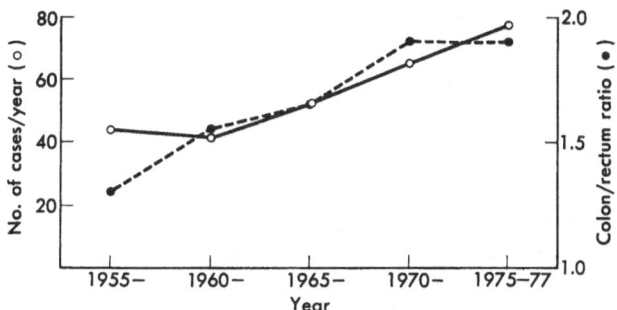

FIG. 4.  Chronological changes in the number of cases of carcinoma of the colon
and rectum and the ratio of carcinoma of the colon to carcinoma of the rectum.
Analysis of materials surgically removed at CIH during 1955–1977.

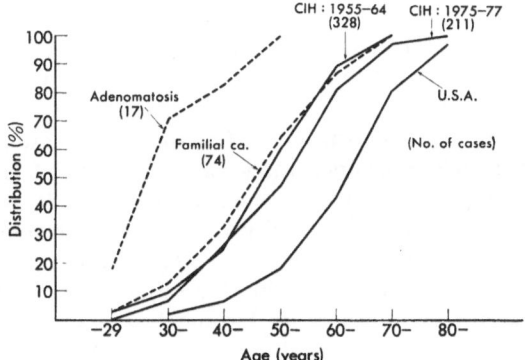

FIG. 5.  The cumulative age incidence of carcinoma cases of the colon and rectum.

figures are surprisingly high when compared to those of Japanese in Japan. It is obvious
that such a high occurrence in Hawaiian Japanese has been caused by the environmental,
probably dietary, change. Therefore, it is presumed that most carcinoma of the colon
and rectum in Japan today belong to basic cancer and those in western countries are
classified as variable cancer. When comparing carcinoma of the colon and rectum, as
American statistics indicate, that of the colon would be more influenced by environmental conditions than that of the rectum.

This presumption is supported by the following finding. Familial or genetic cancer
usually develops in younger ages. In our series, the age incidence of familial cancer of
the colon was found in a bit younger individuals, but was almost the same as that of
carcinoma of the colon and rectum in the period 1955–64 (Fig. 5) (13).

*Acknowledgment*

This work was supported in part by Grants-in-Aid for Cancer Research from the Ministry
of Education, Science and Culture and the Ministry of Health and Welfare of Japan.

REFERENCES

1.  Waterhouse, J., Muir, C., Correa, P., and Powell, J. (eds.) "Cancer Incidence in Five
    Continents," UICC Monogr., Vol. III, pp. 496, 498, 538, 539 (1976). International Agency
    for Research on Cancer, Lyon.

2.  Hanai, A., Fujimoro, I., and Taniguchi, H. Trends of stomach cancer incidence and histological types in Osaka. *In* "Trends in Cancer Incidence," ed. K. Magnus, pp. 143–154, (1982). Hemisphere Publ. Corp., Washington.

3.  Kato, Y., Kitagawa, T., Nakamura, K., and Sugano, H. Changes in histologic types of gastric carcinoma in Japan. *Cancer*, **48**, 2084–2087 (1981).

4.  Kato, Y., Sugano, H., Wada, J., and Nakamura, K. Pathology of carcinoma of the large bowel. *In* "Carcinoma of Large Intestine" (in Japanese), Medical Series No. 30, ed. K. Tsuneoka, pp. 39–58 (1978). Nankodo, Tokyo.

5.  Lauren, P. The two histological main types of gastric carcinoma: Diffuse and intestinal-type gastric carcinoma. *Acta Pathol. Microbiol. Scand.*, **64**, 31–49 (1965).

6.  Muñoz, N. and Asvali, T. Time trends of intestinal and diffuse types of gastric cancer in Norway. *Int. J. Cancer*, **8**, 144–157 (1971).

7.  Muñoz, N. and Connelly, R. Time trends of intestinal and diffuse types of gastric cancer in the United States. *Int. J. Cancer*, **8**, 158–164 (1971).

8.  Nakamura, K. "Pathology of Gastric Cancer, Microcarcinoma and Histogenesis" (in Japanese) (1972). Kinpodo, Kyoto.

9.  Nakamura, K. and Sugano, H. Microcarcinoma of the stomach measuring less than 5 mm in the largest diameter and its histogenesis. 13th Int. Cancer Congr., Research and Treatment, pp. 107–116 (1983).

10. Nakamura, K., Sugano, H., and Takagi, K. Carcinoma of the stomach in incipient phase: its histogenesis and histological appearances. *Gann*, **59**, 251–258 (1968).

11. Nakamura, K., Sugano, H., Takagi, K., and Kumakura, K. Histogenesis of carcinoma of the stomach with special reference to 50 primary microcarcinomas: light- and electron-microscopic, and statistical studies (in Japanese). *Japan. J. Cancer Clin.*, **15**, 627–647, 1967.

12. Stemmermann, G. N. Gastric cancer in the Hawaii Japanese. *Gann*, **68**, 525–535 (1977).

13. Sugano, H. Natural history of cancer (in Japanese). *Trans. Soc. Pathol. Japan*, **69**, 27–57 (1980).

14. Sugano, H. and Nakamura, K. Pathological diagnosis of carcinoma of the large bowel (in Japanese). *In* "Diagnosis and Treatment of Digestive Tract Cancer," ed. T. Kajitani, pp. 190–198 (1973). Medical-Dental-Pharmaceutical Publ., Tokyo.

15. Sugano, H., Nakamura, K., and Kato, Y. Pathological studies of human gastric cancer. *Acta Pathol. Japan*, **32**, Suppl. 2, 329–347 (1982).

16. Sugano, H., Nakamura, K., Kato, Y., and Takagi, K. Early gastric cancer—clinical and morphological aspects. *In* "Digestive Cancer (UICC 1978)," Vol. IX, ed. N. Thatcher, pp. 193–199 (1979). Pergamon Press, Oxford.

# MORPHOGENESIS OF LARGE INTESTINAL CARCINOMA: ITS SIGNIFICANCE IN EARLY DETECTION

A.K.M. Shamsuddin,[*1] Haruo Sugano,[*2] and B. F. Trump[*1][*3]

*Department of Pathology, University of Maryland School of Medicine[*1] and Cancer Institute (JFCR)[*2]*

To date, the prophylaxis of colon carcinoma is based on the polyp-cancer hypothesis whereby the polyps are considered to be the only *precursors* of *colon carcinoma* and the polyps are removed as a prophylactic measure. Preliminary results demonstrate that both in experimental animals and humans, colonic carcinoma may also arise directly from the flat non-polypoid mucosa. These results also suggest that the earliest changes following carcinogen treatment may be expressed as subtle morphological and mucin histochemical changes. It is hoped that identification of such markers may have potential use in early detection and hence prevention of colon cancer in humans.

Large intestinal carcinoma (LIC) is currently one of the most prevalent cancers in the industrialized world (*28*). As in many other cancers, strategies for its detection and prevention depends on the histogenesis of the cancer. However, more than any other cancers, histogenesis of LIC has been a controversial issue. One school of thought holds that most carcinomas arise through a benign polyp stage (*11, 14*). Many pathologists would certainly disagree, since in a good many cancers of the large intestine one may not find any evidence of preexisting polyps. There are others who completely disagree with the " polyp-cancer " hypothesis and hold that all LIC arise directly from the flat mucosa of the large intestine without going through a benign polyp stage (*6, 7*). Histogenetic studies of LIC in animal models have resulted in equally controversial finding. While some investigators reported benign polyps and cancer after chemical induction (*15*), others claim the evolution the LIC directly from the flat mucosa (*12, 13, 20, 31*). This argument regarding histogenesis is more than academic and its resolution has far reaching implications. For, if the " polyp-cancer " hypothesis is the only pathway, we could have a LIC free world by simply removing all the polyps prophylactically. Whereas, if the so-called " *de novo* " hypothesis is correct, then simple removal of the benign polyps will have no effect in preventing LIC.

Clearly, both these hypotheses are much too dogmatic. Since LIC arise from the epithelial cells in the large intestine, there is no reason why these cells would not be transformed following carcinogenic stimuli, irrespective of their location—be it in the polyps, in the flat mucosa or in the diverticula. Indeed, neoplasias in humans have been observed in the flat nonpolypoid mucosa (*8, 14, 17, 23–25, 30, 32*), diverticula (*5, 9*), and certainly polyps (*14*). Studies of carcinogenesis *in vitro* demonstrate that following

---

[*1] Baltimore, Maryland 21201, U.S.A.
[*2] Kami-Ikebukuro, Toshima-ku, Tokyo 170, Japan (菅野晴夫).
[*3] American Cancer Society Professor of Oncology.

carcinogen treatment, epithelial cells from the large intestine show morphological and histochemical changes of neoplasia in explant culture (*21*). Thus, the two primary factors in large intestinal carcinogenesis are the epithelial cells and the proper carcinogenic stimuli. Hence, Shamsuddin (*25*) proposed that LIC may arise both from the polyps as well as from the nonpolypoid mucosa without having to go through the benign polyp stage.

Should this hypothesis be correct, then we are confronted with the question: how can we recognize the early cancers that arise from the nonpolypoid mucosa? Certainly the question, " how do we manage these early cancers? " will also arise.

Recognition of the various changes (morphological, histochemical, biochemical, immunological, *etc.*) during the early stages of carcinogenesis would certainly help us in rationally developing tests for early detection of LIC.

*Animal Studies*

Recognition of the early changes during carcinogenesis in the large intestine must be looked at in a more scientific manner, such as in the context of initiation and promotion (*2*). There is ample evidence that this two-step phenomena is at play during large intestinal carcinogenesis (*1*). The initiated cells may or may not be recognizable morphologically.

Studies of the morphogenesis of LIC in the mouse and rat demonstrate that at least in C57Bl/Ha mice and Fischer 344 rats, the carcinomas arise directly from the flat mucosa without going through a benign polyp stage (*10, 20*). The ICR/Ha mice did show exophytic carcinomas that were less invasive, however, no evidence of adenomatous polyps was seen in any of these animals. Careful evaluation of the morphology of the rodent large intestine reveals that the epithelium is thrown into multiple ridges (*19*). A neoplasm, although arising from the flat mucosa but on the top of the ridge may thus appear misleading (Fig. 1). From the morphological and histochemical point of view, the large intestinal epithelium of the normal rat most closely resembles that of the normal human (*18, 19*). *In vivo* studies of carcinogenesis of the large intestine in rats with azoxymethane demonstrate that one of the earliest changes is dilatation, distortion and branching of the intestinal crypts (*20, 26*). This is accompanied initially by an increase in nor-

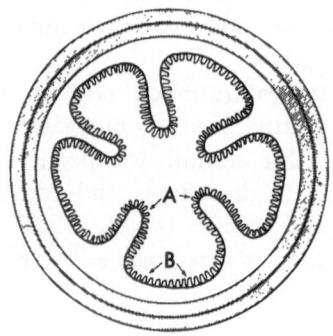

FIG. 1.   Schematic representation of the cross section of rat large intestine.
The mucosa is thrown into multiple folds (*19*). A neoplasm arising from the top of the fold (A) may misleadingly appear as a polyp while the same neoplasm at the bottom (B) may be called "*de novo*" carcinoma.

**Stages in crypt dilatation**

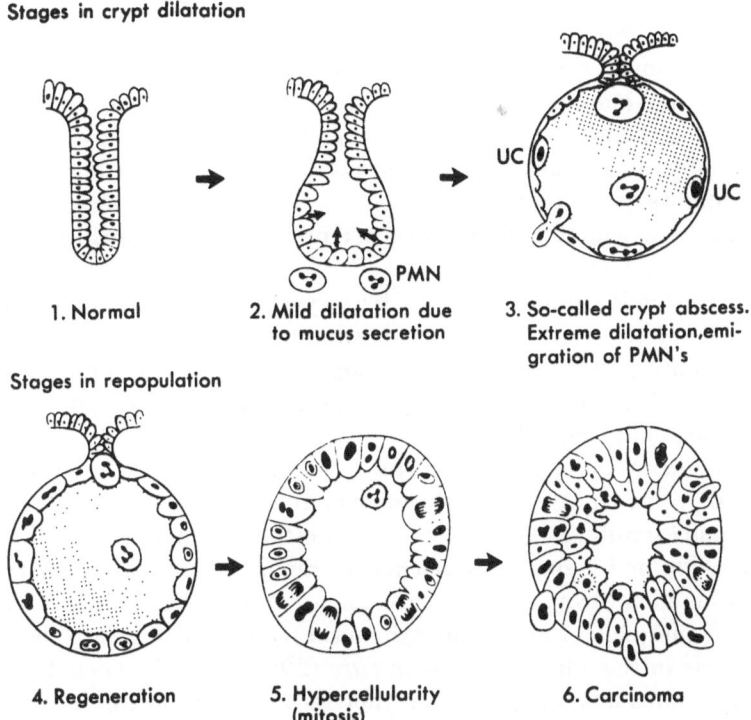

1. Normal

2. Mild dilatation due to mucus secretion

3. So-called crypt abscess. Extreme dilatation, emigration of PMN's

**Stages in repopulation**

4. Regeneration

5. Hypercellularity (mitosis)

6. Carcinoma

FIG. 2. Schematic representation of the steps of morphogenesis of large carcinoma. These have been conceptualized from the data obtained by *in vitro* and *in vivo* experiments (*10, 19–21, 26*). Similarity with the human has been documented (Refs. *18, 22, 24, 25* and Photos 1–4). PMN, polymorphonuclear cell; UC, undifferentiated cell.

mally occurring sulfomucin followed by an increased production of sialomucin. Examination of the large intestinal epithelium in rats at a subsequent time demonstrates basophilic hypercellular crypts that appear neoplastic by light microscopic morphology during which time there is markedly reduced mucus production. Since these neoplastic crypts may be confined within the mucosal layer, one would be hesitant to call these carcinomas. However, ultrastructural examination demonstrates that although the resolution of light microscopy cannot demonstrate invasion, there may very well be invasion of the basement membrane (*20*). Thus, these early neoplasms may very well be carcinomas from their inception.

Results from parallel *in vitro* (*21*) studies of the carcinogenesis of rat large intestine exposed to *N*-methyl-*N'*-nitro-*N*-nitrosoguanidine (MNNG) in explant culture shows a striking resemblance to those of the *in vivo* model. The control untreated explants from rat large intestine demonstrates a **single layer of epithelium with normal sulfomucin**, whereas MNNG-treated explants demonstrate a switch in the production of sialomucin, stratification of cells, and intracellular lumen formation—features typical of adenocarcinoma (*21*). The steps in morphogenesis of LIC as derived from sequential animal experiments (*20, 26*) are schematically represented in Fig. 2.

*Human Studies*

Preliminary comparison of these *in vivo* and *in vitro* animal data with that of the human showed quite interesting parallelism. Since for obvious ethical and moral reasons, one may not inject humans with carcinogens and sequentially study the events leading to cancer, an alternate system for studying the carcinogenesis in humans has been rationalized as follows:

i) It can be presumed that the presence of a LIC in a human represents his/her being exposed to the carcinogen.

ii) Most systemic carcinogen(s) act by way of the field effect whereby the entire target tissue is subjected to the carcinogenic stimuli.

iii) It is quite possible that the carcinogen(s) responsible for LIC may have induced multifocal changes throughout the large intestine, similar to what happens in many other target epithelia.

iv) Of the many initiated sites in the large intestinal epithelium, only one or two may have been promoted to recognizable carcinomas.

Thus, if one carefully examines the large intestinal epithelium in patients with LIC, one could possibly find a spectrum of changes ranging from early dilatation of crypts, sialomucin production through *in situ* carcinomas. Our studies in humans demonstrated the presence of morphological and histochemical features identical to the early changes of carcinogenesis in the animal models *in vitro* (20) and *in vivo* (21). Photos 1–4 show such changes in adenomatous polyps, in mucosa remote from carcinomas, and in carcinomas themselves. Comparison of these morphological and histochemical parameters (in the rat) to those of the human has revealed that in patients harboring colon cancer one can see such morphological and histochemical abnormalities in approximately 100% of colon cases seen in the United States (22). Although one cannot be sure about the reversibility or irreversibility of these morphological and histochemical markers, their presence in patients with colon cancer indicates that they may be related to the generalized field effect of colon carcinogenesis. In other words, the carcinogens that are in our environment, in our diet, or in our feces do not necessarily just select a pre-existing polyp, but rather they do act on the entire large bowel mucosa and randomly induce changes (initiation). Only a few of these initiated foci may become promoted and even fewer of them do progress to what is clinically or pathologically known as carcinoma of the colon.

It is interesting to point out at this time that although such changes have been seen in approximately 100% of patients with cancer of the colon in the U.S., it was only rarely seen in patients in Japan where the incidence of colon cancer is much lower than in the U.S. (28). A striking parallelism was obtained by injecting rats with a low dose of carcinogen (27) as is shown in the following chart. This similarity may shed some light as to the role of initiating or promotional factors in different populations.

Incidence of Early Neoplastic Changes in Carcinoma of Large Intestine

| High-dose azoxymethane rats | ++++ | High-incidence (U.S.) patients |
|---|---|---|
| Low-dose azoxymethane rats | ± | Low-incidence (Japan) patients |

Based on these experiments, it seems that identification of early morphological, histochemical, or immunocytochemical (3) changes may be potentially useful as a screening test. Use of such a marker, based on carcinogenesis studies, may be more meaningful in screening and monitoring high risk individuals than the use of an empirical system such as occult blood tests in feces. It is to be emphasized that fecal occult blood test is based on the coincidence of bleeding in large tumors. Certainly not all tumors bleed and not all bleeding is due to the presence of the tumor. Worst of all, if a cancer is detected when it is already a large tumor that bleeds, obviously it is too late to allow the chance of any real cure to the patient. Thus, there is the need to devise alternate screening tests that can detect the neoplastic transformation prior to the tumor stage. Detection strategies must therefore be devised that can identify the precancerous lesions before the cancer has actually formed, the ideal example being that of the carcinoma of the uterine cervix. Careful analysis of the alteration of mucosal surface may also be useful in endoscopic detection of early *de novo* cancers. These and other scientifically derived rational approaches must be further explored to effectively plan strategies for early detection and prevention of LIC.

## REFERENCES

1. Barthold, S. W. The role of nonspecific injury in colon carcinogenesis. *In* "Experimental Colon Carcinogenesis, " ed. H. Autrup and G. M. Williams, pp. 185–197 (1983). CRC Press, Boca Raton, Florida.
2. Berenblum, I. The mechanism of carcinogenesis: a study of the significance of cocarcinogenic action and related phenomena. *Cancer Res.*, 1, 807–814 (1941).
3. Boland, C. R., Montgomery, C. K., and Kim, Y. S. Alterations in the structure of mucin glycoproteins in colon cancer: a potential new marker of malignancy. *Gastroenterology*, 78, 1143 (1980).
4. Boland, C. R., Montgomery, C. K., and Kim, Y. S. Alterations in human colonic mucin occurring with cellular differentiation and malignant transplantation. *Proc. Natl. Acad. Sci. U.S.*, 79, 2051–2055 (1982).
5. Burkitt, D. P. Epidemiology of cancer of the colon and rectum. *Cancer*, 28, 3–13 (1971).
6. Castleman, B. and Krickstein, H. L. Do adenomatous polyps of the colon become malignant? *New Engl. J. Med.*, 267, 469–475 (1962).
7. Castleman, B. and Krickstein, H. L. Current approach to the polyp-cancer controversy. *Gastroenterology*, 51, 108–112 (1966).
8. Crawford, B. E. and Stromeyer, F. W. Small non-polypoid carcinomas of the large intestine. *Cancer*, 51, 1760–1763 (1983).
9. Hernandez, F. J. and Fernandez, B. B. Mucus-secreting carcinoid tumor in colonic diverticulum. Report of a case. *Dis. Colon Rectum*, 19, 63 (1976).
10. James, J. T., Shamsuddin, A. M., and Trump, B. F. A comparative study of the morphological and histochemical changes induced in the large intestine of ICR/Ha and C5782/Ha mice by 1, 2-dimethyl-hydrazine. *J. Natl. Cancer Inst.*, 71, 955–964 (1983).
11. Lane, N. Precursor tissue of ordinary large bowel cancer. *Cancer Res.*, 36, 2669–2672 (1976).
12. Lev, R. and Herp, A. Pathogenesis of rat colon carcinomas induced by N-methyl-N-nitrosourea. *J. Natl. Cancer Inst.*, 61, 779–786 (1978).
13. Maskens, A. P. Histogenesis and growth patterns of 1, 2-dimethylhydrazine-induced rat colon adenocarcinoma. *Cancer Res.*, 36, 1585–1592 (1976).
14. Muto, T., Bussey, H. J., and Morson, B. C. The evolution of cancer of the colon and rectum. *Cancer*, 36, 2251–2270 (1975).
15. Narisawa, T., Nakano, H., Hayakawa, M., Sato, T., and Sakuma, A. Tumors of the colon

and rectum induced by N-methyl-N'-nitro-N-nitrosoguanidine. *In* "Topics in Chemical Carcinogenesis," ed. W. Nakahara, S. Takayama, T. Sugimura, and S. Odashima, pp. 145–156 (1972). Univ. Park Press, Baltimore.

16. Oohara, T., Ogino, A., Saji, K., and Tohma, H. Studies on the difference of background mucosa among single advanced carcinoma and benign diseases of the large intestine and familial polyposis coli. *Cancer*, **45**, 1637–1645 (1980).

17. Shamsuddin, A.K.M., Bell, H. G., Petrucci, J. V., and Trump, B. F. Carcinoma *in situ* and "microinvasive" adenocarcinoma of colon. *Pathol. Res. Pract.*, **167**, 374–379 (1980))

18. Shamsuddin, A. M., Phelps, P. C., and Trump, B. F. Human large intestinal epithelium: light microscopy, histochemistry and ultrastructure. *Hum. Pathol.*, **13**, 790–803 (1982).

19. Shamsuddin, A. M. and Trump, B. F. Colon epithelium. I. Light microscopic, histochemical and ultrastructural features of normal colon epithelium of male Fischer 344 rats. *J. Natl. Cancer Inst.*, **66**, 375–388 (1981).

20. Shamsuddin, A. M. and Trump, B. F. Colon epithelium. II. *In vivo* studies of colon carcinogenesis. Light microscopic, histochemical and ultrastructural studies of histogenesis of azoxymethane induced colon carcinomas in Fischer 344 rats. *J. Natl. Cancer Inst.*, **66**, 389–401 (1981).

21. Shamsuddin, A. M. and Trump, B. F. Colon epithelium. III. *In vitro* studies of colon carcinogenesis in Fischer 344 rats. N-Methyl-N'-nitro-N-nitrosoguanidine induced changes in rat colon epithelium in explant culture. *J. Natl. Cancer Inst.*, **66**, 403–411 (1981).

22. Shamsuddin, A. M., Weiss, L., Phelps, P. C., and Trump, B. F. Colon epithelium. IV. Human colon carcinogenesis. Changes in human colonic mucosa adjacent to and remote from carcinomas of the colon. *J. Natl. Cancer Inst.*, **66**, 413–419 (1981).

23. Shamsuddin, A. M. and Elias, E. G. Rectal mucosa: malignant and premalignant changes following radiation. *Arch. Pathol. Lab. Med.*, **105**, 150–151 (1981).

24. Shamsuddin, A. M. and Phillips, R. M. Preneoplastic and neoplastic changes in colonic mucosa of Crohn disease. *Arch. Pathol. Lab. Med.*, **105**, 283–286 (1981).

25. Shamsuddin, A. M. Microscopic intraepithelial neoplasia in large bowel mucosa. *Hum. Pathol.*, **13**, 510–512 (1982).

26. Shamsuddin, A. M. Morphogenesis of colon carcinoma. Ultrastructural studies of azoxmethane-induced early lesions in colon epithelium of Fischer 344 rats. *Arch. Pathol. Lab. Med.*, **106**, 140–144 (1982).

27. Shamsuddin, A. M. and Hogan, M. L. Large intestinal carcinogenesis. II. Histogenesis and unusual features of low dose azoxymethane-induced carcinomas in Fischer 344 rats. *J. Natl. Cancer Inst.*, **73**, 1293–1296 (1984).

28. Shamsuddin, A. M., Kato, Y., and Sugano, H. Large intestinal carcinogenesis. III. Studies in low incidence (Japanese) patients. *J. Natl. Cancer Inst.*, **73**, 1307–1310 (1984).

29. Silverberg, E. Cancer statistics 1982. *Ca.—A Cancer Journal for Clinicians*, **32**, 15–31 (1982).

30. Snover, D. C., Gilbertsen, V. A., and Niratvongs, S. Minute adenocarcinoma of the colon arising in flat mucosa: five cases asking the question: "does *de novo* colon carcinoma exist?" (Abstr.), *Lab. Invest.*, **46**, 78A–79A (1982).

31. Ward, J. M. Morphogenesis of chemically induced neoplasms of the colon and small intestine in rats. *Lab. Invest.*, **30**, 505–513 (1974).

32. Woda, B. A., Forde, K., and Lane, N. A unicryptal colonic adenoma. The smallest colonic neoplasm yet observed in a non-polyposis individual. *Am. J. Clin. Pathol.*, **68**, 631–632 (1977).

## EXPLANATIONS OF PHOTOS

PHOTO 1.  Normal human large intestine. Hematoxylin-Eosin stain (H-E). ×375.

PHOTO 2.  Large intestinal mucosa remote from a carcinoma in the lumen. Note dilated, distorted, and branched crypts. H-E. ×150.

PHOTO 3.  Human adenomatous polyp. Note distored, dilated, and branched crypts. H-E. ×150.

PHOTO 4.  Human large intestinal carcinoma. Note similar crypt changes and striking resemblance to the conceptual model (Fig. 2) derived from experimental carcinogenesis (26). H-E. ×150.

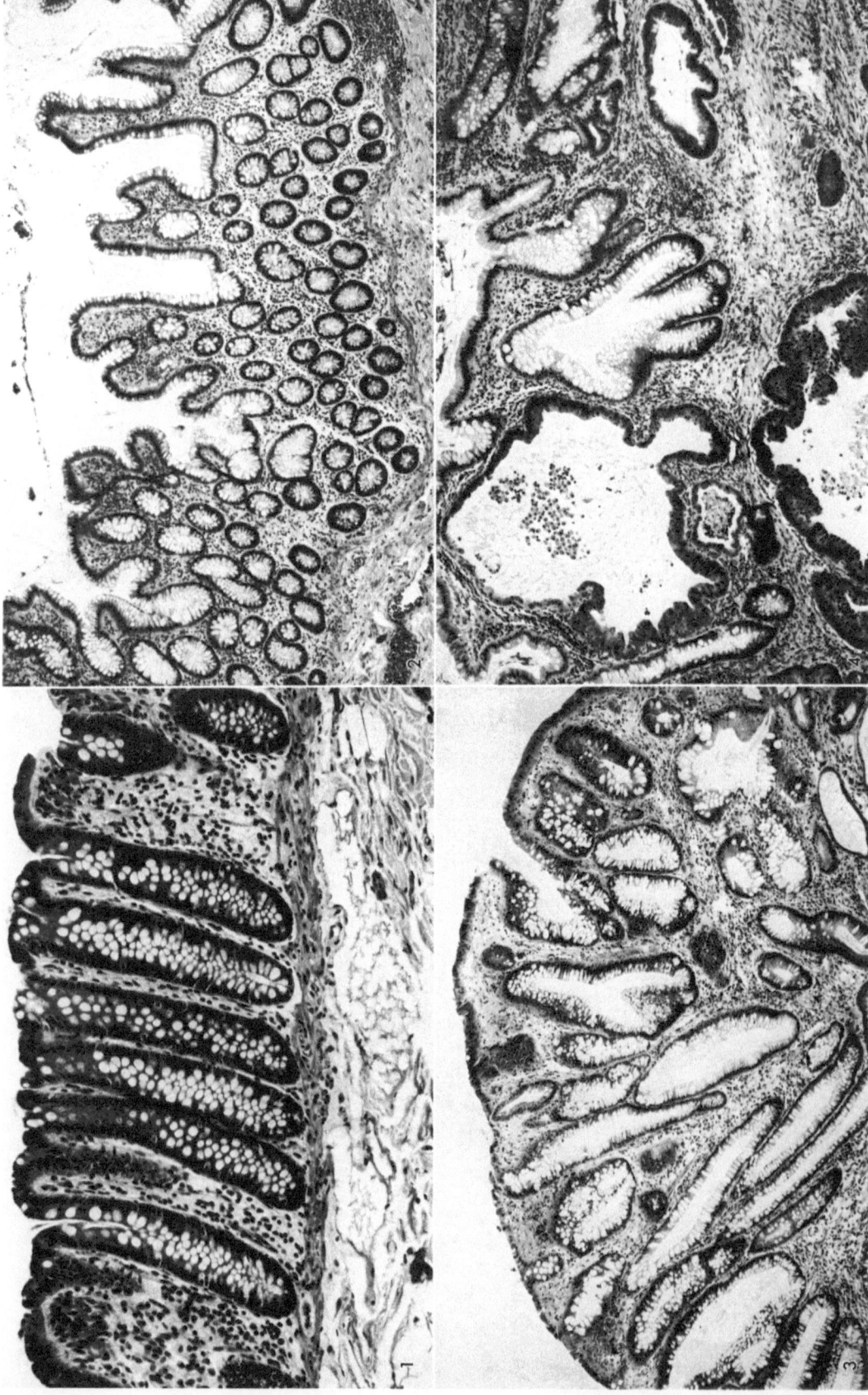

# PATHOLOGY OF PRIMARY LIVER CANCER AND CLINICAL RELEVANCE

Kunio OKUDA

*First Department of Medicine, Chiba University School of Medicine**

Gross new anatomical classification of hepatocellular carcinoma (HCC) is proposed and histopathology of HCC in relation to its clinical features is discussed.

In most countries, including Japan, more than 80% of HCC patients have cirrhosis at the time they develop HCC. HCC tends to be more poorly differentiated in the absence of cirrhosis and grows fast, whereas, as is often the case in Japan, it tends to be well differentiated in highly cirrhotic livers.

Histopathology of HCC has significant bearing on the clinical features, treatment, and prognosis. Therefore, it is important to determine the pathological characteristics of the carcinoma at the time of diagnosis.

Primary liver cancers are divided pathologically into hepatocellular carcinoma (HCC), cholangiocellular carcinoma, combined hepatocholangiocarcinoma, and other rare varieties. Of these, HCC is by far the most common in Japan where the ratio to cholangiocellular carcinoma is roughly 10: 1. This ratio is greater in areas where HCC is more frequent, and smaller where it is less common. The incidence of HCC varies greatly with the global area, and is about 500 times more frequent among males in Mozambique than in Norway. The differences in frequency are perhaps related to the leading etiologic factors in these areas of which hepatitis B virus infection is an important one. In this presentation, I will mainly discuss the histopathology of HCC in relation to its clinical features, because the latter seem to be closely related to the former.

## Gross Anatomical Classification of HCC

There has been no satisfactory gross anatomical classification. The one proposed by Eggel (6) was based mainly on tumor size and not applicable to the small HCCs frequently diagnosed in Japan in recent years. Nakashima (9) and Okuda, et al. (18) have maintained that it be based on growth pattern. Okuda et al. (18) have compared HCCs in Japan, Los Angeles, and Pretoria, South Africa, and have proposed a new classification which divides these carcinomas into I, expanding type—subdivided into encapsulated and non-encapsulated; II, spreading type—lobular, pseudolobular, and invasive; III, multifocal—not diffuse and diffuse; IV—a combination of these; V, other types—sclerosing, fibrolamellar, mainly intravascular, mainly intraductal, and hemorrhagic; and VI—indeterminate. There is a considerable difference in relative frequencies of these gross types among the above three areas of the world.

---

* Inohana 1-8-1, Chiba 280, Japan (奥田邦雄).

*Histopathology of HCC and Relation to Cirrhosis*

Typical HCC cells look like hepotocytes with eosinophilic cytoplasm. Edmondson and Steiner (5) graded HCC cells and growth patterns into four grades according to the degree of differentiation in 1954, although they did not have cases of Grade I, or a highly differentiated one not readily distinguishable from normal hepatocytes or hepatic cell adenoma. Steiner (22) compared cirrhosis and HCC seen among sub-Saharan Bantus and Americans in Chicago, and found that HCC in African blacks tended to be more poorly differentiated with less frequent associated cirrhosis, and that the liver bearing HCC had less inflammatory reactions compared to the counterparts in Chicago. In most countries including Japan, more than 80% of HCC patients have cirrhosis, usually

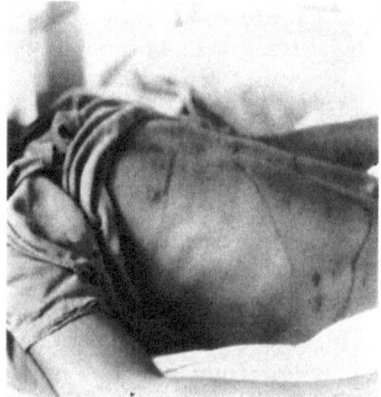

FIG. 1. Young gold miner from Mozambique.

He was robust on arrival at the mine, but when he came to the dispensary complaining of abdominal pain, cancer was already very advanced.

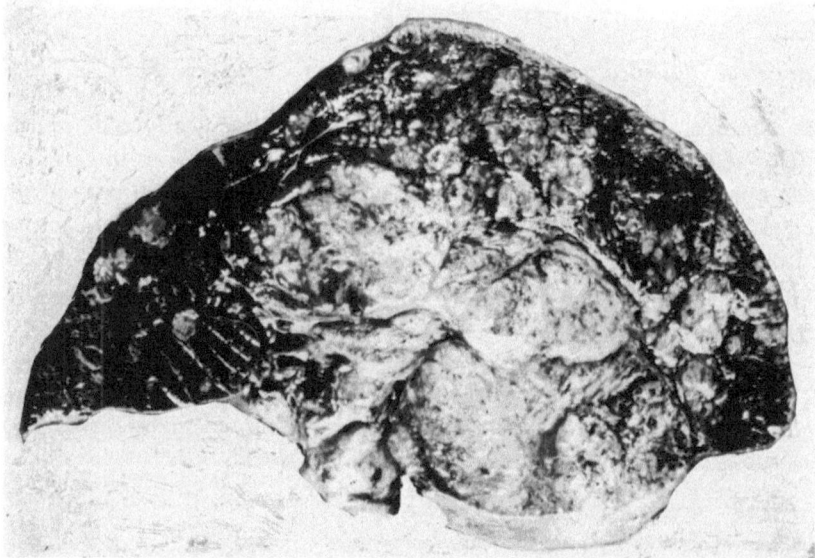

FIG. 2. Hepatocellular carcinoma arising in a non-cirrhotic liver seen in Johannesburg.

macro- or mixed macro- and micronodular cirrhosis at the time they develop HCC, whereas this incidence is about 40% among Bantus. In Japan, cirrhosis is often advanced when HCC arises, the liver is shrunk, and the patient dies from cirrhosis rather than from HCC; HCC is rather small in such cirrhotic livers at the time of autopsy. In contrast, cirrhosis is much milder and often of a different variety grossly in South Africa as this authors found in studies there. The liver weight at the time of autopsy is about 2 kg on average in Japan, whereas it is about 4 kg according to Berman (1) who studied HCC among mostly young South African Bantu blacks (Fig. 1). This difference may be explained on the basis of more frequent advanced cirrhosis among Japanese HCC patients and more frequent noncirrhotic livers (Fig. 2) in South Africa. With a good liver function, the patient will live till cancer grows to a huge size replacing most of the normal liver tissue. Furthermore, we have found that HCC tends to be more poorly differentiated in the absence of cirrhosis, growing fast, whereas it tends to be well differentiated in highly cirrhotic livers; this is often the case in Japan (15). These two opposite or different features of HCC will account for the twofold difference in liver weight between these two areas of the world.

## Clinical Types

Berman (1) classified his patients among gold miners in Johannesburg into frank cancer, acute abdominal cancer, febrile cancer, occult cancer, and metastatic cancer according to the clinical features. However, acute abdominal cancer presenting as acute abdomen or sudden loss of blood into the abdominal cavity, and febrile cancer are rare in other parts of the world, although nearly half of all patients have bloody ascites at the time of death. In Japan, a considerable proportion of patients present as cirrhosis, and die from hepatic failure rather than from cancer (19). Febrile cancer or patients who present with high fever and leukocytosis are difficult to distinguish from liver abscess clinically. In such patients, cancer cells are usually very poorly differentiated and grow fast (11). The following histopathological types of HCC are clinically distinct, if not diagnosable by clinical features alone.

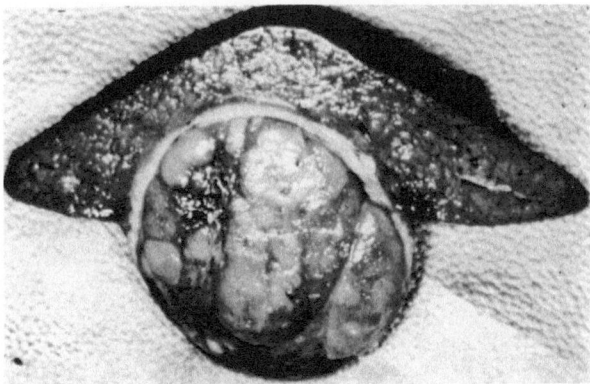

FIG. 3.  Encapsulated hepatocellular carcinoma commonly seen in Japan.
For reasons yet unclear, the frequency of encapsulated HCC varies considerably with the area.

*Encapsulated HCC (Okuda, 1977)*

Hepatocellular carcinoma with a thick fibrous capsule is rather common in Japan in contrast to South Africa and Los Angeles where it is a rarity. A slowly expanding HCC tends to acquire a capsule (Fig. 3), and one with a thick capsule suggests a slow growth, hence a long survival. Intravascular invasion is relatively infrequent and late in this type (*13*).

*Intraductal Growth*

If HCC invades a major bile duct near the porta hepatis, the clinical manifestations are similar to those in obstructive jaundice, such as right upper quadrant pain and jaundice. A necrotic tumor mass may be detached and lodged at the end of the common bile duct. According to Kojiro *et al.* (*7*), this occurred in 9% of all autopsy cases. Hemobilia was seen in one out of five cases of intraductal growth. At autopsy, tumor invasion in the major portal vein was seen in the majority of patients, and often invasion started from the intraportal tumor growth.

*Intravascular Growth*

Hepatocellular carcinoma is known for its propensity to invade the venous sytem, particularly the portal vein. In our study of 232 autopsies, tumor growth was seen in the major portal vein system in 64.7%, and in a large hepatic vein in 23.3%. The tumor was seen reaching the right atrium in 11 of 232 cases (*9*). Although intravascular invasion entails no distinct clinical signs, it signifies a grave consequence. Intraportal growth contraindicates surgery, and intravenous growth causes pulmonary metastases. Diagnosis of vascular tumor invasion is not difficult with the modern imaging techniques (*10, 12, 14*).

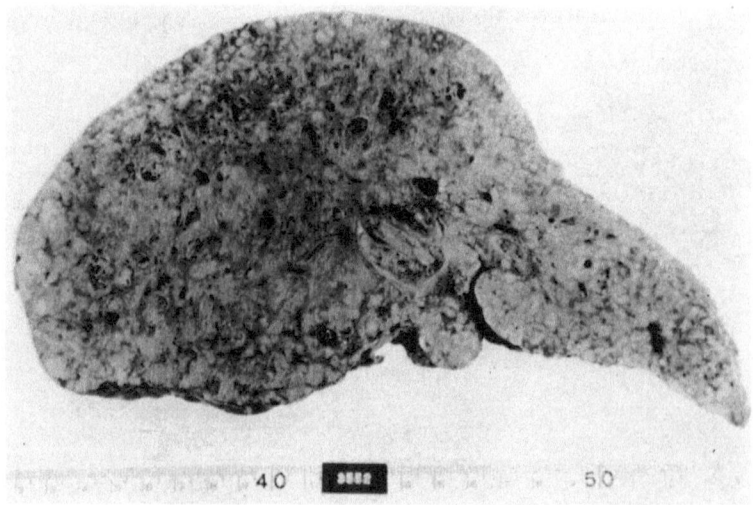

Fig. 4.  Diffuse type hepatocellular carcinoma.
Note that the right portal vein is filled with cancer thrombus.

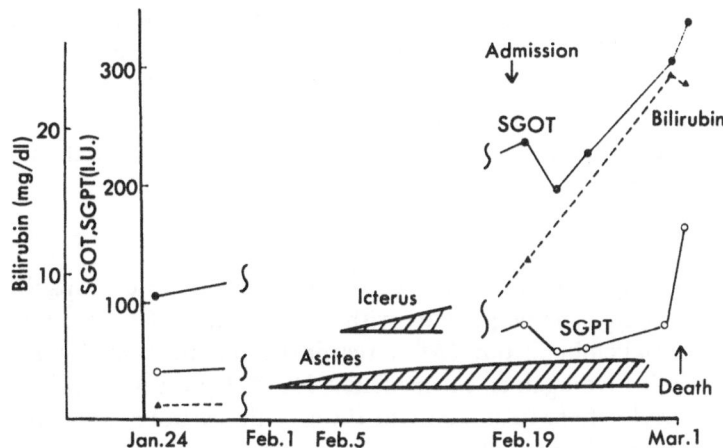

FIG. 5. The clinical course of a 54-year-old patient with diffuse type HCC.
He died within one month after admission from rapidly progressive jaundice,
ascites, and hepatic failure.

## Diffuse Type HCC

Although this was one of the three major gross types in Eggel's classification, in a strict sense it is rather uncommon (Fig. 4). In our experience, it is usually a sequela to intraportal tumor spread occurring throughout the liver within a short span of time. The clinical course of the patient is quickly downhill (Fig. 5), manifested by rapid increase in serum bilirubin and development of hepatic failure (16).

## Sclerosing HCC (Omata, 1981)

This type of HCC is characterized by intense fibrosis in which the tubular neoplastic structures are embedded. Although sometimes superficially resembling peripheral cholangiocarcinoma, most such tumors are of apparent hepatocyte origin. For reasons which are unclear, hypercalcemia not due to bone metastasis is very common in this tumor (20).

## Fibrolamellar HCC (Craig, 1980)

Craig et al. in 1980 described 23 patients with a variant histologic type characterized by deeply eosinophilic neoplastic cells, many of which contained intracytoplasmic inclusions, and fibrosis arranged in a lamellar fashion around cancer cells. The average age was 26.4 years, and survival was considerably longer than in HCC patients with ordinary HCC (3). More recently, it was found that these patients have very high serum vitamin $B_{12}$ levels as a result of increased production of transcobalamin I by cancer cells (21).

## Clear Cell HCC

Occasionally there will be a predominance of clear cells that are almost indistinguishable from clear cell carcinoma of the kidney and adrenal. In the series studied by

Buchannan and Huvos (2), clear cells constituted 30 to 100% of tumor cells in 13 out of 150 cases. Although Edmondson (4) suggested a favorable prognosis with less frequent distant metastases, and Lai *et al.* (8) reported a 50% survival rate at 14 weeks without treatment in contrast to 3 weeks for the same survival in patients without clear cells, it is still undetermined whether clear cell HCC has a better prognosis than ordinary HCC.

*Therapeutic Implications*

Expanding HCC, particularly those which acquire a thick capsule, grow slowly and are relatively benign. Some patients with encapsulated HCC may live several years. Transcatheter arterial embolization (23), a recent therapeutic modality popular in Japan, may prove very effective against encapsulated HCC. However, once tumor cells have penetrated the capsule, those in and outside the capsule are not readily killed by cessation of arterial blood supply. Transcatheter arterial embolization is not as effective for spreading type HCC as it is for expanding HCC. Surgical removal of the cancer, or hepatic resection, is meaningless if HCC arises multicentrically. Fortunately, in Japan and the Far East, unicentrical or oligocentrical tumorigenesis is more common, and survival of patients with successful resection is better than that of medically treated patients (17).

## REFERENCES

1.  Berman, C. "Primary Carcinoma of the Liver. A Study in Incidence, Clinical Manifestations, Pathology and Aetiology" (1951). Lewis, London.
2.  Buchannan, T. F., Jr. and Huvos, A. G. Clear-cell carcinoma of the liver. *Am. J. Clin. Pathol.*, **61**, 529–539 (1974).
3.  Craig, J., Peters, R. L., Edmondson, H. A., and Omata, M. Fibrolamellar carcinoma of the liver: a tumor of adolescent and young adults with distinctive clinicopathologic features. *Cancer*, **46**, 372–379 (1980).
4.  Edmondson, H. A. "Tumor of the liver and Intrahepatic Bile Ducts," Section VII, Facicle 25 (1958). Armed Forces Institute of Pathology, Washington, D.C.
5.  Edmondson, H. A. and Steiner, P. E. Primary carcinoma of the liver. A study of 100 cases among 48,900 necropsies. *Cancer*, **7**, 462–503 (1954).
6.  Eggel, H. Ueber das primäre Carcinoma der Leber. *Beitr. Pathol. Anat.*, **30**, 506–604 (1901).
7.  Kojiro, M., Kawabata, K., Kawano, Y., Shirai, F., Takemoto, N., and Nakashima, T. Hepatocellular carcinoma presenting as intrabile duct tumor growth. A clinicopathologic study of 24 cases. *Cancer*, **49**, 2144–2147 (1982).
8.  Lai, C. L., Wu, P. C., Lam, K. C., and Todd, D. Histologic prognostic indicators in hepatocellular carcinoma. *Cancer*, **44**, 1677–1684 (1979).
9.  Nakashima, T., Okuda, K., Kojiro, M., Jimi, A., Yamaguchi, R., Sakamoto, K., and Ikari, T. Pathology of hepatocellular carcinoma in Japan. 232 consecutive cases autopsied in ten years. *Cancer*, **51**, 863–877 (1983).
10. Nakayama, T., Hiyama, Y., Ohnishi, K., Tsuchiya, S., Kohno, K., Nakajima, Y., and Okuda, K. Arterioportal shunts on dynamic computed tomography. *Am. J. Roentgenol.*, **140**, 953–957 (1983).
11. Okuda, K. Clinical aspects of hepatocellular carcinoma—analysis of 134 cases. *In* "Hepatocellular Carcinoma," ed. K. Okuda and R. L. Peters, pp. 387–436 (1976). Wiley, New York.
12. Okuda, K. Advances in hepatobiliary ultrasonography. *Hepatology*, **1**, 662–672 (1981).
13. Okuda, K., Musha, H., Nakajima, Y., Kubo, Y., Shimoka, Y., Nagasaki, Y., Sawa, Y., Jinnouchi, S., Kaneko, T., Obata, H., Hisamitsu, T., Motoike, Y., Okazaki, N., Kojiro,

M., Sakamoto, K., and Nakashima, T. Clinicopathological features of encapsulated hepatocellular carcinoma. A study of 26 cases. *Cancer*, **40**, 1240–1245 (1977).

14. Okuda, K., Musha, H., Yoshida, T., Kanda, Y., Yamazaki, T., Jinnouchi, S., Moriyama, M., Kawaguchi, S., Kubo, Y., Shimokawa, Y., Kojiro, M., Kuratomi, S., Sakamoto, K., and Nakashima, T. Demonstration of growing cats of hepatocellular carcinoma in the portal vein by celiac angiography: the thread and streaks sign. *Cancer*, **117**, 303–309 (1975).

15. Okuda, K., Nakashima, T., Sakamoto, K., Ikara, T., Hidaka, H., Kubo, Y., Sakuma, K., Motoike, Y., Okuda, H., and Obata, H. Hepatocellular carcinoma arising in noncirrhotic and highly cirrhotic livers: a comparative study of histopathology and frequency of hepatitis B markers. *Cancer*, **49**, 450–455 (1982).

16. Okuda, K., Noguchi, T., Kubo, Y., Shimokawa, Y., Kojiro, M., and Nakashima, T. A clinical and pathological study of diffuse type hepatocellular carcinoma. *Liver*, **1**, 280–289 (1981).

17. Okuda, K., Obata, H., Nakajima, Y., Ohtsuki, T., Okazaki, N., and Ohnishi, K. Prognosis of primary hepatocellular carcinoma. *Hepatology*, **4**, 3S–6S (1984).

18. Okuda, K., Peters, R. L., and Simson, I. Gross anatomical features of hepatocellular carcinoma from three disparate geographic areas—proposal of new classification. *Cancer*, **54**, 2165–2173 (1984).

19. Okuda, K., Suzuki, N., Kubo, Y., and Obata, H. Clinical aspects of hepatocellular carcinoma. *In* "Advances in Medical Oncology, Research and Education," Vol. 9, "Digestive Cancer," ed. N. Thatcher, pp. 133–140 (1979). Pergamon, Oxford.

20. Omata, M., Peters, R. L., and Tatter, D. Sclerosing hepatic carcinoma: relationship to hypercalcemia. *Liver*, **1**, 33–49 (1981).

21. Paradinas, F. J., Melia, W. M., Wilkinson, M. L., Portmann, B., Johnson, P. J., Murray-Lyon, I. M., and Williams, R. High serum vitamin $B_{12}$ binding capacity as a marker of the fibrolamellar variant of hepatocellular carcinoma. *Br. Med. J.*, **2**, 840–842 (1982).

22. Steiner, P. E. Cancer of the liver and cirrhosis in trans-Saharan Africa and the United States of America. *Cancer*, **13**, 1085–1166 (1960).

23. Takayasu, K., Moriyama, N., Muramatsu, Y., Suzuki, M., Yamada, T., Kishi, K., Hasegawa, H., and Okazaki, N. Hepatic arterial embolization for hepatocellular carcinoma. Comparison of CT scans and resected specimens. *Radiology*, **150**, 661–665 (1984).

# CLASS I AND CLASS II HLA ANTIGENS IN COLORECTAL AND LIVER CARCINOMAS

S. Ferrone,[*1] T. Fukusato,[*2] M. A. Gerber,[*2] T. G. Pullano,[*1]
D. J. Ruiter,[*3] S. H. Thung,[*2] and H. F. van den Ingh[*3]

*Department of Microbiology and Immunology, New York Medical College,[*1] Department
of Pathology, Mount Sinai School of Medicine and City Hospital Center at
Elmhurst,[*2] and Department of Pathology, University Medical Center[*3]*

Information about the distribution of Class I and Class II HLA
antigens in normal colon-rectum and liver and about changes in the expression of the antigens associated with malignant transformation is
reviewed. Immunohistochemical staining of surgically removed tissues
with monoclonal antibodies has shown that Class I HLA antigens are
expressed by normal mucosa of colon and rectum, but are not detectable
in hepatocytes. Class I HLA antigens appear on the majority of tumor
cells in hepatomas, but are detectable only in a low percentage of tumor
cells in mucinous and signet-ring cell carcinomas.

As far as Class II HLA antigens is concerned, HLA-DQ antigens
are not detected in colon and rectum, whereas HLA-DR antigens are
weakly expressed in colon. Neither type of Class II HLA antigens is
detected in hepatocytes. Class II HLA antigens may appear on colorectal
carcinomas and hepatomas.

Class I and Class II HLA antigens represent the major types of human histocompatibility antigens. Class I HLA antigens, the classical transplantation antigens, comprise
the gene products of the A, B, and C loci located in the major histocompatibility complex
(MHC) region. They consist of a 45K molecular weight (M.W.) polymorphic glycopolypeptide nonconvalently associated with $\beta_2$-microglobulin ($\beta_2$-$\mu$) (for review, see Ref. *28*).
Class II HLA antigens comprise the gene products of the DP, DQ, and DR loci located
in the MHC region (*5*). On the cell surface Class II HLA antigens are composed of
two noncovalently associated glycopolypeptides with the approximate M.W. of 34K
and 29K. During cytoplasmic assembly and processing the two subunits are noncovalently
bound to a glycopolypeptide with the approximate M.W. of 32K (*4*).

Because of the potential role of abnormalities in the expression of Class I and Class
II HLA antigens in the escape of tumor cells from immune surveillance, characterization
of their HLA phenotype has been the subject of several investigations. The information
from these studies will also contribute to our understanding of the effect of malignant
transformation of cells on the structural and functional properties of cellular components.

**In the early 1970's** Takasugi and Terasaki (*33*) reported that certain human tumor
cell lines in long term culture may display abnormal reactivity with anti-Class I HLA

---

[*1] Valhalla, New York 10595, U.S.A.
[*2] New York, New York 10003, U.S.A.
[*3] Leiden, The Netherlands.

alloantisera in serological assays. Similar results were obtained by us in 1976 when analyzing the HLA phenotype of fibroblasts transformed with SV40 (26). Although similar findings were described in a variety of model systems (for review, see Ref. 3), these observations were accepted with a certain skepticism because of the limited specificity of anti-HLA alloantisera and because of the lack of information about the molecular basis of these unexpected serological findings. Furthermore, at the time it was not possible to determine whether the abnormal serological findings reflected *in vitro* artifacts or were paralleled by similar *in vivo* phenomena, since the available alloantisera with their limited specificity were not suitable for immunohistochemical analysis of surgically removed tissues. These limitations have been overcome by the development of monoclonal antibodies to HLA antigens which have facilitated the application of immunohistochemical techniques to characterize the expression of Class I and Class II HLA antigens in surgically removed tissues.

In this paper we will review the available information about the distribution of Class I and Class II HLA antigens in normal colon-rectum and liver and about changes in the expression of these antigens associated with malignant transformation of cells, after having briefly described the methodology used in these studies.

*Methodology*

Both indirect immunofluorescence and immunoperoxidase have been used to characterize the tissue distribution of Class I and Class II HLA antigens. The substrates have been frozen sections, since the available monoclonal antibodies elicited and selected for reactivity with native Class I and Class II HLA antigens do not react with paraffin embedded tissues. The denaturation occurring during the fixation procedure changes the antigenic profile of Class I and Class II HLA antigens so that they do not react with antibodies to native HLA antigens, but acquire reactivity with antibodies elicited with denatured HLA antigens.

*1.  Distribution of Class I and Class II HLA antigens in normal colon, rectum, and liver*

Class I HLA antigens are expressed by the histologically normal mucosa of colon and rectum (18, 35). Among Class II HLA antigens HLA-DQ antigens have been detected in neither organ, while HLA-DR antigens have not been detected in rectum but have a faint and variable expression in colon (22, 25, 35). No information is available about the expression of HLA-DP antigens in these organs.

In liver, bile duct epithelia, vascular endothelia, and sinusoidal lining cells express Class I HLA antigens (9, 18). In man, as in mice (27, 32), the information about the expression of Class I HLA antigens by hepatocytes is controversial. While Barbatis et al. (1), Fleming et al. (8), and Natali et al. (18) have not detected these antigens on hepatocytes, Montano et al. (17) have reported these antigens on the hepatocyte plasma membrane, although in low density. In our recent studies (9) we have not detected Class I HLA antigens by staining frozen sections of normal liver from fetuses and adult donors utilizing a battery of monoclonal antibodies to distinct monomorphic determinants of the Class I HLA molecular complex. This conclusion has also been confirmed by immunoperoxidase staining of paraffin embedded liver tissue with a xenoantiserum elicited against denatured Class I HLA antigens (Fig. 1).

There is general agreement about the distribution of Class II HLA antigens in

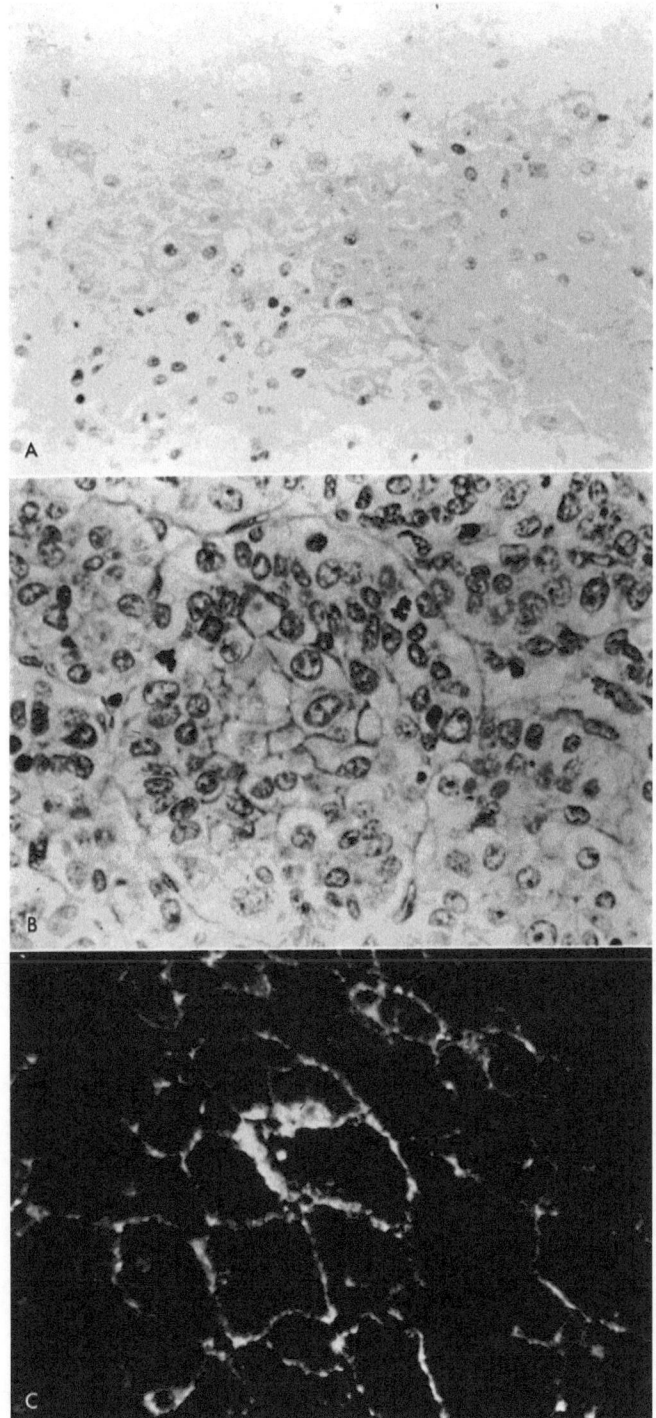

Fig. 1. Staining with a xenoantiserum to denatured Class I HLA antigens of paraffin sections of a normal liver (panel A), of a hepatocellular carcinoma (panel B) utilizing the avidin-biotin-peroxidase method, and with the anti Class I HLA monoclonal antibody CR-1 of a frozen section of a hepatocellular carcinoma (panel C) utilizing the indirect immunofluorescence method.

Class I HLA antigens are not detected in normal liver, but are expressed by hepatocytes which have undergone malignant transformation.

liver: both HLA-DR and DQ antigens are expressed by Kupffer cells, but are not detected on hepatocytes (*9, 22, 25*).

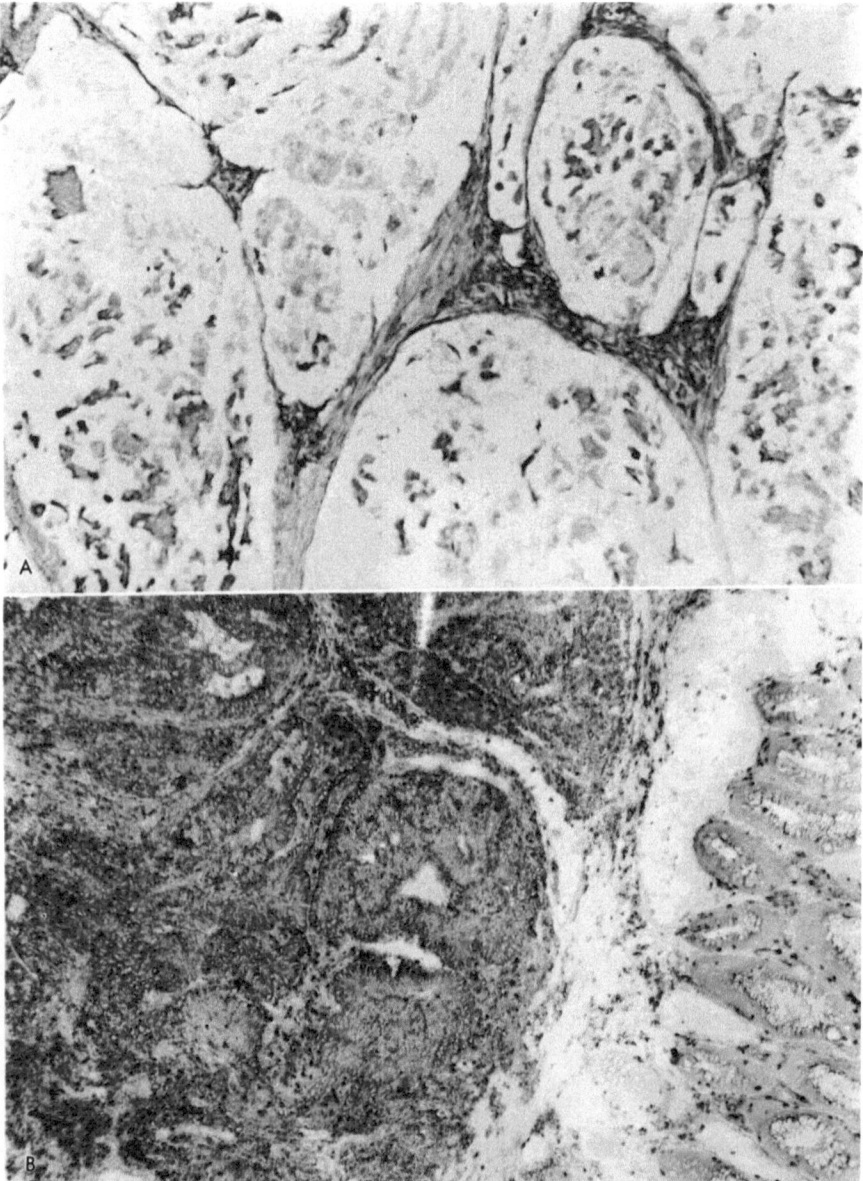

FIG. 2. Staining of a frozen section of a mucinous colorectal carcinoma (panel A) with the anti Class I HLA monoclonal antibody W6/32 and of a colorectal carcinoma (panel B) with the anti Class II HLA monoclonal antibody Q5/13, utilizing the avidin-biotin-peroxidase method.

The expression of Class I HLA antigens is low in the mucinous colorectal carcinoma; expression of Class II HLA antigens is high in the colorectal carcinoma.

## 2. Changes in the expression of Class I HLA antigens associated with malignant transformation of cells

Class I HLA antigens are expressed by the majority of tumor cells in colorectal adenocarcinomas, but are detectable only in a small percentage of tumor cells in mucinous carcinomas and in signet-ring cell carcinomas (35). Representative results are shown in Fig. 2.

In 9 out of 11 hepatomas tested (9, 18) malignant transformation of hepatocytes has been found to be associated with the appearance of Class I HLA antigens. Representative results are shown in Fig. 1. The gene products of the HLA-B locus appear to be less susceptible to modulation by the malignant process than those of the other loci, since hepatoma cells display a markedly lower reactivity with the monoclonal antibody Q6/64 to a determinant restricted to HLA-B locus antigens than with monoclonal antibodies to determinants expressed also on the gene products of the HLA-A and HLA-C loci. It is likely that Class I HLA antigens are synthesized by tumor cells and not absorbed from the milieu, since they have been found also on 5 hepatoma cell lines in long term culture (9).

Like other types of surgically removed tumors of various embryological origin (2, 10, 16, 18, 20, 23, 24, 30, 31) and colorectal carcinoma and hepatoma cell lines in long term culture (9, 14), surgically removed colorectal carcinomas and hepatomas are heterogeneous in their expression of Class I HLA antigens both among cells within a lesion and among lesions isolated from different patients. Furthermore, tumor cells display differential reactivity with monoclonal antibodies to distinct monomorphic determinants of Class I HLA antigens. This heterogeneity is detectable even when the level of expression

TABLE I. Effect of Recombinant Immune Interferon on the Reactivity of Liver
Carcinoma Cell Lines with Monoclonal Antibodies to Monomorphic
Determinants of HLA Antigens

| Monoclonal antibody | Specificity | Cell lines | | | |
|---|---|---|---|---|---|
| | | Hep G2 | | SK-Hep I | |
| | | −[a] | +[b] | − | + |
| CR11-115 | Class I HLA | 0.660[c] | 1.490 | 1.821 | >2.0 |
| CR11-463 | Class I HLA | 0.632 | 0.735 | 1.706 | >2.0 |
| Q1/28 | Class I HLA | 0.541 | 1.024 | 1.345 | >2.0 |
| W6/32 | Class I HLA | 0.728 | 1.598 | >2.0 | >2.0 |
| Q5/13 | HLA-DR+DP | 0.533 | 0.499 | 1.217 | >2.0 |
| B2 | HLA-DQ | 0.676 | 0.658 | 0.643 | 0.856 |

[a] Controls.

[b] Cells were incubated with recombinant immune interferon (250 U/ml) for 72 hr at 37°.

[c] The enzyme linked immunosorbent assay (ELISA) was performed in a 96 well, U bottomed plate (Falcon 3911, Becton Dickson Labware, Oxnard, CA) precoated with Hanks balanced salt solution containing 1% bovine serum albumin (Hanks/BSA). Target cells ($1 \times 10^5$) were incubated with 100 μl of antibody solution diluted with Hanks/BSA for 60 min at 4°C. Following three washings with Hanks/BSA, cells were incubated with 100 μl of an appropriate dilution of horseradish peroxidase conjugated anti-mouse Ig xenoantibodies. At the end of a 60-min incubation, cells were washed four times and incubated with a freshly prepared substrate solution containing 0.05% o-phenylenediamine and 0.0075% hydrogen peroxide in McIlvain's buffer, pH 6.0. After a 30-min incubation at room temperature, absorbance of each test well was read at 405 nm on a Titertek Multiscan plate reader (Flow Laboratories, Inc., McLean, VA).

of Class I HLA antigens on the cell membrane has been increased. As shown in Table I, *in vitro* treatment of the hepatoma cell line Hep G2 with recombinant immune interferon results in a marked increase in their reactivity with the monoclonal antibodies CR11-115, Q1/28, and W6/32 to distinct monomorphic determinants of Class I HLA antigens, but does not affect that with the monoclonal antibody CR11-463. Finally, tumor cells may display a higher reactivity with monoclonal antibodies to the Class I HLA molecular complex than with monoclonal antibodies to $\beta_2$-microglobulin.

### 3. Changes in the expression of Class II HLA antigens associated with malignant transformation of cells

Appearance of Class II HLA antigens in colorectal carcinomas (Fig. 2) has been described by several investigators (*6, 11, 14, 19, 21, 29, 34, 35*), the frequency of the phenomenon ranging between almost 30% and almost 100% of the surgically removed lesions and between 0% and about 30% of the cell lines analyzed (Table II). The reasons for these differences are not known and may include biological variables (such as degree of differentiation of tumors, anatomic site of lesion, effect of therapy) and technical variables (such as specificity and affinity of antibodies, sensitivity of assays, interpretation of results).

Malignant transformation of hepatocytes may be associated with the appearance of Class II HLA antigens. The phenomenon is markedly less frequent than in other types of malignant tumors of non-lymphoid origin (for review, see Ref. *19*) since Class II HLA antigens have been detected in only 1 out of the 17 surgically removed hepatomas analyzed and only on 1 of the 5 long term liver carcinoma cell lines tested (*9, 19*).

Like Class I HLA antigens, Class II HLA antigens are heterogeneous in their expression on both colon carcinomas and hepatomas. Their level of expression can be modulated by recombinant immune interferon. The gene products of the various loci of the HLA-D region appear to differ in their susceptibility to modulation by immune interferon. As shown in Table I, *in vitro* incubation of the hepatoma cell line SK-Hep 1 with recombinant immune interferon has a much more marked effect on HLA-DR antigens than on HLA-DQ antigens. The data shown in Table I also indicates that immune interferon does not induce Class II HLA antigens in a liver carcinoma cell line, Hep G2, which lacks them.

TABLE II.   Expression of Class II HLA Antigen in Colorectal Carcinomas

|  | No. tested | No. positive |
|---|---|---|
| Surgically removed lesions |  |  |
| Natali *et al.* (1981) | 16 | 8 |
| Daar *et al.* (1982) | 15 | 8 |
| Thompson *et al.* (1982) | 9 | 7 |
| Rognum *et al.* (1983) | 33 | 30 |
| van den Ingh *et al.* (1985) | 14 | 4 |
| Natali *et al.* (1985) | 24 | 9 |
| Cell lines |  |  |
| Howe *et al.* (1981) | 2 | 0 |
| MacLean *et al.* (1982) | 16 | 5 |

## DISCUSSION

The present study has shown that changes in the expression of Class I and Class II HLA antigens may be associated with malignant transformation of hepatocytes and of epithelial cells of colon and rectum.

These changes are not specific to the malignant process, since appearance of Class I HLA antigens on hepatocytes occurs in a variety of liver diseases including viral, auto immune, and alcoholic hepatopathies (9). Appearance of Class II histocompatibility antigens in colonic epithelium has been described in graft-*versus*-host disease in rats (15).

As far as the mechanism(s) for the above described changes is concerned, the susceptibility to modulation of HLA antigens by interferon suggests a potential mechanism for their appearance on hepatomas and colorectal carcinomas. The loss of Class I HLA antigens by mucinous colorectal carcinomas may reflect a variety of reasons such as i) masking of molecules by overlying membrane-bound mucoproteins and/or auto antibodies; ii) lack of transcription of genes coding for the heavy chain and/or for $\beta_2$-$\mu$, iii) decreased stability of HLA-A, B, C heavy chain and/or $\beta_2$-$\mu$ mRNA; iv) defects in post-transcriptional processing of HLA-A, B, C heavy chain and/or $\beta_2$-$\mu$ mRNA; and/or v) abnormalities in the assembly of the 2 subunits of Class I HLA antigens, their transport to or insertion into the plasma membrane.

The clinical significance of the changes in the HLA profile of colorectal carcinomas and hepatomas is not known. It is noteworthy that the expression of Class I HLA antigens is lower in mucinous colon carcinomas than in non-mucinous ones and that the latter have a better prognosis than the former ones (36). Furthermore, the differential expression of the gene products of the loci coding for Class I HLA antigens is noteworthy, since in mice the lack of expression of gene products of the K and/or D loci by tumor cells has been reported to play a role in their metastatic ability and in their degree of malignancy (7, 12, 13). If additional studies on a large number of samples detect a correlation between expression of Class I and Class II HLA antigens by hepatomas and colorectol carcinomas and clinical parameters of the disease, then anti-Class I and anti-Class II HLA monoclonal antibodies, especially those reacting with paraffin embedded tissues, will become useful reagents in surgical pathology.

*Acknowledgments*

This work was supported by the National Institutes of Health Grants AI21384, CA38469, and AM30854, by a grant-in-aid from the American Heart Association: Westchester / Putnam Chapter, and by a grant from the Cancer Research Institute, New York, NY. The authors wish to acknowledge the expert secretarial assistance of Mrs. Edwina L. Jones, Miss Donna Jones, and Mrs. Vicky Temponi.

## REFERENCES

1. Barbatis, C., Woods, J., Morton, J. A., Fleming, K. A., McMichael, A., and McGee, J. Immunohistochemical analysis of HLA-(A, B, C) antigens in liver disease using a monoclonal antibody. *Gut*, **22**, 985–991 (1981).
2. Bhan, A. K. and DesMarais, C. L. Immunohistologic characterization of major histocompatibility antigens and inflammatory cellular infiltrate in human breast cancer. *J. Natl. Cancer Inst.*, **71**, 507–516 (1983).

3.  Bortin, M. M. and Truitt, R. L. (eds.) Alien histocompatibility antigens. *Transplant. Proc.*, **13**, 1751 (1981).

4.  Charron, D. J. and McDevitt, H. O. Characterization of HLA-D-region antigens by two-dimensional gel electrophoresis molecular genotyping. *J. Exp. Med.*, 152, 18s (1980).

5.  Crumpton, M. J., Bodmer, J. G., Bodmer, W. F., Heyes, J. M., Lindsay, J., and Rudd, E. Biochemistry of class II antigens; workshop report. *In* "Histocompatibility Testing," ed. E. Albert and W. Mayr (1984), in press. Springer-Verlag, Heidelberg.

6.  Daar, A. S., Fuggle, S. V., Ting, A., and Fabre, J. W. Anomalous expression of HLA-DR antigens on human colorectal cancer cells. *J. Immunol.*, **129**, 447–449 (1982).

7.  Dennis, J. W., Donaghue, T. P., Carlow, D. A., and Kerbel, R. S. Demonstration of a correlation between tumor cell H-2 antigen content immunogenicity and tumorigenicity using lectin-resistant tumor variants. *Cancer Res.*, **41**, 4010–4019 (1981).

8.  Fleming, K. A., McMichael, A., Morton, J. A., Woods, J., and McGee, J. Distribution of HLA class 1 antigens in normal human tissue and mammary cancer. *J. Clin. Pathol.*, **34**, 779–784 (1981).

9.  Fukusato, T., Gerber, M. A., Thung, S. N., Ferrone, S., and Schaffner, F. Aberrant expression of HLA class I antigens on hepatocytes in liver disease (1985), submitted.

10. Holden, C. A., Sanderson, A. R., and MacDonald, D. M. Absence of human leukocyte antigen molecules in skin tumors and some cutaneous appendages: evidence using monoclonal antibodies. *J. Am. Acad. Dermatol.*, **9**, 867–871 (1983).

11. Howe, A. J., Seeger, R. C., Molinaro, G. A., and Ferrone, S. Analysis of human tumor cells for Ia-like antigens with monoclonal antibodies. *J. Natl. Cancer Inst.*, **66**, 827–829 (1981).

12. Katzav, S., De Baetselier, P., Tartokovsky, B., Feldman, M., and Segal, S. Alterations in major histocompatibility complex phenotypes of mouse cloned T10 sarcoma cells: association with shifts from nonmetastatic to metastatic cells. *J. Natl. Cancer Inst.*, **71**, 317–324 (1983).

13. Katzav, S., Segal, S., and Feldman, M. Immuno-selection *in vivo* of H-2D phenotypic variants from a metastatic clone of sarcoma cells results in cell lines of altered metastatic competence. *Int. J. Cancer*, **33**, 407–415 (1984).

14. MacLean, G. D., Seehafer, J., Shaw, A.R.E., Kieran, M. W., and Longenecker, B. M. Antigenic heterogeneity of human colorectal cancer cell lines analyzed by a panel of monoclonal antibodies. I. Heterogeneous expression of Ia-like and HLA-like antigenic determinants. *J. Natl. Cancer Inst.*, **69**, 357–363 (1982).

15. Mason, D. W., Dallman, M., and Barclay, A. N. Graft-*versus*-host disease induces expression of Ia antigen in rat epidermal cells and gut epithelium. *Nature*, **129**, 150–151 (1981).

16. Mauduit, G., Turbitt, M., and MacKie, R. M. Dissociation of HLA heavy chain and light chain ($\beta_2$ microglobulin) expression on the cell surface of cutaneous malignancies. *Br. J. Dermatol.*, **109**, 377–381 (1983).

17. Montano, L., Miescher, G. C., Goodall, A. H., Wiedmann, K. H., Janossy, G., and Thomas, H. C. Hepatitis B virus HLA antigen display in the liver during chronic hepatitis B virus infection. *Hepatology*, **2**, 557–561 (1982).

18. Natali, P. G., Bigotti, A., Nicotra, M. R., Viora, M., Manfredi, D., and Ferrone, S. Distribution of human class I (HLA-A-B-C) histocompatibility antigens in normal and malignant tissues of non lymphoid origin. *Cancer Res.*, **44**, 4679–4687 (1984).

19. Natali, P. G., Bigotti, A., Russo, C., Sakaguchi, K., Igarashi, M., and Ferrone, S. Monoclonal antibodies to human histocompatibility antigens. *In* "The Handbook of Monoclonal Antibodies: Applications in Biology and Medicine," ed. S. Ferrone and M. P. Dierich (1985). Noyes Publications, Park Ridge, NJ, in press.

20. Natali, P. G., Cavaliere, R., Bigotti, A., Nicotra, M. R., Russo, C., Ng, A. K., Giacomini, P., and Ferrone, S. Antigenic heterogeneity of surgically removed primary and autologous metastatic human melanoma lesions. *J. Immunol.*, **130**, 1462–1466 (1983).
21. Natali, P. G., De Martino, C., Quaranta, V., Bigotti, A., Pellegrino, M. A., and Ferrone, S. Changes in Ia-like antigen expression on malignant human cells. *Immunogenetics*, **12**, 409–413 (1981).
22. Natali, P. G., De Martino, C., Quaranta, V., Nicotra, M. R., Frezza, F., Pellegrino, M. A., and Ferrone, S. Expression of Ia-like antigens in normal non-lymphoid tissues. *Transplantation*, **31**, 75–78 (1981).
23. Natali, P. G., Giacomini, P., Bigotti, A., Imai, K., Nicotra, M. R., Ng, A. K., and Ferrone, S. Heterogeneity in the expression of HLA and tumor associated antigens by surgically removed and cultured breast carcinoma cells. *Cancer Res.*, **43**, 660–668 (1983).
24. Natali, P. G., Viora, M., Nicotra, M. R., Giacomini, P., Bogotti, A., and Ferrone, S. Antigenic heterogeneity of skin tumors of nonmelanocyte origin. Analysis with monoclonal antibodies to tumor-associated antigens and to histocompatibility antigens. *J. Natl. Cancer Inst.*, **71**, 439–447 (1983).
25. Natali, P. G., Segatto, O., Ferrone, S., Tosi, R., and Corte, G. Differential tissue distribution and ontogeny of DC-1 and HLA-DR antigens. *Immunogenetics*, **19**, 109–116 (1984).
26. Pellegrino, M. A., Ferrone, S., Brautbar, C., and Hayflick, L. Changes in HLA antigen profiles on SV40 transformed human fibroblasts. *Exp. Cell Res.*, **97**, 340 (1976).
27. Ponder, B.A.J., Wilkinson, M. M., Wood, M., and Westwood, J. H. Immunohistochemical demonstration of H2 antigens in mouse tissue sections. *J. Histochem. Cytochem.*, **31**, 911–919 (1983).
28. Reisfeld, R. A. and Ferrone, S. "Current Trends in Histocompatibility" (1981). Plenum Press, New York-London.
29. Rognum, T. O., Brandtzaeg, P., and Thorud, E. Is heterogeneous expression of HLA-DR antigens and CEA along with DNA-profile variations an evidence of phenotypic instability and clonal proliferation in human large bowel carcinomas? *Br.J.Cancer*, **48**, 543–551 (1983).
30. Ruiter, D. J., Bergman, W., Welvaart, K., Scheffer, E., van Vloten, W. A., Russo, C., and Ferrone, S. Immunohistochemical analysis of malignant melanomas and nevocellular nevi with monoclonal antibodies to distinct monomorphic determinants of HLA antigens. *Cancer Res.*, **44**, 3930–3935 (1984).
31. Ruiter, D. J., Bhan, A. K., Harrist, T. J., Sober, A. J., and Hihm, M. C., Jr. Major histocompatibility antigens and mononuclear inflammatory infiltrate in benign nevomelanocytic proliferations and malignant melanoma. *J. Immunol.*, **129**, 2808–2815 (1982).
32. Saunders, D.A., Beals, T. F., and Schultz, J.S. Qualitative and quantitative evaluation of indirect immunofluorescent H-2 stain on tissue sections. *Tissue Antigens*, **14**, 73–85 (1979).
33. Takasugi, M. and Terasaki, P. I. Detection of HL-A and other cell-surface antigens on cultured cells by a cytotoxic plating inhibition test. *J. Natl. Cancer Inst.*, **49**, 1229–1237 (1972).
34. Thompson, J. J., Herlyn, M. F., Elder, D. E., Clark, W. H., Steplewski, Z., and Koprowski, H. Expression of DR antigens in freshly frozen human tumors. *Hybridoma*, **1**, 161–168 (1982).
35. **van den Ingh, H. F., Ruiter, D. J., Griffioen, G., and Ferrone, S.** Human major histocompatibility complex antigens in colorectal adenomas **and carcinomas** (1985), submitted.
36. Wolfman, E. F., Astler, V. B., and Coller, F. A. Mucoid adenocarcinomas of the colon and rectum. *Surgery*, **42**, 846–852 (1957).

# NEW TRENDS IN CANCER DIAGNOSIS

# EARLY GASTRIC CARCINOMA: ANALYSIS
# OF ITS GROWTH PATTERNS

Kiyoshi INOKUCHI

*Department of Surgery II, Faculty of Medicine, Kyushu University\**

In our investigations on the natural history of gastric malignancy, we arrived at the following conclusions. There are at least two types of gastric cancers: a rapidly growing penetrating type (Pen) and a slow growing superficial type (Super). It seems that the Super type early cancer progresses to a Funnel shaped, non-Borrmann advanced type of cancer of a lesser incidence, and the Pen type leads to the most advanced cancer of Borrmann type. A slow growing Super type cancer is more likely to be detected because it remains at the early stage for a longer period. Conversely, the rapidly growing Pen type cancer is less likely to be detected until it has reached an advanced stage. Ulcer symptoms accompanying the Super type seem to create a detection bias, and the chance of detection is increased. A rough estimation of the occurrence rate of slow and rapidly growing cancers is 1: 2 or 1: 3. Considerable effort should be directed to studies on rapidly growing gastric cancer, and the early detection of Pen type cancer is of top priority. The focus of our inspection in future should be directed to differentiation of "type oriented early cancer."

Recent advances in diagnostic techniques have greatly facilitated the detection of "early gastric cancer." Its ratio to the total cases of gastric cancer treated in most clinics has reached an average of 20% and 30 to 40% in clinics with a well organized gastroenterology team. It is the general opinion that such an inclining trend is undoubtedly a triumph of modern medicine, since patients with detected early gastric cancer can expect a long survival after surgery. Nevertheless, gastric cancer still remains a leading cause of death in Japan: in 1980, the annual mortality rates were 54.0 per 100,000 males and 33.2 in females. Since statistics show that the decrease in male numbers has been only 3.9 during the last decade, we looked for the pitfalls, if any, hidden behind the routine detection and treatment of early gastric cancer.

This report is an analysis of the biological behavior of early gastric cancer, and the relationship between early and advanced gastric cancer will also be discussed. An agreement at the Japanese Research Society for Gastric Cancer in 1963 defined early gastric carcinoma as a lesion with an invasion limited to the mucosa and submucosa regardless of the presence of lymph node metastasis. The designation " early " has been commonly used to mean a cancer which can be cured.

*Extreme Cases of Slow and Rapid Recurrence of Early Gastric Cancer*

Table I shows the incidence of gastric cancer detected in periodical examinations. Although early gastric cancer was found in more than 60% of the individuals examined,

\* Fukuoka 812, Japan (井口　潔).

TABLE I.   Gastric Cancer in Japan Detected by Periodic Examination

| Depth | Interval | |
|---|---|---|
| | 1 year (Nationwide, 1980) | 1 year (Fukuoka district) |
| m | 26.5% (143) | 29.6% (21) |
| sm | 29.3% (159) | 25.4% (18) |
| pm | 13.8% (75) | 19.7% (14) |
| s | 20.4% (165) | 18.3% (13) |
| Inoperable | | 7.0% (5) |

m, mucosal; sm, submucosal; pm, proper muscle; s, serosal.

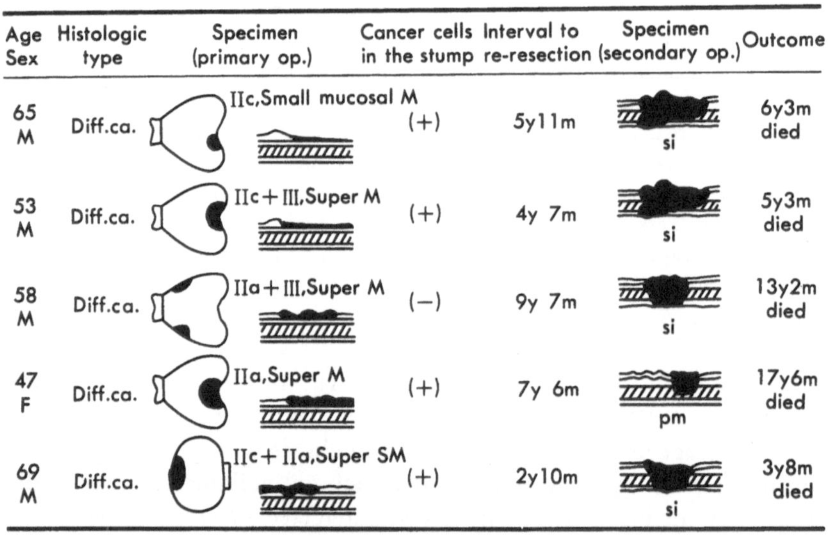

FIG. 1.   Late recurrence of early gastric cancer.

advanced carcinoma was detected in 20 to 30%. This strongly suggests that gastric cancer involves very diverse growth patterns ranging from very slow to rapid growth. Although the overall prognosis of early gastric cancer is excellent, there are a small but definite number of recurrences. An analysis of recurrences should provide insight into the growth pattern of this cancer; extreme cases of slow and rapid recurrence are cited.

Figure 1 demonstrates cases with late recurrence. All were a mucosal carcinoma with a wide extension of several square centimeters; cancer cells had been left behind at the oral gastric stump at the time of the primary operation. An effective re-resection was done about 4 to 9 years after the primary operation. These findings indicate to us that a superficial mucosal carcinoma has extremely slow growth.

Figure 2 shows descriptions of five other cases with an early recurrence; all had an elevated lesion with a papillary adenocarcinoma located at the antrum. Liver recurrence occurred relatively soon after the surgery.

There are two types of recurrence of early gastric carcinoma, early and late. We attempted to identify the two types by differentiating their growth patterns as well as by clinical factors.

| Age | Sex | Histologic type | Specimen | Lymph node metastasis | Site of recurrence | Outcome |
|-----|-----|-----|-----|-----|-----|-----|
| 54 | M | Ac.pap. | IIa + IIc, Pen A | (−) | Liver | 1y10m died |
| 68 | F | Ac.pap. | I, Pen A | (+) | Liver | 2y11m died |
| 58 | M | Ac.pap. | IIa + IIc, Pen A | (+) | Liver | 1y4m died |
| 62 | M | Ac.pap. | I, Pen A | (−) | Liver | 2y6m died |

Fig. 2.  Early recurrence of early gastric cancer.

## Our Classification of Growth Patterns (3)

Growth patterns of early gastric carcinoma were classified according to the histologic appearance of the cut surface of the entire tumor as illustrated in Fig. 3. The superficially spreading (Super) type was designated as one with a diameter of over 4.0 cm and either confined to the mucosa (Super m subtype) or only partly invading the submucosa (Super sm subtype). A lesion with a diameter of less than 4.0 cm and which invaded the submucosa in a wide penetrating fashion was designated as Pen type. This type was further divided into two subtypes according to the mode of invasion through the muscularis mucosae: a carcinoma growing expansively with complete destruction of the muscularis mucosae (Pen A subtype), and a carcinoma growing downward infiltratively with the fenestration of the muscularis mucosae (Pen B subtype). A carcinoma with a diameter

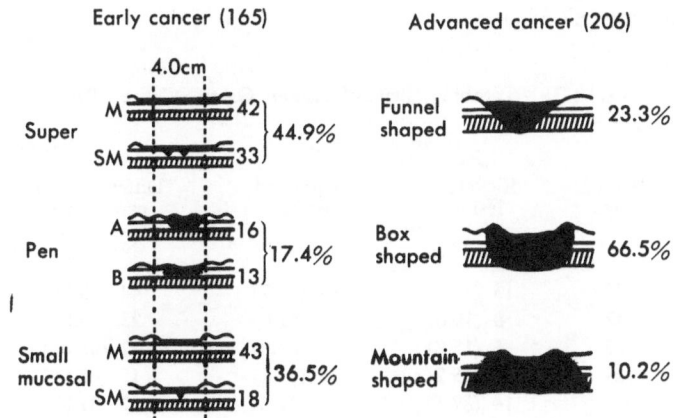

Fig. 3.  Growth patterns of early and advanced cancers.
● recurrence in the remnant stomach; ▲ recurrence in the liver; ■ recurrence in the bones; ○ unknown patterns of recurrence. * Cancer cells in the stump of the resected specimen.

of less than 4.0 cm with intramucosal invasion or slight submucosal invasion was designated as a small mucosal type which can be classed as neither Super or Pen.

The classification of growth patterns was extended to advanced carcinoma invading the proper muscle or the serosa, according to the shape of the cut surface of the whole tumor. Funnel, Box, and Mountain shaped types are advanced cancers.

*Characteristics of the Respective Growth Patterns in Early Carcinoma*

One hundred and sixty-seven cases of early gastric carcinoma and a solitary lesion resected during the 22 years from 1951 to 1972 in the Second Department of Surgery, Kyushu University Hospital, were analyzed according to their characteristics. Carcinoma confined to the mucosa numbered 85 and those invading the submucosa accounted for 82.

*1. Incidence*

The small mucosal type accounted for 36.5%, the Super type 44.9%, and the Pen type 17.4% (Table II, Fig. 3).

*2. Age and sex*

The mean age of the patients was 53.9 in the small mucosal, 52.2 in the Super type and 59.9 in the Pen type. The male to female ratio was 3:1 in the Super type, 3:2 in the Pen A subtype, 2:1 in the Pen B subtype and 3:1 in the small mucosal type.

*3. Location*

The stomach was separated equally into upper, middle and lower areas. The Super type dominantly located in the middle and the next preponderance was in the lower third. The Pen A mostly located in the lower third, while Pen B was more often found in the middle third.

*4. Gross appearance*

Depressed lesions dominated in the Super subtype (82.7%), Pen B subtype (84.6%), and the small mucosal carcinoma (73.8%), while elevated lesions were more numerous in the Pen A subtype (87.5%).

TABLE II.   Pathology Data of Various Gastric Cancer Types

| Growth pattern | No. of cases | Gross appearance | | Histologic type | |
|---|---|---|---|---|---|
| | | Elevated lesion | Depressed lesion | Differentiated carcinoma | Poorly diff. carcinoma |
| | | No. (%) | No. (%) | No. (%) | No. (%) |
| Super | 75 | 13 (17.3) | 62 (82.7) | 44 (58.7) | 31 (41.3) |
| m | 42 | 8 (19.0) | 34 (81.0) | 23 (54.8) | 19 (45.2) |
| sm | 33 | 5 (15.2) | 28 (84.8) | 21 (63.6) | 12 (36.5) |
| Pen | 29 | 16 (55.2) | 13 (44.8) | 18 (62.1) | 11 (37.8) |
| A | 16 | 14 (87.5) | 2 (12.5) | 13 (81.3) | 3 (18.7) |
| B | 13 | 2 (15.4) | 11 (84.6) | 5 (38.5) | 8 (61.5) |
| Small mucosal | 61 | 16 (26.2) | 45 (73.8) | 44 (72.1) | 17 (27.9) |
| m | 43 | 13 (30.2) | 30 (69.8) | 32 (74.4) | 11 (25.6) |
| sm | 18 | 3 (16.7) | 15 (83.3) | 12 (66.7) | 6 (33.3) |

TABLE III. Vessel Invasion and Lymph Node Metastasis

| Growth pattern | No. of cases | Lymphatic permeation | Lymph node metastasis | Venous permeation |
|---|---|---|---|---|
| | | No. (%) | No. (%) | No. (%) |
| Super | 75 | 14 (18.7) | 8 (10.7) | 0 (0) |
| m | 42 | 6 (14.3) | 3 (7.1) | 0 (0) |
| sm | 33 | 8 (24.2) | 5 (15.2) | 0 (0) |
| Pen | 29 | 11 (37.9) | 5 (17.2) | 4 (13.8) |
| A | 16 | 7 (43.8) | 4 (25.0) | 4 (25.0) |
| B | 13 | 4 (30.8) | 1 (7.7) | 0 (0) |
| Small mucosal | 61 | 3 (4.9) | 2 (3.3) | 0 (0) |
| m | 43 | 2 (4.7) | 1 (2.3) | 0 (0) |
| sm | 18 | 1 (5.6) | 1 (5.6) | 0 (0) |

## 5. Histologic type

The small mucosal type was primarily composed of differentiated carcinoma (72.1%), whereas the Super type was almost equally divided between differentiated carcinoma (58.7%) and poorly differentiated carcinoma (41.3%). Differentiated carcinoma with frequent papillotubular structures characterized the Pen A subtype (81.3%), but poorly differentiated carcinoma was more common (61.5%) in the Pen B subtype.

## 6. Vessel invasion and lymph node metastasis

Only 4.9% of the small mucosal type showed lymphatic invasion. The Super type demonstrated a somewhat higher incidence of 18.7%. A much higher invasion rate was seen in the Pen type: 43.8% in Pen A, and 30.8% in Pen B subtype (Table III).

The incidence of lymph node metastasis was relatively low (3.3%) in the small mucosal type and was 10.7% in the Super type. The highest rate of metastasis was seen in Pen A subtype, 25.0%, while it was 7.7% in Pen B subtype. Venous invasion was noted in 4 cases, all of which were Pen A subtype (25.0%). In three of these cases, recurrence in the form of liver metastasis was later confirmed.

## 7. Accompanying peptic ulcer

Rate of accompanying peptic ulcer varied, depending on the growth pattern. We found that 62.5% of Super type carcinomas were accompanied by a peptic ulcer, while in the Pen A type the rate was only 10%. Pen B subtype had an accompanying ulcer in 24% and in the small mucosal type the rate was 50%.

## 8. Recurrence

Thirty postoperative deaths were confirmed. Of these, 13 patients died of a recurrence of cancer and 17 of various other diseases (Fig. 4). Late recurrence in the remnant stomach was common in the Super type, while early recurrence in the liver was more often seen in the Pen A subtype. In the small mucosal type, 3 cases of recurrence were found in the remnant stomach, liver and an unknown site, respectively.

## 9. Outcome

Postoperative survival curves were calculated and grouped according to the growth patterns. Two patients were lost to follow-up and the 16 who died of other diseases were

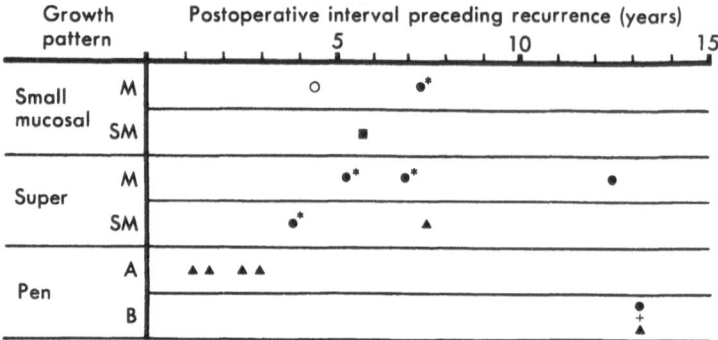

FIG. 4. Mode and postoperative interval of recurrence in early gastric cancer according to growth patterns.

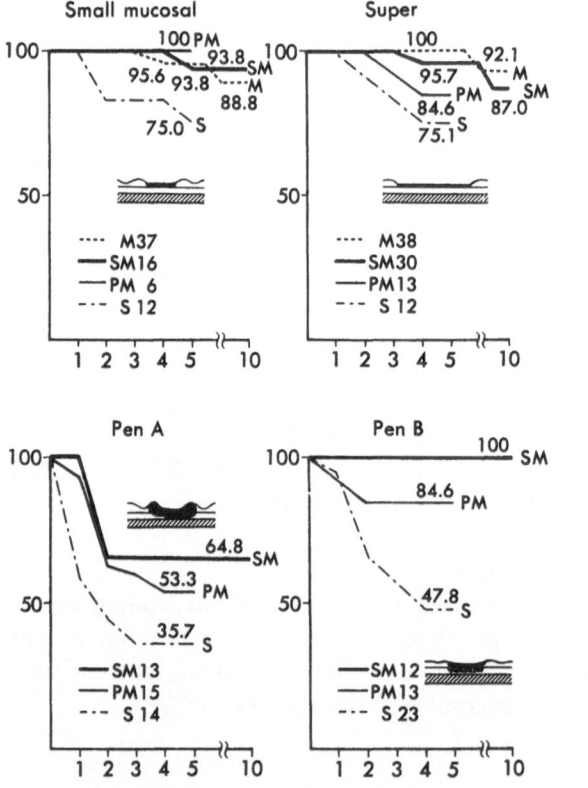

FIG. 5. Postoperative survival curves and growth patterns.
Ordinate, survival rate (%); abscissa, postoperative time (years).
m, mucosal; sm, submucosal; pm, proper muscle; s, serosal.

excluded. The small mucosal, Super, and Pen B types have excellent outcomes, the 10 year survival rate being about 90%. In contrast, the 5 year survival rate of Pen A submucosal cancer was quite poor at 64.8%.

Postoperative survival curves of the 146 patients with early carcinoma and the 108 patients with advanced carcinoma of various growth patterns are illustrated in Fig. 5.

TABLE IV. Duration of Ulcer Symptoms in Each Gastric Cancer Growth Pattern

| Growth pattern | Ulcer history | No. of cases | Duration of symptoms (months) | | | | | | | | |
|---|---|---|---|---|---|---|---|---|---|---|---|
| | | | −3 | −6 | −12 | −24 | −36 | −48 | −60 | −72 | 72− |
| Super | (−) | 16 | 6 | 7 | 1 | 2 | | | | | |
| | (+) | 19 | | 1 | 4 | 4 | 2 | 1 | 3 | 3 | 1 |
| Pen A | (−) | 10 | 10 | | | | | | | | |
| | (+) | 0 | | | | | | | | | |
| Pen B | (−) | 4 | 3 | 1 | | | | | | | |
| | (+) | 2 | | 1 | | | | | 1 | | |
| Small mucosal | (−) | 28 | 12 | 11 | 4 | 1 | | | | | |
| | (+) | 24 | 1 | 1 | 5 | 7 | 3 | 3 | 1 | 3 | |

Three operative deaths were excluded from this evaluation. The 5 year survival rates were over 75% in the small mucosal pm and -s, and the Super pm and -s subtypes. In the advanced Pen A type, the survival time was shorter in cases of a deep invasion of the lesion, 53.3% in pm and 35.5% in s. In the advanced Pen B type, the survival rate was favorable when the lesion was confined to pm (84.6%), however serosal invasion resulted in a much poorer rate (47.8%).

### 10. Speed of growth in Super and Pen type cancers

As to the speed of growth of Super and Pen type cancers, Okabe's report (4) is informative. He reached the conclusion after investigation of duration of symptoms and follow-up of endoscopic findings that two forms of gastric cancer exist: one is rapid growing and presents an elevated appearance (IIa+IIc), and the other is slow growing with a depressed lesion (IIc, IIc+III). His conclusions lend support to our idea of the Pen and Super growth patterns.

Table IV shows the duration of symptoms in each group pattern according to the ulcer history (I. Kusaba, personal communication). In the Super type, particularly in the ulcer history, the symptoms lasted 60 months or more, whereas in Pen A type there was no patient with a history of ulcer and clinical symptoms were of only 3 months duration. In Pen B subtype, findings were similar to the cases of the Pen A type. This table strongly suggests that the speed of growth is quite slow in the Super type and rapid in the Pen type.

In the case of small mucosal cancer, the duration of the symptoms was relatively short in those with no ulcer history, while it was considerably long in those with such a history. It is thus presumed that a prototype of the Super or the Pen type of carcinoma is included in the small mucosal type of cancer.

### 11. Summary of growth pattern characteristics

Depressed lesions are common in the Super and Pen B types. These lesions usually show a slight tendency toward vessel invasion and metastasis and the postoperative prognosis is good. In particular, the prognosis of the Super type is good even when the lesion extends to the proper muscle layer and/or the serosa. An elevated lesion, however, is frequently seen in the Pen A type cancer growing downwards and expansively. This type of cancer is associated with a less favorable prognosis, which is ascribed to the propensity for invasion of the lymphatics and veins, spreading to the liver during the postoperative period.

TABLE V.   Characteristics of the Super, Pen A, and Pen B
Types in Early Gastric Carcinoma

| Features | Super type | Pen A type | Pen B type |
|---|---|---|---|
| Most common site | Middle third | Lower third | Middle third |
| Gross type | Depressed lesion (IIc, IIc+III) | Elevated lesion (IIa, IIa+IIc) | Depressed lesion (IIc, IIc+IIa) |
| Histologic type | Differentiated and poorly differentiated carcinoma | Differentiated and particularly papillary carcinoma | Differentiated and poorly differentiated carcinoma |
| Lymphogenous metastasis | Low incidence | High incidence | Low incidence |
| Hematogenous metastasis | Very rare | Rather frequent | Rare |
| Recurrence | Remnant stomach more than 5 years after surgery | Liver within 3 years | Rare |
| Prognosis | Excellent | Poor | Favorable |
| Progression | Slow | Rapid | Rapid |

In the Pen B type cancer growing downwards and in an infiltrative fashion, the outcome after surgery is excellent if the lesion is confined to the proper muscle layer, but the prognosis is poor when the lesion reaches the serosa. It appears that the spread of growth is quite slow in the Super type, while it is rapid in the Pen type (Table V).

## Cytophotometric DNA Analysis of Early Carcinoma

One hundred and seven cases of early gastric cancer were subjected to cytophotometric DNA analytical study (1). Ten micron-thick paraffin sections were made from the portion just adjacent to the HE stained section. Feulgen stained specimens were examined to obtain the cell nuclear DNA content. The DNA histogram pattern was graded into Types I, II, III, and IV, according to the degree of dispersion shown. Types I, II and Types III, IV are designated as low ploidy and high ploidy, respectively.

DNA distribution types in terms of growth pattern of early gastric carcinoma are summarized in Table VI. The majority of the Super type lies in Type II, low ploidy. This propensity was similar in the small mucosal and Pen B subtypes. On the other hand, more than 80% of Pen A subtype showed types III or IV, the high ploidy. Differences

TABLE VI.   Growth Patterns in DNA Distribution of Early Carcinoma

| Growth pattern | No. of cases | Low ploidy | | High ploidy | |
|---|---|---|---|---|---|
| | | I | II | III | IV |
| Super | 19 | 2 | 14 | 1 | 2 |
| | | 84.2% | | 15.8% | |
| Pen A | 17 | 0 | 3 | 6 | 8 |
| | | 17.7% | | 82.3% | |
| Pen B | 10 | 0 | 7 | 1 | 2 |
| | | 70.0% | | 30.0% | |
| Small mucosal | 62 | 5 | 40 | 5 | 12 |
| | | 72.6% | | 27.4% | |
| Normal mucosa | 5 | 5 | 0 | 0 | 0 |

TABLE VII. Growth Patterns in DNA Distribution of Advanced Carcinoma

| Growth pattern | No. of cases | Low ploidy | | High ploidy | |
|---|---|---|---|---|---|
| | | I | II | III | IV |
| Funnel | 25 | 2 | 18 | 2 | 3 |
| | | 80.0% | | 20.0% | |
| Box | 30 | 0 | 6 | 14 | 10 |
| | | 20.0% | | 80.0% | |
| Mountain | 12 | 0 | 5 | 1 | 6 |
| | | 41.7% | | 58.3% | |

of DNA distribution patterns between the Super and Pen A, or Pen A and Pen B were significant. All the normal gastric mucosa showed Type I. It is to be noted that the DNA pattern reflects well the malignancy of the Pen A subtype.

DNA patterns of advanced cancer in terms of extended growth patterns are also shown in Table VII. Funnel shaped advanced cancer has a low ploidy DNA pattern similar to the Super type early cancer. The majority of Box and Mountain-shaped advanced carcinomas had a high ploidy DNA pattern.

The DNA distribution pattern showed a lack of correlation with the histologic types, except that Types III and IV were less frequent in cases of poorly differentiated adenocarcinoma.

### Determining the Relation between Early and Advanced Carcinoma

#### 1. Consistency of DNA distribution patterns according to growth of tumor

To determine the relationship of early to advanced cancer, it is essential to know whether the DNA distribution pattern is consistent as the cancer grows. In 9 patients, each of whom had undergone re-resection of the lesion due to a recurrence, five had the same DNA pattern in the primary and recurrent lesions, while three of 4 cases with Type IV in the primary lesion followed Type III, and the other one Type II, at the time of recurrence. These findings support the consistency of the DNA pattern during the

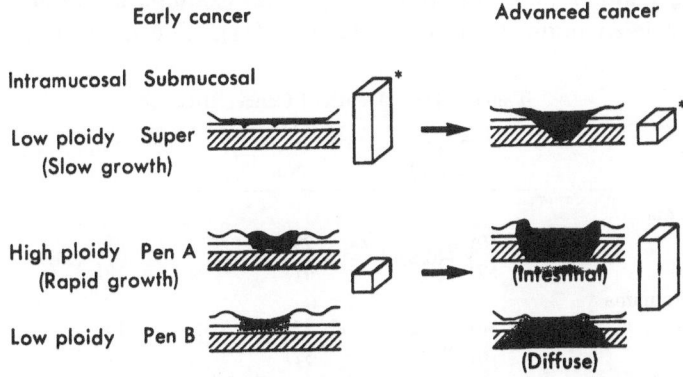

FIG. 6. Possible relationship between early and advanced gastric cancer.

* Columns illustrated roughly express the rate of detection of each growth pattern on an arbitrary scale.

growth of cancer from the early to the advanced stage. The DNA distribution pattern seems to be a legitimate tool for assessing the relationship between early and advanced cancers.

### 2. Postulated correlation between early and advanced cancer

From various clinicopathological features and from the similarity in DNA pattern, it is probable that the Super type early cancer progresses to the Funnel shaped advanced cancer which is often designated as "early cancer simulating advanced cancer," or as the non-Borrmann type cancer. It can thus be deduced that the Pen A and Pen B early cancers will lead to advanced cancer with a Box and Mountain shape, respectively.

Figure 6 illustrates the possible relationship between early and advanced gastric cancer.

## Why the Pen Type is Detected Less Frequently in the Early Stage

It seems paradoxical that the Pen type cancer is less detectable in the early stage, even though this type leads to most of the advanced cancer cases. The reason may be that the Pen type grows rapidly and develops into an advanced cancer in a short time, and hence detection is less frequent. On the other hand, the Super type may often be detected in the early stage because it grows so slowly. The discrepancy of true occurrence and detection may be large in case of cancer with a rapid growth, yet relatively less in case of slow growing cancer.

As the Super type cancer is more often accompanied by a peptic ulcer than is the Pen type, this may pose a detection bias in patients of the former who visit the hospital more often than do patients afflicted with the latter.

## How to Detect Pen Type More Frequently in the Early Stage

The only way toward a better detection rate of the Pen type cancer in the early stage would be to perform periodic examinations at short intervals. In 267 patients with gastric carcinoma detected in mass surveys in the Fukuoka district from 1964 to 1980 (2) the rate of detection was 0.08%. Of 267 cases, 196 were detected at the first examination (Group A) and another 71 at an annual sequential examination after two or more examinations had been done (Group B) (Table VIII). The distribution of the growth

TABLE VIII. Depth of Cancer Invasion

| Depth of cancer invasion | Total No. (%) | Group A No. (%) | Group B No. (%) | p value |
|---|---|---|---|---|
| Early carcinoma | | | | |
| Mucosa | 50 } (40.8) | 29 } (35.7) | 21 } (54.9) | <0.01 |
| Submucosa | 59 | 41 | 18 | |
| Advanced carcinoma | | | | |
| Muscularis | 36 } (39.7) | 22 } (40.3) | 14 } (38.0) | |
| Serosa | 70 | 57 | 13 | |
| Far advanced[a] | 52 (19.5) | 47 (24.0) | 5 (7.1) | <0.01 |
| Total | 267 | 196 | 71 | |

[a] Far advanced cases included those not operated on or in which only an exploratory laparotomy was done.

TABLE IX. Yearly Examination Facilitates the Detection of Pen Type Cancer

| Growth pattern | | Group A (first exam.) No. of cases (%) | Group B (sequential exam.) No. of cases (%) | $p$ value |
|---|---|---|---|---|
| Super | m | 12⎫ 32.9 | 1⎫ 7.7 | <0.01 |
| | sm | 11⎭ | 2⎭ | |
| | | 26.8 (11/41, sm)[a] | 11.1 (2/18, sm)[a] | |
| Pen (sm) | A | 6⎫ 11.4 | 5⎫ 23.1 | <0.2 |
| | B | 2⎭ | 4⎭ | |
| | | 19.5 (8/41, sm)[b] | 50.0 (9/18, sm)[b] | <0.05 |
| Small | m | 17 24.3 | 20 51.3 | <0.01 |
| Mucosal | sm | 16 22.9 | 7 17.9 | |
| Mixed | | 6 8.6 | 0 | |
| Total | | 70 100.0 | 39 100.0 | |

Rate of Super type[a] and Pen type[b] in submucosal cancers.

patterns in early carcinoma is summarized in Table IX. The ratio of Super type was 32.9% in Group A, such being higher than the 7.7% in Group B ($p<0.01$). The Super sm was also 26.8% in Group A, being higher than 11.1% in Group B, albeit not statistically significant. On the other hand, the ratio of the Pen type was 23% in Group B which was higher than 11.4% in Group A in overall cases, and it was 50.0% in Group B which was significantly higher than 19.5% in Group A, in cases of submucosal cancer. The small mucosal m was 51% in Group B, this rate being higher than the 24% in Group A.

Therefore, the annual periodic examination is useful for detection of the Pen type, however, shorter intervals of examination are recommended.

## REFERENCES

1. Inokuchi, K., Kodama, Y., Sasaki, O., Kamegawa, T., and Okamura, T. Differentiation of growth patterns of early gastric carcinoma determined by cytophotometric DNA analysis. *Cancer*, **51**, 1138–1141 (1983).
2. Kodama, Y., Inokuchi, K., Kamegawa, T., Okamura, T., Matsuura, K., Enjoji, M., Nakamura, Y., and Kusaba, I. Growth patterns of gastric carcinoma detected by mass survey. *Jpn. J. Surg.*, **14**, 366–370 (1984).
3. Kodama, Y., Inokuchi, K., Soejima, K., Matsusaka, T., and Okamura, T. Growth patterns and prognosis in early gastric carcinoma. Superficially spreading and penetrating growth types. *Cancer*, **51**, 320–326 (1983).
4. Okabe, H. Growth of early gastric cancer. Clinical study of growth and invasion patterns of early gastric cancer: its position in the natural history of gastric cancer. *GANN Monogr. Cancer Res.*, No. 11, 67–79 (1971).

# AN EVALUATION OF BALLOON CYTOLOGY IN THE EARLY DETECTION OF CARCINOMA OF THE ESOPHAGUS

Guo-Jun HUANG[*1] and Qiong SHEN[*2]

*Department of Surgical Oncology, Cancer Institute and Hospital, Chinese
Academy of Medical Sciences[*1] and Department of Pathoanatomy,
Henan Medical College[*2]*

Balloon cytology has been extensively used in China since 1961 both in high-incidence areas of esophageal carcinoma as a means of mass screening for the detection of this malignancy and for detection and follow-up of esophageal dysplasia; it has also been used in general clinics as a diagnostic method for esophageal carcinoma.

By balloon cytology the rate of accurate diagnosis among cases with esophageal carcinoma of all stages is comparable to those by roentgenography, fiberesophagoscopy, or endoscopic biopsy. In stage I esophageal carcinoma, however, the accuracy by balloon cytology is superior to the other three techniques.

As a result of mass screening by balloon cytology in high-incidence areas a large number of very early cases of esophageal carcinoma have been discovered, the extensive surgical treatment of which, in turn, created valuable resources for the study and control of this disease.

Balloon cytology is of great value when used in mass screening in high-incidence areas for the detection of cases with precancerous changes including marked dysplasia of esophageal epithelium. It helps to identify high-risk subjects to whom interruption treatment may be given in an attempt to prevent cancer development. Periodic follow-up balloon cytologic studies of these high-risk subjects can lead to the discovery of early carcinoma, and is a good means to check the effect of interruption treatment.

The limitations of balloon cytology include: 1) as a means of mass screening it is only practicable in high-incidence areas, 2) it is not precise enough in determining the site and extent of the lesion, and 3) despite the rarity of false positives, false negatives do exist.

Early cases of carcinoma of the esophagus are seen only occasionally in hospitals. Huang (2) in China reported a series of 1,647 cases of esophageal carcinoma treated surgically over a period of 21 years in which only 0.5% of the patients had stage I disease, whereas about 80% of them had stages III and IV diseases. Endo and associates (1) in Japan reported a 3.3% of early cases among 846 resected cases of esophageal carcinoma over a period of 14 years. Absence of marked symptoms and lack of awareness of the disease on the part of the patients as well as the medical profession may account for the rarity in the discovery of early esophageal carcinoma.

---

[*1] Beijing, People's Republic of China.
[*2] Henan, People's Republic of China.

Technically the diagnosis of advanced esophageal carcinoma is relatively easy. The diagnosis of this disease in its early stage, however, may be quite difficult, since the mild superficial mucosal changes of early esophageal carcinoma may escape detection by either roentgenography or fiberesophagoscopy.

Methods to improve the condition of early diagnosis of esophageal carcinoma have been the subject of intensive investigation. Abrasive cytology using a balloon catheter, or so-called balloon cytology, has been extensively used in China since 1961 both in high-incidence areas of esophageal carcinoma as a means of mass screening for the detection of this malignancy and for the detection and follow-up study of esophageal dysplasia; it has also been used in general clinics as a useful technique for diagnosing carcinoma of the esophagus and gastric cardia.

The purpose of this communication is to present an evaluation of balloon cytology both in general clinics and in high-incidence areas of China.

## The Apparatus and Technique

The balloon catheter is either a double lumen tube made of rubber and plastic or a single lumen semirigid plastic tube, both of which are about 65 cm in length and 25 mm in diameter and graduated every 5 cm. The distal end of the tube is connected to an inflatable balloon about 5 cm long and 2.5 cm wide covered with a cotton mesh net, which is used for abrasion of the esophageal epithelium.

The subject to be examined is asked to come to the clinic usually in the morning in a fasting state and is instructed to swallow the tube with the balloon deflated until it passes through the cardia of the stomach. It is then inflated with about 30 ml of air and then slightly deflated so that it can be pulled back past the cardia. When the balloon comes up into the lower segment of the esophagus, it is redistended to obtain good contact with the mucosal surface. The tube is then slowly withdrawn until the 20-cm mark is reached, when the balloon should be deflated completely and drawn out of the mouth.

Direct smears are made from the material collected on the mesh over the balloon and stained by Papanicolaou's method. Throughout the staining procedure the slides should be kept wet.

In screening the smear, the cytologic picture as a whole should be carefully analyzed. The characteristics of the normal, hyperplastic, and dysplastic cells are all important in the interpretation of pathologic conditions reflected in the smear. The diagnosis of carcinoma is established by finding of definite cancer cells and is usually confirmed at a second examination.

## Use of Balloon Cytology in Clinics

Balloon cytology has become an indispensable diagnostic tool in many clinics in China. It is used in patients suspected to have carcinoma of the esophagus or gastric cardia. When balloon cytology is positive for carcinoma of usual cell types and X-ray shows definite filling defects of the esophagus or the gastric cardia, the diagnosis is established and treatment may be planned without resorting to esophagoscopy. In patients with symptoms but where barium swallow examination fails to show any abnormality, balloon cytology is indicated and should be followed by fiberesophagoscopy. A negative

TABLE I. Diagnostic Rates by Stages in 220 Cases of Carcinoma of the
Esophagus by Four Different Techniques

| Stage | No. cases examined | Balloon cytology | | Roentgeno-graphy | | Esophago-scopy | | Endoscopic biopsy | |
|-------|---------|-----|------|-----|------|-----|-------|-----|------|
| | | (+) | % | (+) | % | (+) | % | (+) | % |
| I | 24 | 23 | 95.8 | 15 | 62.5 | 20 | 83.3 | 21 | 87.5 |
| II | 57 | 54 | 94.7 | 52 | 91.2 | 54 | 94.7 | 54 | 94.7 |
| III | 84 | 76 | 90.5 | 80 | 95.2 | 84 | 100.0 | 79 | 94.0 |
| IV | 55 | 39 | 70.9 | 52 | 94.5 | 50 | 90.9 | 49 | 89.1 |
| Total | 220 | 192 | 87.3 | 199 | 90.5 | 208 | 94.5 | 203 | 92.3 |

D. Y. Xu *et al.* (5).

esophagoscopic finding may not rule out early esophageal carcinoma unless repeated cytology is also negative.

Xu and associates (5) collected 220 cases of esophageal carcinoma of all stages in whom preoperative examinations by balloon cytology, roentgenography, fiberesophagoscopy, and endoscopic biopsy had all been done, and found an accurate diagnostic rate of 87.3% by balloon cytology, which was comparable to those by X-ray (90.5%), fiberesophagoscopy (94.5%), and endoscopic biopsy (92.3%). In stage I esophageal carcinoma, however, the accurate diagnostic rate by balloon cytology was 95.8%, which was superior to all those by X-ray (62.5%), fiberesophagoscopy (83.3%), and endoscopic biopsy (87.5%) (Table I). Huang (2) reported in a group of 80 patients with stage I esophageal carcinoma primarily detected by balloon cytology, the positive diagnostic rate by X-ray was only about 50%, and by fiberesophagoscopy, 75%.

It can be seen from the foregoing that balloon cytology is a sensitive diagnostic method in the detection of early esophageal carcinoma, and is clinically as indispensable as are roentgenography, fiberesophagoscopy, and endoscopic biopsy.

## Balloon Cytology in Mass Screening

Balloon cytology has been used extensively in China since 1961 as a means of mass screening in high-incidence areas of esophageal carcinoma, such as Linxian of Henan province, not only for the detection of carcinoma, but also for the detection and follow-up study of esophageal dysplasia.

### 1. Early detection

It is the result of mass screenings by balloon cytology in the high-incidence areas that a large number of very early cases of esophageal carcinoma have been discovered. The extensive surgical treatment of these early cases, in turn, has created invaluable resources for the pathologists, cytologists, epidemiologists, radiologists, both diagnostic and therapeutic, and other workers in the broad field of cancer prevention and research, and made important contributions to the study and control of carcinoma of the esophagus.

It is interesting to note that screening by balloon cytology in different populations shows different discovery rates of carcinoma (all stages) in which the proportion of early (stage I) cases varies. For instance, in a group of 8,528 hospital cases screened, carcinoma

TABLE II.  Detection of Early (Stage I) Esophageal Carcinoma
by Balloon Cytology Screening (Linxian)

| Source of data | People examined | Carcinoma all stages | | Carcinoma stage I | |
|---|---|---|---|---|---|
| | | No. | % | No. | % |
| Hospital cases (1967–1970) | 8,528 | 3,122 | 36.6 | 212 | 6.8 |
| Screening of people with symptoms (1963–1969) | 7,686 | 510 | 6.6 | 86 | 16.9 |
| Screening of people over age 30 (1970–1972) | 11,564 | 136 | 1.2 | 96 | 70.6 |

From Ref. *3*.

of the esophagus was found in 3,122, or 36.6% of the cases, in which only 212, or 6.8%, were stage I cases. In contradistinction to the mass screening of 11,564 subjects over the age of 30, however, carcinoma was found in only 136, or 1.2% of the cases, of which 96, or 70.6%, were stage I cases (*3*) (Table II).

With experience the rate of correct diagnosis by balloon cytology in mass screenings is usually over 90%. It may be calculated by dividing the number of carcinomas found in the survey by that number plus those found in the same group of subjects during the next 2 years (*3*). With experience it is possible to tell in a good percentage of cases by balloon cytology whether the carcinoma is early or late, small or large.

## 2. Detection and follow-up study of esophageal dysplasia

Balloon cytology is of unique value when used in mass screening in high-incidence areas of esophageal carcinoma for the detection of cases with precancerous changes, including marked dysplasia of the esophageal epithelial cells which are known to develop into carcinoma in a high percentage of cases. Mass screening by this means at different areas in China has shown a close correlation between the incidence of esophageal carcinoma and that of esophageal dysplasia.

Shu and associates (*4*) in a follow-up study of 530 cases with marked esophageal dysplasia and 530 cases with mild esophageal hyperplasia each for 1 to 12 years, found 79 cases (14.9%) of carcinoma in the first group and only 5 cases (0.9%) in the second group. In their control study of 477 cases with normal cytology followed for 1 to 5 years, however, no carcinoma was found.

It is obvious, therefore, that balloon cytology is of value in identifying high-risk subjects to whom interruption treatment may be given with the hope that cancerous changes may be prevented. Periodic follow-up balloon cytologic examinations of the high-risk subjects can lead to the discovery of carcinoma at its very early stage.

In a recent mass screening by this method of 17,388 subjects between 40 and 65 years of age in Linxian county, normal cytology was found in 32%, mild hyperplasia in 37%, marked dysplasia in 26.4%, near-carcinoma in 2%, and carcinoma in 2.3%, or approximately 400 cases, of the series. It is estimated that 60–70% of the latter group would be early cases of esophageal carcinoma. Based on these findings, a pilot interruption treatment study for subjects with marked esophageal dysplasia is under way. The effects of this treatment can be checked by periodic balloon cytology and esophagoscopy.

## An Efficient and Safe Method

Balloon cytology is a simple, inexpensive, efficient, and safe method of examination which has stood the test of time. To date it has been used in China in mass screenings for over 150,000 subjects with no serious complications except in one patient with early esophageal carcinoma who had bleeding from the lesion after the procedure. He was then operated upon with resection of the carcinoma followed by uneventful recovery.

## Limitations

Balloon cytology, however, has its limitations in that as a means of mass screening it is only practicable in high-incidence areas where cases of early esophageal carcinoma and dysplastic changes of esophageal epithelial cells are present in sufficiently large numbers to warrant its use. Even so, it necessitates a great deal of manpower in mobilization and organization of the mass and in screening the great number of cytologic smears. Although balloon cytology is quite sensitive in detecting superficial esophageal carcinoma, it is not precise enough in determining the site and extent of the lesion, and therefore has to be backed up by roentgen examination, esophagoscopy, and other techniques of investigation for these purposes. Further, despite the rarity of false positives by balloon cytology, false negatives do exist.

## REFERENCES

1. Endo, M., Yamada, A., Ide, H., Yoshida, M., Hayashi, T., and Kakayama, K. Early cancer of the esophagus: diagnosis and clinical evaluation. *Int. Adv. Surg. Oncol.*, 3, 49–71 (1980).
2. Huang, G. J. Early detection and surgical treatment of esophageal carcinoma. *Japan. J. Surg.*, 11, 399–405 (1981).
3. Shen, Q. Diagnostic cytology and early detection. *In* "Carcinoma of the Esophagus and Gastric Cardia," ed. G. J. Huang and Y. K. Wu, p. 176 (1984). Springer-Verlag, Berlin-Heidelberg-New York-Tokyo.
4. Shu, Y. J., Yang, X. Q., and Jin, S. P. Further investigation of the relationship between dysplasia and cancer of the esophagus (in Chinese). *Chin. Med. J.*, 60, 39–41 (1980).
5. Xu, D. Y., Zhang, D. Y., Li, D., and Niu, W. H. A comparison of diagnostic rates in 220 cases of esophageal carcinoma by balloon cytology, roentgenography, fiberesophagoscopy, and endoscopic biopsy (in Chinese). *Cancer Res. Prev. Treat.*, 12, 162–164 (1985).

APPENDIX

# NEW MEASURES FOR EARLY DETECTION OF CARCINOMA OF THE ESOPHAGUS

Kin-ichi Nabeya

*Second Surgical Department, Kyorin University
School of Medicine**

The capsulated brushing cytology is a simple method where the patient feels no pain and anesthesia of any kind is unnecessary. The diagnostic rate was 95% in 118 cases of esophageal carcinoma. Viewing these by radiologic types, the diagnostic rate was 100% in serrated type carcinoma and 86.8% in superficial type carcinoma.

The Lugol-staining endoscopy has made it possible to make detection of minute carcinomas measuring approximately 5 mm. This method is also effective for detections of early carcinomas and ill-defined carcinomas. The Lugol-staining is also applied to resected specimens which assists in the observation of minute lesions.

The main methods for detection of carcinoma of the esophagus are radiologic, endoscopic, and cytologic examinations. For the detection of early carcinoma of the esophagus by cytology, there is a report by Imbriglia and Lopusniak (*1*) made in 1949. Lugol-staining endoscopy was reported by Torie *et al.* (*6*) in 1975, and by many other authors.

However, in Japan, the total number of early carcinoma reported in the past 15 years amount to only 245 cases (*3*) indicating unsatisfactory results. In this paper, as new measures for early detection of carcinoma of the esophagus, our capsulated brushing cytology and Lugol-staining endoscopy will be presented.

## Capsulated Brushing Cytology

### 1. Instrument and method (4)

The instrument consists of an abrasive brush and a capsule to enclose the compressed brush with a long string attached to it. The brush is a ball made from polyurethane sponge and the brush sizes vary from 20 to 27 mm in diameter to fit every need, although generally the 27 mm size brush is used. Lead has recently been attached to this brush so that passage of the brush can be confirmed by X-ray (Fig. 1).

Examination is made when the stomach is empty. Sedatives or anesthesia of any kind are unnecessary. The capsule is swallowed with 200 ml of water. Approximately 10 min later, the capsule will melt and the brush will expand. When the string is pulled out slowly, the brush will collect the cells from esophageal mucosa on its way out. The pulled-out brush is washed in 30 ml of physiologic saline solution so the collected cells will float in it. Three Papanicolau-staining specimens and one Giemsa-staining specimen are made and cytologic diagnosis is made.

---

* Shinkawa 6-20-2, Mitaka 181, Japan (鍋谷欣市).

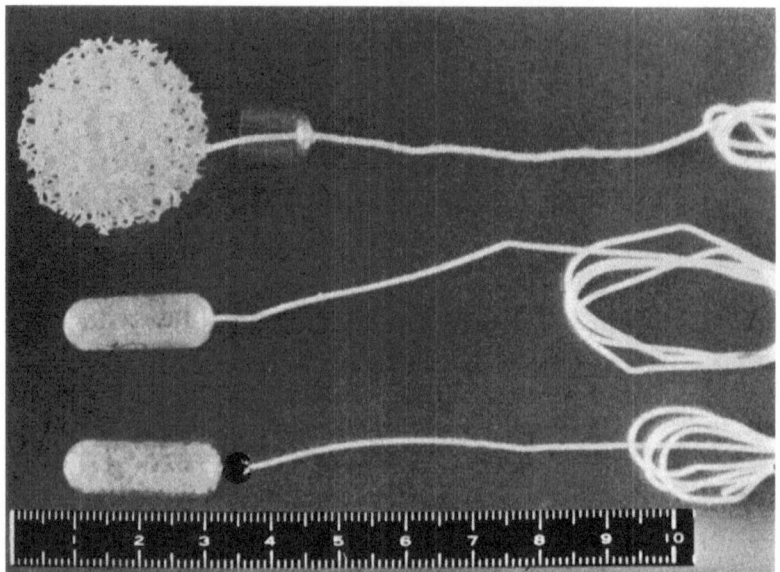

Fig. 1.   Instrument for capsulated brushing cytology
The brush is a polyurethane sponge ball with a long string attached to it. Lead
attached to the brush is shown in the lower sponge.

## 2.   Results

Examinations were made on 10 persons with normal esophagus and the average
number of cells collected with one capsulated brushing cytology with a brush of 25 mm
was approximately 100,000.

In the cases of normal esophagus and benign esophageal diseases, only one case
showed falsely positive. In esophageal carcinoma, the diagnostic rate of Class IV plus
Class V (positive rate) was 78.8%, and when suspicious cases in Class III were included,
the diagnostic rate was 95%. The diagnostic rate of cardia carcinoma was over 60%.
Mass screening for esophageal carcinoma was performed on nearly 4,000 people and
one case of advanced carcinoma was detected (Table I).

By radiologic types in 118 cases of esophageal carcinoma, the highest ranking diagnostic rate of 100% was in the serrated type, followed by 91.7% in the tumorous type
and 86.7% in the superficial type. The spiral and funnelled types showed a trend of
having more suspicious cases (Table II).

TABLE I.   Results of Capsulated Brushing Cytology for Esophageal Diseases

| Diseases | Cases | Class | | | | | Diagnostic rate (%) | |
|---|---|---|---|---|---|---|---|---|
| | | I | II | III | IV | V | IV+V | III+ IV+V |
| Normal esophagus and benign esophageal disease | 216 | 78 | 132 | 5 | 1 | | — | |
| Esophageal carcinoma | 118 | | 6 | 19 | 51 | 42 | 78.8 | 95.0 |
| Cardia carcinoma | 29 | | 9 | 2 | 10 | 2 | 62.1 | 69.1 |
| Postoperative recurrence cases of esophageal or gastric carcinoma | 4 | | | 2 | 1 | 1 | 50.0 | 100.0 |
| Mass screening for esophageal carcinoma | 3,682 | 2,380 | 1,286 | 15 | 1 | | — | |

TABLE II. Results of Capsulated Brushing Cytology for Esophageal
Carcinoma by Radiologic Types

| Radiologic types | Cases | Class | | | | | Diagnostic rate (%) | |
|---|---|---|---|---|---|---|---|---|
| | | I | II | III | IV | V | IV+V | III+IV+V |
| Superficial | 15 | | 2 | | 8 | 5 | 86.7 | 86.7 |
| Tumorous | 12 | | 1 | | 6 | 5 | 91.7 | 91.7 |
| Serrated | 14 | | | | 5 | 9 | 100.0 | 100.0 |
| Spiral | 67 | | 3 | 15 | 29 | 20 | 73.1 | 95.5 |
| Funnelled | 10 | | | 4 | 3 | 3 | 60.0 | 100.0 |
| Total | 118 | | 6 | 19 | 51 | 42 | 78.8 | 95.0 |

In Japan, early esophageal carcinoma is defined as carcinoma where invasion is superficially limited to the submucosal layer and is without lymph node metastasis. Based on this definition, we treated 14 early esophageal carcinoma cases in which six cases demonstrated intraepithelial carcinoma, a comparatively high ratio. Of these 14 cases, the capsulated brushing cytology was applied to 13 and the diagnostic rate was 84.6%. Two cases of intraepithelial minute carcinomas were negative in Class II. However, these two cases were detected with Lugol-staining endoscopy and positive biopsies were obtained.

*Lugol-Staining Endoscopy*

*1. Method*

The normal esophageal mucosa contains glycogen which reacts to iodine by dyeing brown. However, when carcinoma is present, the normal epithelium is destroyed and the lesion will resist dyeing. An endoscopic examination is made after a Lugol solution is scattered on the esophageal cavity. We usually use a solution of 2% (iodine 10 g, potassium iodine 20 g, water 1,500 ml). After the operation, the Lugol-staining is repeated on the resected specimen, but at this time a diluted solution of 0.4% is used.

*2. Results*

On the 14 cases of early esophageal carcinoma, unstained regions were recognized with Lugol-staining in every case. Biopsy was made from each lesion and positive cells were obtained. Generally, unstained regions measuring over 5 to 10 mm can be detected

TABLE III. Color Classification in Lugol-Staining (90 Lesions in 22 Esophagectomy Cases)

| Color | Lesion | | | | | |
|---|---|---|---|---|---|---|
| | Invasive carcinoma | *In situ,* mucosal carcinoma | Submucosal extension metastasis | Dysplasia | Parakeratosis | Normal |
| A-5 (dark brown) | | | | | | 6 |
| A-4 (deep brown) | | | 1 | 1 | | 14 |
| A-3 (brown) | | 2 | 2 | 2 | | 11 |
| A-2 (light brown) | 8 | 3 | 2 | 4 | 3 | 1 |
| A-1 (dark yellow) | 5 | 3 | 1 | 5 | 4 | |
| A-0 (yellow, unstained) | 6 | 6 | | | | |
| Total | 19 | 14 | 6 | 12 | 7 | 32 |

as carcinoma but when these regions measure less than 5 mm there are times when differentiation of carcinoma or dysplasia becomes difficult by coloring alone, particularly when the two exist together.

The color tones of Lugol-staining resected specimens were divided into six grades from A-5 (dark brown) to A-0 (yellow, unstained) (Table III). All invasive carcinomas were less than A-2. Of *in situ* and intramucosal carcinomas, A-3 was recognized in two of the 14 lesions and detection was difficult. In submucosal extension and metastasis, completely unstained lesions (A-0) were nonexistent and some even showed staining close to normal A-4 and A-3. In normal regions, one A-2 part was found but the majority were A-4.

## DISCUSSION

Every year 5,000 people die from esophageal carcinoma in Japan, however, only about 30 cases of early esophageal carcinoma are detected. The duration of illness, from natural history, is estimated to be 2 to 3 years from the early stage until death. Therefore, the detection of asymptomatic early carcinoma is an urgent problem. We are now studying mass screening (2) but many social problems still remain. If the capsulated brushing cytology is used more widely in mass screening, it will be effective in the early detection of esophageal carcinoma and will lead to good treatment results.

In viewing the results of 13 cases of early carcinoma, two minute carcinomas were negative by the capsulated brushing cytology. The diameter of the carcinoma lesions was approximately 10 mm and this may be the limit of capsulated brushing cytology ability, though we are not yet sure. We are contemplating using a larger brush and combining this method with other examinations.

In China (5), the carcinoma cells were counted in 100 cases of early carcinoma where balloon cytology was applied. Three specimens were made from every case and examined. Cases where carcinoma cells amounted to less than 10 accounted for more than 1/3 of the total. This figure is practically identical to our capsulated brushing cytology figure.

In Lugol-staining endoscopy, the solution concentration differs with every reporter. From our experience, we usually use a 2% solution, as a solution of comparatively thinner consistency is sometimes more favorable in observation. Comparisons between Lugol-staining coloring and histologic lesions cannot be made with endoscopic figures alone and this is why further investigations were made by repeating Lugol-staining on the resected specimens.

In minute lesion detections, as in intraepithelial carcinomas, it is our desire to gain experience with more cases and to make further examinations.

## REFERENCES

1.  Imbriglia, J. E. and Lopusniak, M. S. Cytologic examination of sediment from the esophagus in a case of intra-epithelial carcinoma of the esophagus. *Gastroenterology*, **13**, 457–463 (1949).
2.  Nabeya, K. Markers of cancer risk in the esophagus and surveillance of high-risk groups. *In* "Precancerous Lesions of the Gastrointestinal Tract", ed. P. Sherlock, B. C. Morson, L. Barbara, and U. Veronesi, pp. 71–86 (1983). Raven Press, New York.

3.  Nabeya, K., Arai, Y., Kawahara, T., Miura, F., and Hiramatsu, K. Early esophageal cancer (in Japanese). *Surg. Ther.*, **49**, 63–70 (1983).

4.  Nabeya, K., Onozawa, K., and Ri., S. Brushing cytology with capsule for esophageal cancer. *Chir. Gastroenterol.*, **13**, 101–107 (1979).

5.  The Co-Ordinating Group for the Research of Esophageal Carcinoma, Chinese Academy of Medical Sciences and Honan Province. The early detection of carcinoma of the esophagus. *Sci. Sin.*, **16**, 457–463 (1973).

6.  Torie, S., Kohli, Y., Akasaka, Y., and Kawai, K. New trial for endoscopical observation of esophagus by dye-scattering method. *Endoscopy*, **7**, 75–79 (1975).

# THE ENDOSCOPIC DIAGNOSIS OF EARLY GASTRIC CANCER

Yanao OGURO*¹ and Takao SAKITA*²

*Department of Internal Medicine, National Cancer Center Hospital*¹
*and Department of Internal Medicine, Showa General Hospital*²

Recent advances in endoscopic diagnosis of early gastric cancer in Japan are of two kinds at the macroscopic level and biopsy diagnosis at the microscopic level. These advances are due chiefly to the remarkable development of endoscopic instruments in this country and to the increased diagnostic abilities of our specialists. We refer to the popularization and development of panendoscopes, the significance of the side-viewing fiberscope in diagnosis of early gastric cancer (especially the GTF types), and advances in gastrofiberscopic biopsy recognition of the early form of the disease which simulates gastritis.

Recent advances in the endoscopic diagnosis of early gastric cancer can be classified into two types, that at the macroscopic level and biopsy diagnosis at the microscopic level. These advances are due to the remarkable development of endoscopic instruments in Japan and to the increased abilities of the country's specialists.

## Frequency of Early Gastric Cancer in Japan

Early gastric cancer in Japan has been studied twice, in 1971 and 1981 (6). The first study covered 8,316 cases during the 10 year period between 1962 and 1971, an average of 831.6 cases a year; 9,143 lesions were of record. During the 9 years from 1972 to 1980, 15,933 cases (an annual average of 1,770.3) and 17,212 lesions were noted. Figure 1 shows the annual incidence of early gastric cancer detection from 1962 to 1980. The frequency of detection is seen to have increased rapidly and reached 2,400 cases in 1980. During the second period studied, cases were reported from 110 major hospitals and institutes. According to follow-up studies after surgery for early gastric cancer in the National Cancer Center Hospital, Tokyo, the 5-year survival rate was 97.7% ($p < 0.01$), the 10-year rate was 96.4% ($p < 0.01$), and the 15-year rate was 96.4%. One of the main reasons for this recent decrease in mortality in Japan is the high incidence of early detection and subsequent successful treatment.

## Popularization and Development of the Panendoscope

The panendoscope is a fiberscope which allows forward and oblique observation of the entire upper gastrointestinal tract, from the esophagus, the stomach and to the duodenum. With the improved capability of this instrument, the frequency of panendo-

*¹ Tsukiji 5-1-1, Chuo-ku, Tokyo 104, Japan (小黒八七郎).
*² Tenjin-cho 2-450, Kodaira, Tokyo 187, Japan (﨑田隆夫).

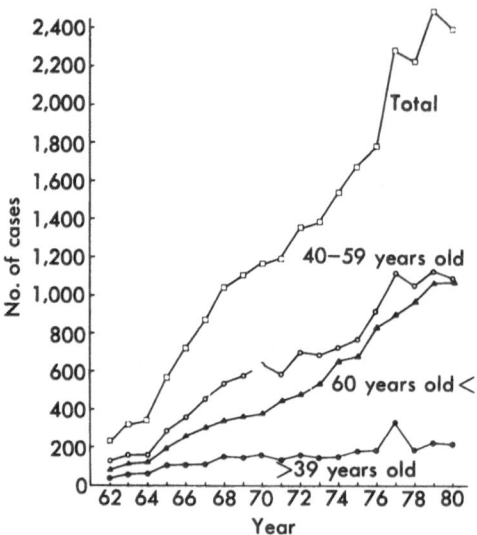

FIG. 1.   Annual incidence of early gastric cancer detection (1962–1980).
    Frequency of the disease's detection increased rapidly and reached 2,400 cases in
1980.

TABLE I.   Specifications of Panendoscopes in Japan (Nov. 1984)

| | | View angle (°) | Working length (mm) | Diameter tube (mm) | Up | Down | r/l | Max. | Channel (mm) | Comment |
|---|---|---|---|---|---|---|---|---|---|---|
| | | | | | | Angulation (°) | | | | |
| **Forward view** | | | | | | | | | | |
| Small | | | | | | | | | | |
| GIF-XP10 | Olympus | 100 | 1,025 | 7.9 | 210 | 90 | 100 | 240 | 2.0 | |
| GIF-P10 | Olympus | 100 | 1,025 | 9.0 | 210 | 90 | 100 | 240 | 2.0 | |
| FGI-SD50 | Machida | 80 | 1,030 | 9.8 | 180 | 90 | 120 | 200 | 2.6 | |
| UGI-FP | Fujinon | 105 | 1,110 | 9.5 | 190 | 90 | 90 | | 2.7 | |
| FG-28B | Pentax | 93 | 1,050 | 9.5 | 180 | 180 | 100 | | 2.4 | |
| GIF-XQ10 | Olympus | 100 | 1,025 | 9.8 | 210 | 90 | 100 | 240 | 2.8 | |
| Middle | | | | | | | | | | |
| GIF-Q10 | Olympus | 120 | 1,030 | 11.0 | 210 | 90 | 100 | | 2.8 | |
| FGI-D50 | Machida | 100 | 1,030 | 11.2 | 180 | 60 | 90 | | 2.8 | |
| UGI-F2 | Fujinon | 105 | 1,110 | 11.0 | 210 | 90 | 90 | | 2.8 | |
| FG-34A | Pentax | 95 | 1,050 | 11.5 | 180 | 180 | 180 | | 3.5 | |
| Large | | | | | | | | | | |
| GIF-D4 | Olympus | 70 | 1,110 | 12.4 | 210 | 90 | 100 | 240 | 2.8 | Foc. 10 × mag. |
| GIF-HM | Olympus | 70 | 1,135 | 12.5 | 180 | 90 | 100 | 200 | 2.8 | Foc. 35 × mag. |
| GIF-1T10 | Olympus | 100 | 1,025 | 12.6 | 180 | 90 | 100 | | 3.7 | |
| GIF-2T | Olympus | 100 | 1,110 | 12.6 | 180 | 90 | 100 | 200 | 2.8 × 2 | 2 channels |
| TGF-2D | Olympus | 64 | 1,110 | 14.4 | 180 | 90 | 100 | | 2.8, 3.7 | 2 channels |
| UGI-CT | Fujinon | 105 | 970 | 12.0 | 180 | 90 | 90 | | 3.7 | |
| **Oblique view** | | | | | | | | | | |
| GIF-K10 | Olympus | 100 | 1,035 | 11.4 | 180 | 100 | 100 | 210 | 2.8 | 30° oblique |
| UGI-G | Fujinon | 125 | 1,110 | 11.3 | 150 | 130 | 100 | | 2.8 | 45° oblique |

Foc., focusing; mag., magnified.

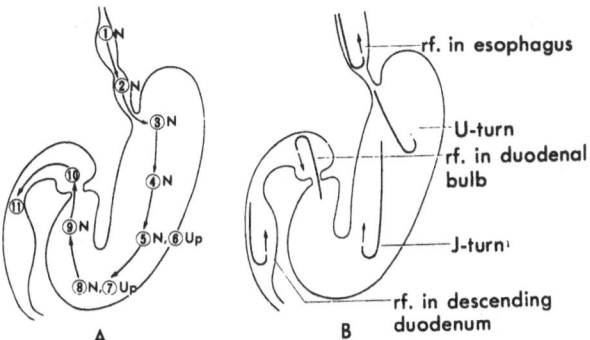

FIG. 2.   Panendoscopic examination.
A, routine; B, retroflexion (rf.).

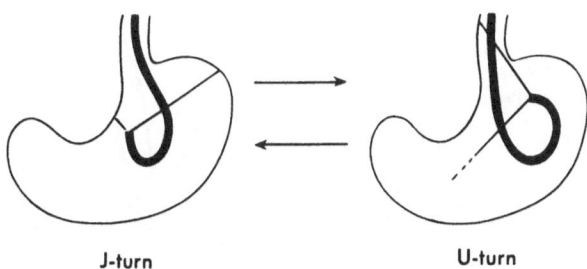

J-turn                                    U-turn

FIG. 3.   Alteration of retroflected panendoscope in the stomach, from J-turn to
U-turn and *vice versa*.

scopy examination has increased remarkably and is now used in preference to fluoroscopy for upper gastrointestinal examinations. Improvement of the panendoscope and its popularization has contributed to the detection and accurate diagnosis of early gastric cancer.

The intrument has four extreme angulations (Table I), so that it allows observation of the upper gastrointestinal tract with almost no blind site, for example, the esophagus, esophago-gastric junction, cardia, greater curvature of the gastric body, the pyloric channel, duodenal bulb, and the second portion of the duodenum in a normal condition (Fig. 2). Even a pathological deformity or stricture of the tract is visible, which was very difficult or impossible to observe or pass through with the side-viewing fibergastroscope. As Table I shows, the panendoscope has three tube diameter classifications: small, less than 10 mm; middle, between 10 and 12 mm; and large, greater than 12 mm. Small panendoscopes are frequently used because they cause the patient less pain, allow excellent visualization and can be used in biopsy; this small size is thus currently in greatest demand.

The small instrument also has extreme angulation upward with narrow curvature, so that alteration from a J-turn to a U-turn or *vice versa* in a strong Up-angulation in the upper stomach can be done smoothly and without patient pain (Fig. 3). Even with this small panendoscope, all endoscopic treatments are possible, such as endoscopic polypectomy and laser endoscopic treatment.

*Significance of Side-Viewing Fiberscope in Diagnosis of Early Gastric Cancer, Especially GTF Types*

With panendoscopes, the cavity of the upper gastrointestinal tract can be observed obliquely from the oral ward, especially the lesser curvature of the stomach where a gastric cancer most frequently occurs. However, such examination, as stated, requires strong Up-angulation, and can sometimes result in observation difficulty because of the closeness to the portion being viewed and, as a result, make biopsy harder (Fig. 4).

With a side-viewing fiberscope, the lesser curvature of the stomach, especially the gastric angle, can be observed from the front with optimum distance and an exact biopsy can be performed there. Observation and biopsy with this instrument are much easier

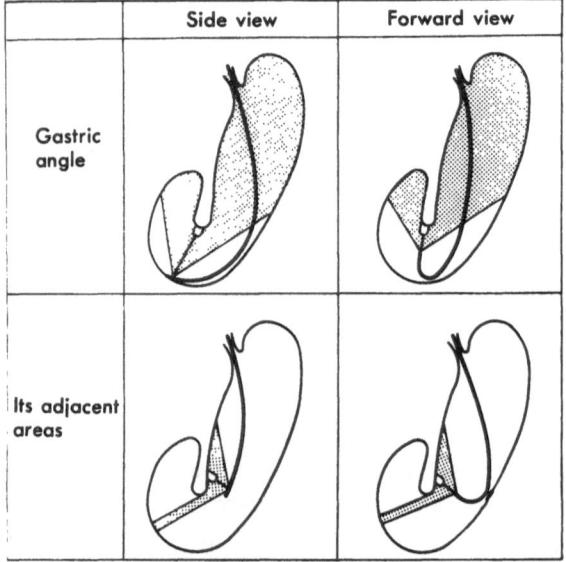

FIG. 4.   Observation and biopsy for the gastric angle and its adjacent areas with side- and forward-viewing fiberscopes.

For observation and biopsy, a side-viewing fiberscope is much more accurate than a forward-viewing fiberscope.

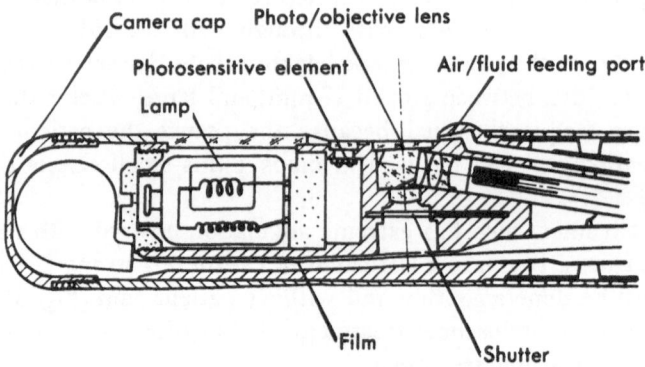

FIG. 5.   Distal lens of GTF type B2, single-lens reflex gastrocamera with biopsy.

for examination of the posterior body of the stomach, but are more difficult for the middle and lower greater curvature of the gastric body.

The gastrocamera was invented in Japan in 1950 and had a miniature camera part at the tip but, in those days, no fiberscope. In 1964 the fiberscope was introduced into the gastrocamera and was called a gastrocamera with a fiberscope, or GTF. Examination with the gastrocamera or GTF is referred to as intragastric photography, because it is a direct picture through the lens in the stomach, not through a fiber bundle as is an ordinary fiberscope; excellent pictures by the gastrocamera and GTF have contributed greatly to the establishment and detection of early gastric cancer. In 1972, a biopsy device was introduced to GTF, and the improved instrument was called GTF type B. It was modified and improved to GTF type B2 in 1974 (Fig. 5) and the latest model (1982) is type B3. Observation, photography and biopsy with GTF types have contributed not only to the detection, but also to a much more detailed analysis of early gastric cancer, including the extent and depth of the carcinoma. A GTF picture is now essential not only in the detection and analysis of early gastric cancer, but also in endoscopic research and our knowledge of gastric lesions.

While a marked increase in the use of panendoscopic examinations has taken place in Japan and throughout the world, the significance of the GTF examination lies in the fact that it is a side-viewing fiberscopic examination resulting in high quality photographs made by the camera situated at the tip. The GTF types are used strictly for the stomach, but the panendoscope can be used for all of the upper GI tract. At times, lesions left undetected during GTF fiberscopic observation are discovered later by a detailed reading of outstanding photographs taken by GTF, and therefore, the reading of these photographs is essential, especially to detect minute or indistinct types of early gastric cancer. Although panendoscopic pictures have improved recently, examinations using this means tend to lay emphasis on diagnosis during the observation, which may be affected by operator fatigue or concern with a particularly distinct lesion, rather than the search for an obscure malignancy. As panendoscopic examination is easy to perform, it is rapidly replacing the X-ray and GTF examination. However, the GTF should be applied in order to assure a more detailed diagnosis as well as for follow-up (4).

*Advances in Gastrofiberscopic Biopsy and Early Gastric Cancer Simulating Gastritis*

For the past several years the macroscopic features of early gastric cancer have been changing to flatter, smaller, more obscure lesions. It is our opinion that such an alteration has been the result of improved endoscopic diagnosis and, especially, by popularization of fiberscopic biopsy. According to our study, retrospectives of endoscopic photographs, especially by gastrocameras or GTFs, have made it possible to clearly recognize the initial features of early gastric cancer and its natural history. We have found that the early characteristics of this cancer simulate those of gastritis in many cases.

We performed fiberscopic biopsies on many such lesions and were able to detect **an almost indistinguishable carcinoma of the stomach. We call these lesions early** gastric cancers which endoscopically simulate gastritis, and believe that these are earlier cancer which precede early gastric cancer with clear malignant findings, macroscopically. We have classified early gastric cancer into three types, polypoid, ulcerative, and that simulating gastritis. The polypoid and ulcerative types used to show so-called malignant features. As shown in Fig. 6, of the three types, incidences of that simulating gastritis

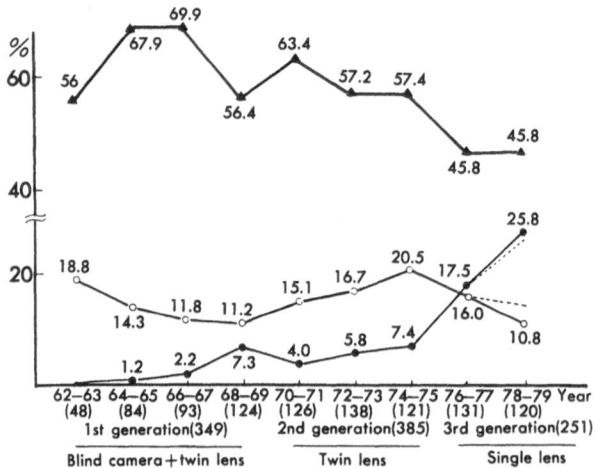

FIG. 6.  Annual change of endoscopic features in early gastric cancer in the National
Cancer Center Hospital (1962–1979).

▲ ulcerative type; ○ polypoid type; ● gastritis like type. ( ) number of cases.

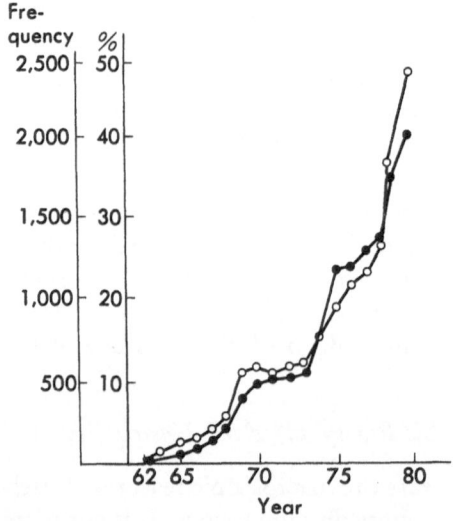

FIG. 7.  Frequency and ratio of biopsy to upper GI endoscopy in the National
Cancer Center Hospital (1962–1980).

● frequency; ○ ratio.

have been increasing rapidly while the other two types have decreased proportionately.
We assume this phenomenon to be caused by the great improvements in subsequent
popularity of fiberscopic biopsy (Fig. 7). Endoscopic examination which includes fiberscopic biopsy can detect early gastric cancer at a much earlier stage than that based on
malignant findings, proposed in 1962.

*Other Advances in the Diagnosis of Early Gastric Cancer*

Other new methods of detection and diagnosis of early gastric cancer have also been studied recently. For enlarged endoscopy, GIF-D4 and GIF-HM (Olympus) are available; the latter can enlarge a lesion up to 35 times its actual size, and the former 10 times. As a prototype, an enlargement fiberscope with 160 times capacity is being studied. With such instruments, mucosal patterns including capillary vessels are clearly distinguishable from benign, adenomatous, and malignant lesions. Pigment endoscopy is proving to be a useful adjuvant method to observe lesions and thereby detect and differentiate malignancies. According to our study on pigment-spraying endoscopy using indigo carmine, the borderline of a slightly elevated lesion or a slight converging are apparent, thus giving very accurate information, especially for the detection, diagnosis and detailed observation of early gastric cancer.

Since 1973 we have performed endoscopic polypectomies using high frequency electric current for elevated lesions of the gastrointestinal tract, not only benign, but also malignant lesions. After removal of a polypectomied lesion, pathohistological study is performed on the entire lesion, so that this method is called excisional biopsy or total biopsy. In 1971, histological critera for a biopsy specimen of the stomach were established in Japan. Degrees of malignancy were classified into five groups: Group I is benign, Group II is a benign lesion with slight atypia, Group III corresponds usually to gastric adenoma, Group IV corresponds to a lesion strongly suspicious for malignancy, and Group V is malignant. According to our study on 46 lesions of IIa type of early gastric cancer which were very difficult to differentiate from gastric adenoma endoscopically, the first biopsy results showed that 12 lesions (26.1%) were of Group III, 10 lesions (21.7%) were of Group IV, and 24 lesions (52.2%) were of Group V. Thus ordinary biopsy results are not always correct and excisional biopsy is necessary for elevated lesions. In 1980, fluorescence from some types of resected gastric cancer was discovered by argon laser. Recently, a fluorescent endoscopy system for the detection of early gastric cancer was devised. Ultrasonic endoscopy is now being used to study gastric and upper abdominal lesions. According to our investigations, cases of deep invasion of gastric cancer, submucosal tumor of the stomach or extra-gastric compression from pancreatic cancer are revealed by this means much more clearly than by ordinary ultrasonic examination.

## REFERENCES

1. Fukutomi, H., Kawakita, I., Nakahara, A., Kasimura, H., Sai, S., Kumagaya, H., and Sakita, T. Diagnosis of cancer by laser beam (in Japanese). *Igakunoayumi*, 124 (5), 389–394 (1983).
2. Oguro, Y. Endoskopische und bioptische Verlaufuntersuchungen über die Entstehung und Entwicklung des Magenfrühkarzinom. *In* "Das Magenkarzinom, Frühdiagnose und Therapie," ed. H. G. Beger, W. Bergemann, and H. Oshima, pp. 124–132 (1980). Georg Thieme Verlag, Stuttgart.
3. Oguro, Y. Early gastric cancer simulating gastritis. *In* "Stomach Disease," ed. Y. M. F. van Mercke, E. M. J. van Moer, and P. A. R. Pelckmans, p. 194 (1981). Excerpta Medica, Amsterdam.
4. Oguro, Y. The role of the GTF type of gastrocamera in gastric endoscopy (in Japanese with English abstract). *I to Cho*, **19**(1), 35–46 (1984).

5.  Oguro, Y. "Development of Endoscopic Apparatus for Diagnosis and Treatment of Cancer with Laser Fluorescence" (in Japanese) (1983). Foundation for Development of Medical Techniques and Research, Tokyo.

6.  Sakita, T. Study on early gastric cancer throughout Japan (in Japanese). *Gastroenterological Endoscopy*, **25**(2), 317–343 (1983).

# ENDOSCOPIC DIAGNOSIS AND MANAGEMENT OF EARLY CARCINOMA OF THE COLON

Tetsuichiro Muto, Junjiro Kamiya, Toshio Sawada, Fumio Konishi, Miki Adachi, Yoshiro Kubota, and Yasuhiko Morioka

*Department of Surgery 1, School of Medicine University of Tokyo\**

The usefulness of colonoscopic polypectomy was described in the treatment of early carcinoma of the colon. Histological examination of the removed polyps showed that small adenomas under 2 cm in diameter have much higher malignant potential than previously thought. Moreover, small flat adenomas with focal carcinoma are detectable colonoscopically. The role of these lesions in the adenoma-carcinoma sequence and their relationship to "*de novo*" carcinoma is briefly discussed.

Recent advances in endoscopy and endoscopic polypectomy now offer us quick and accurate diagnosis of early carcinoma of the colon. Colonoscopic polypectomy is well recognized as a successful treatment in most colonic early carcinomas, however, the question remains unanswered how to treat invasive carcinoma (*2, 9*). This paper will review the usefulness of colonoscopy and colonoscopic polypectomy in the diagnosis and treatment of early carcinoma of the colon, and will report the detection of a new type of early carcinoma. Early carcinoma is defined here as that confined to the mucosa or the mucosa and submucosa only, the former being termed mucosal carcinoma and the latter invasive carcinoma.

Many suggestions have been made on methods to detect early carcinoma such as the dyeing method, irregularity of the surface, white spots on the surrounding mucosa (*8*), *etc.*, however, none of these is entirely reliable. Carcinomatous focus may be patchy in the adenoma and forceps biopsy does not provide us enough tissue to make a correct diagnosis of early carcinoma. Colonoscopic polypectomy is therefore required of a polyp whenever feasible in order to correctly diagnose the presence or absence of carcinomatous tissue. Excised polyps should be carefully prepared in order to make proper histological slides with good orientation (*4*).

*Histology of Removed Polyps in Relation to Adenoma-Carcinoma Sequence*

Among 878 polyps in 561 patients colonoscopically removed in Tokyo University Hospital, 833 were retrieved and 765 of these were histologically examined. The patients were 397 males and 164 females, a sex ratio of 2.4:1. Most polyps less than 5 mm in diameter were destroyed by hot-biopsy technique and were not included in this study. About 70% of the removed polyps were neoplastic and, among these, early carcinomas were detected in 15%. A similar trend was also experienced at St. Mark's Hospital, London, where early carcinomas were found in 10.6% of 1,242 neoplastic polyps colono-

\* Hongo 7-3-1, Bunkyo-ku, Tokyo 113, Japan (武藤徹一郎, 上谷潤二郎, 沢田俊夫, 小西文雄, 安達実樹, 久保田芳郎, 森岡恭彦).

scopically removed (3). Malignancy rate increases with increasing size in a polypectomy series as shown by previously surgically resected specimens (5) (Table I). However, it is interesting to note that the middle-sized early carcinoma is the most prevalent in actual

TABLE I.　Malignancy Rate of Removed Polyps by Size

| Size | Grade of atypia | | | | | Malig. rate (%) |
|---|---|---|---|---|---|---|
| | Mild | Moderate | Focal ca. | Invasive ca. | Total | |
| ~9 mm | 363 | 29 | 20 | 3 | 415 | 5.5 |
| 10~19 | 107 | 31 | 40 | 12 | 190 | 27.4 |
| 20~ | 12 | 6 | 18 | 7 | 43 | 58.1 |
| Total | 482 | 66 | 78 | 22 | 648 | 15.4 |

The rate increases with increasing size but middle-sized early carcinomas are greatest in actual number.

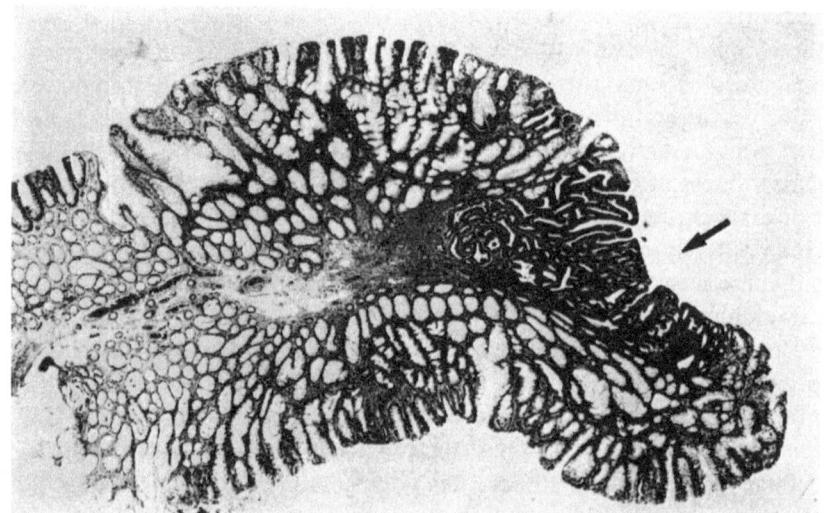

FIG. 1.　A small adenoma with a short stalk (6 mm in diameter) showing severe atypia or focal carcinoma (arrow).

TABLE II.　Early Carcinoma of the Colon (Size Distribution and Malignancy Rate)

| | | | ~1 cm | 1~2 cm | 2 cm~ | Total |
|---|---|---|---|---|---|---|
| Frümorgen | (1973) | $n=179$ | 1 (1.0) | 6 (11.5) | 7 (26.9) | 14 ( 7.8) |
| Shinya | (1979) | $n=6,942$ | 103 (5.0) | 549 (16.9) | 535 (32.9) | 1,187 (17.1) |
| Sulser | (1979) | $n=581$ | 1 (0.3) | 10 ( 8.6) | 19 (26.0) | 30 ( 5.2) |
| Bergoz | (1980)[a] | $n=262$ | 6 (5.1) | 22 (22.9) | 16 (33.3) | 44 (16.8) |
| Konishi | (1980)[a] | $n=1,242$ | 38 (4.4) | 76 (23.2) | 18 (31.0) | 132 (10.6) |
| Cronstedt | (1981) | $n=104$ | 4 (8.2) | 9 (25.0) | 7 (36.8) | 20 (19.2) |
| Funada | (1978) | $n=181$ | 3 (3.4) | 23 (30.3) | 8 (47.1) | 34 (18.8) |
| Muto | (1981) | $n=448$ | 23 (5.5) | 52 (27.4) | 25 (58.1) | 100 (15.4) |
| Kobayashi (enquête 1980) | | $n=2,366$ | 80[a] | 163[b] | 53[c] | 296 (12.5) |

Malignancy rate increases with increasing size and middle-sized early carcinomas are those most frequently found.

[a] ≦1 cm.　[b] >1 cm≦2 cm.　[c] >2 cm. ( ): malignancy rate.

number, and even small adenomas under 1 cm in diameter seem to have much higher malignant potential than previously thought (6) (Fig. 1). Seventy-five percent of early carcinomas removed colonoscopically are less than 2 cm in diameter. The trend of finding more early carcinomas under 2 cm in a polypectomy series is also seen in other countries, with minor differences in frequency (3, 9) (Table II). It is also true in early carcinomas found in adenomasosis coli, in which much smaller lesions are seen than in a polypectomy series (6). These observations make it apparent that the origin of colonic carcinoma is not only large adenomas but that adenomas under 2 cm in diameter may well play an important role in the adenoma-carcinoma sequence. To support this possibility, transformation from a small or middle-sized adenoma to an ulcerating carcinoma in a fairly short period of time has also been reported (7). Ninety percent of these early carcinomas colonoscopically removed histologically showed both adenomatous and carcinomatous components in a polyp, strong evidence to support the view of the adenoma-carcinoma sequence previously reported (5, 6). Realizing that even small adenomas can contain carcinomas, it is reasonable to assume that these small lesions may well be a source of so-called "*de novo*" carcinomas, and a carcinoma under 2 cm across lacking adenomatous tissue is no longer definite evidence of a "*de novo*" carcinoma (10).

## Management of Invasive Carcinoma

Whenever a carcinoma invades the submucosa there is a potential risk of node metastasis; however, the risk differs according to the different features of the invasion. There seem to be two different trends of management for invasive carcinoma, based on the experiences of different institutions, one suggesting colonic resection in almost every case (1), and the other avoiding additional major surgery as much as possible (4). The risk factors of node metastasis from invasive carcinoma are thought to be as follows: 1) submucosal lymphatic invasion, 2) poorly differentiated adenocarcinoma, and 3) massive invasion close to the cut end. Following this criteria, 9 out of 22 invasive carcinomas were submitted to additional surgery with one residual carcinoma and one lymphatic invasion in the perirectal tissue. Seven cases showed no carcinoma present either in the colon or regional lymph nodes; the remaining 13 patients have been doing well after up to 8 years follow-up without local recurrence. The reason of additional surgery required was mostly massive invasion close to the cut end. Although frequency of metastasis from such lesions is rather low, there is a certain risk as shown by the many examples reported during a study in Japan. Shape of the carcinoma is also taken into consideration as a risk factor: a broad based carcinoma seems to invade the submucosa more easily and widely. Even though lymphatic permeation of the submucosa is present, the risk of metastasis is not 100%, and therefore the decision of further treatment should be carefully and individually considered taking into account the age and general condition of the patient and the tumor site.

## Small Flat Elevation—a New Type of Lesion in Adenoma-Carcinoma Sequence?

During the course of colonoscopy and histologic examination of surgically resected specimens we have encountered very small, flat lesions which contain a high percentage of focal carcinoma (Fig. 2). Colonoscopically the lesion usually is rather flat with a slight elevation and occasionally has a reddish surface color. A central depression is visible

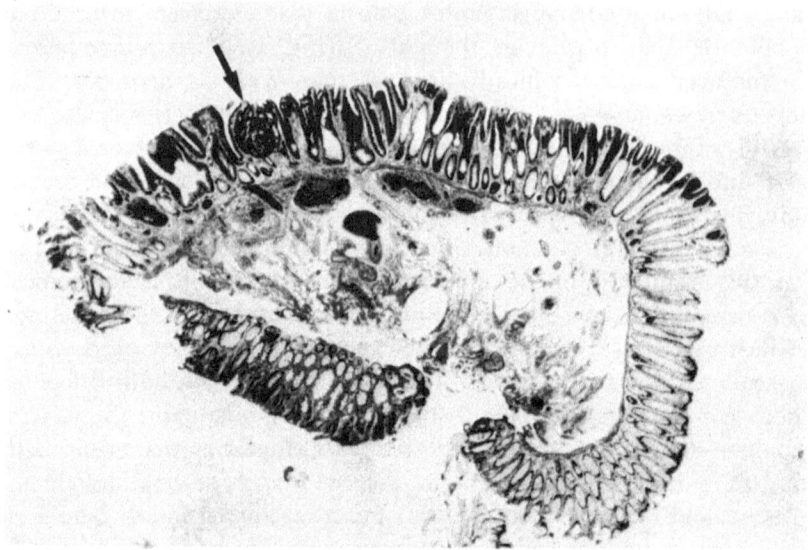

FIG. 2.  A small flat adenoma (7 mm in diameter) showing severe atypia of focal carcinoma (arrow).

Note adenomatous tissue spreading laterally and thin muscularis mucosae.

TABLE III.  Histology of Small "Flat Elevation" and Malignancy Rate by Size

| Size (mm) | Grade of atypia | | | | Total | Malig. rate (%) |
|---|---|---|---|---|---|---|
| | Mild | Moderate | Severe (=focal ca.) | Invasive carcinoma | | |
| 1–2 | 2 | 0 | 0 | 0 | 2 | 25.0 |
| 2.1–4 | 4 | 0 | 2 | 0 | 6 | |
| 4.1–6 | 3 | 3 | 3 | 0 | 9 | 45.5 |
| 6.1–8 | 4 | 2 | 5 | 2 | 13 | |
| 8.1–10 | 1 | 0 | 4 | 1 | 6 | 83.3 |
| Total | 14 | 5 | 14 | 3 | 36 | 47.2 |
| av. size (mm) | 5.4 | 6.0 | 7.0 | 7.7 | 6.3 | |
| av. age | 56.9 | 55.2 | 66.5 | 57.0 | 57.6 | |

Note the high malignancy rate which increases with increasing size.

when not too much air is insufflated. On histology the tumor tends to spread laterally forming a very slight elevation with flat and thin muscularis mucosae. Tumor height does not exceed twice the thickness of the surrounding normal mucosa. Making a differential diagnosis between a focal carcinoma and a benign adenoma on colonoscopy is quite difficult, and therefore the term "flat elevation" is proposed.

To date we have collected 36 "flat elevations" in 34 patients, 6 being detected in surgically resected specimens and all others by colonoscopy and snare polypectomy. Twenty-five males, 7 females, and 2 unknown sex were involved with a mean age of 57.6 years. There were 10 lesions in the rectum, 11 in the sigmoid, 3 in the descending, 3 in the transverse, 6 in the ascending colon, and 3 of unknown locations. All lesions were under 1 cm in diameter and were histologically examined. Associated lesions found were colonic carcinoma in 2, adenoma in 2, and both carcinoma and adenoma in 4 cases. There were 14 adenomas with mild atypia, 5 adenomas with moderate, 14 focal carcinomas confined to the mucosa, and 3 invasive carcinomas (Table III). All adenomatous components had a tubular growth pattern. It is striking to note that the overall malignancy rate is 47% and increases with increasing lesion size.

These lesions can be missed in radiology and careful colonoscopy with snare polypectomy is the treatment of choice, because the tumor is small and the muscularis mucosae is thin. A flat carcinoma arising in a flat adenoma can easily destroy the surrounding tissue and invade the submucosa, forming a small ulcerated growth which could be erroneously diagnosed as a "*de novo*" carcinoma. Although our experiences are limited, it is assumed that these "flat elevations" play some important role in the adenoma-carcinoma sequence. Our observations based on histological examination of snared polyps suggest that a diagnosis of "*de novo*" carcinoma must be carefully made by ruling out the possibility of transformation from small adenomas or small flat adenomas; there are, however, a few definite examples of "*de novo*" carcinoma in Japanese literature (*11*).

## REFERENCES

1. Colacchio, T. A., Forde, K. A., and Scantleburg, V. P. Endoscopic polypectomy. Inadequate treatment for invasive colorectal carcinoma. *Ann. Surg.*, **194**, 704–707 (1981).
2. DeCosse, J. J. Malignant colorectal polyp. *Gut*, **25**, 433–436 (1984).
3. Konishi, F. and Morson, B. C. Pathology of colorectal adenomas: a colonoscopic survey. *J. Clin. Pathol.*, **35**, 830–841 (1982).
4. Morson, B. C., Whiteway, J. E., Jones, E. A., Macrane, F. A., and Williams, C. B. Histopathology and prognosis of malignant colorectal polyps treated by endoscopic polypectomy. *Gut*, **25**, 437–444 (1984).
5. Muto, T., Bussey, H.J.R., and Morson, B. C. The evolution of cancer of the colon and rectum. *Cancer*, **36**, 2251–1170 (1975).
6. Muto, T., Kamiya, J., Sawada, T., Kusama, S., Itai, Y., Ikenaga, T., Yamashiro, M., Hino, Y., and Yamaguchi, S. Colonoscopic polypectomy in diagnosis and treatment of early carcinoma of the large intestine. *Dis. Colon Rectum*, **23**, 68–75 (1980).
7. Muto, T., Kamiya, J., and Umeda, N. Rapid evolution of colon cancer from a polyp: report of two cases. Am. J. Proctol. Gastroenterol. *Colon Rectal Surg.*, **33**, 15–24 (1982).
8. Muto, T., Kamiya, J., Sawada, T., Sugihara, K., and Morioka, Y. Clinico-pathological study on "white-spots" of the colonic mucosa around polyps with special reference to the endoscopic diagnosis of early carcinoma. *Gastrointest. Endosc.*, **30**, 231–233 (1984).
9. Shinya, H. and Wolff, W. I. Morphology, anatomic distribution and cancer potential of colonic polyps. *Ann. Surg.*, **190**, 679–683 (1979).
10. Spratt, J. S., Jr. and Ackerman, L. V. Small primary adenocarcinoma of the colon and rectum. *J. Am. Med. Assoc.*, **179**, 337–346 (1962).
11. Tsujinaka., Y., Tsuchiya, S., Ooki, S., Oomi, Y., Kaneko, H., Eguchi, H., and Kikyo, S. IIc (depressed) type of early carcinoma of the rectum originating "*de novo*." Report of a case (in Japanese). *I to Cho*, **18**, 211–217 (1983).

# NEW TRENDS IN THE DIAGNOSIS OF HEPATOCELLULAR CARCINOMA

Michael C. Kew

*Department of Medicine, University of the Witwatersrand
Medical School and Johannesburg and Baragwanath Hospitals**

Many of the more important new advances in the diagnosis of hepatocellular carcinoma have been concerned with its early recognition. Long-term surveillance programmes of individuals at high risk of developing hepatocellular carcinoma are being carried out in an attempt to detect tumours at an early stage. Serial estimation of serum $\alpha$-fetoprotein (AFP) levels has proved to be a useful although not infallible means of recognising small tumours. A sustained rise in the level of AFP occurs in about 50% of cases. However, in up to 30% of patients the value remains within the normal range and in the remainder the value is raised but not to a diagnostic level. AFP monitoring must therefore be undertaken in conjunction with a sensitive imaging technique. Real-time linear array or sector ultrasonography is currently the screening procedure of choice: it is capable of detecting most small tumours, and is safe, convenient, and quick. Conventional or dynamic computed tomography and infusion hepatic arteriography are used in selected cases.

The search for new tumour markers of hepatocellular carcinoma continues. Tumour-specific isoenzymes of $\gamma$-glutamyl transferase are present in about 60% of patients and can profitably be used in conjunction with AFP. Carcino-embryonic antigen, tissue polypeptide antigen, and tumour-specific isoferritins have proved to be of little diagnostic value. Des-$\gamma$-carboxy prothrombin is an exciting new marker but this observation needs to be confirmed.

Because hepatocellular carcinoma (HCC) is insidious in onset and runs a silent course during its early stages, patients with this tumour frequently seek medical attention late in the natural history of the disease. The absence of pathognomonic symptoms or signs, even at this late stage, further delays diagnosis. Advanced HCC is rarely resectable and responds poorly to irradiation and cancer chemotherapy. Moreover, this tumour has a particular propensity to vascular invasion and haematogenous spread. For all these reasons, as well as the frequent coexistence of cirrhosis, HCC carries an especially grave prognosis. Understandably, therefore, more and more attention has been focused during recent years on the detection of HCC at an early stage when the tumour is still amenable to surgical resection or, if not, at least more responsive to conservative modalities of treatment. Consequently, many of the more important new developments in the diagnosis of this tumour have been concerned with its early recognition.

Major recent advances in the diagnosis of HCC may conveniently be considered under the headings: "Tumour Markers" and "Imaging Techniques".

---

* Johannesburg, South Africa.

Before considering these two subjects in detail, brief mention will be made of some recent clinical observations which have a bearing on diagnosis. The usual clinical presentations of HCC have been adequately described. Less well known are several unusual modes of presentation which have recently received attention in the literature. Without an awareness of these, the diagnosis of HCC may sometimes be missed or, at least, delayed. The more important of these presentations include hypoglycaemia, acute abdominal crisis, obstructive jaundice, bone pain, and growth of the tumour into the inferior vena cava (and even the right atrium).

Hypoglycaemia occurs in about 6% of patients with HCC (4). Two forms are apparent (4). The more common is a modest and easily controllable fall in blood sugar concentration in the last few weeks of life. The second and more severe variety manifests early in the course of the disease and necessitates the continuous administration of large quantities of intravenous glucose; it is unresponsive to steroids, glucagon, thiazides, and diazoxide. It presents with an acute neuropsychiatric disturbance, confusion, convulsions, or coma.

Rupture of a HCC producing an acute haemoperitoneum and manifesting as an acute abdominal crisis is a rare but important initial presentation of this tumour, e.g., it occurred in two of 508 Thai patients (1) and in three of 211 Hong Kong Chinese (10). Rupture is usually spontaneous or follows inapparent trauma, but in two of our patients it followed obvious blunt trauma to the abdomen. By contrast, tumour rupture is a frequent preterminal event, at least in Oriental and African patients: this complication occurred in 18.6% of 296 rural southern African Blacks (5) and in 17% of 211 Hong Kong Chinese (10).

Mild or moderate degrees of jaundice are present in approximately 1/4 of patients with HCC when they are first seen. A small proportion of these patients show the features of severe obstructive jaundice. This usually results from invasion of the biliary system by the tumour; in rare cases the malignant plug may extend into the common hepatic duct and even the common bile duct (9). Alternatively, malignant glands in the porta hepatis or the tumour itself may compress the common hepatic duct.

Occasionally, HCC may present with the consequences of hepatic venous obstruction (Budd-Chiari syndrome) or inferior vena caval obstruction. Tumour invasion of the hepatic veins is not infrequently seen at post-mortem examination, and the tumour may grow into the inferior vena cava and may even extend into the right atrium (3). Patients with the Budd-Chiari syndrome present with ascites and hepatomegaly; with vena caval obstruction there is, in addition, swelling of the legs. Finally, bone pain caused by skeletal metastases may rarely precede the more typical symptoms of HCC. The vertebrae are most often affected, but other reported sites include the cranium, ribs, hip, and jaw.

HCC is responsible for a large number of paraneoplastic phenomena (in this regard it is probably second only to bronchogenic carcinoma), some of which have proved to be invaluable in its diagnosis. However, one system which has seemed in the past either not to be affected or to be rarely affected by non-metastatic manifestations is the skin.

Pityriasis rotunda is known to occur in Japanese and African patients with tuberculosis, malignant disease, and various other chronic diseases. It has previously been described in only three Black patients with HCC. During the past 2 years we have seen 9 Black patients with pityriasis rotunda who proved to have this tumour. The rash consists of more than one circular hyperpigmented patch of scales, ranging in size from

0.5 to 28 cm in diameter. The edge is sharply demarcated. The lesions occur mainly on the trunk. They have the histological appearance of icthyosis vulgaris.

### Tumour Markers

#### 1. α-Fetoprotein (AFP)

AFP remains the most useful marker of HCC; it is the "gold standard" against which all new markers must be compared.

Although there have been no major new developments in its use in the diagnosis of advanced HCC, this onco-foetal protein has in recent years proved to be valuable in the detection of "small" (defined as a solitary tumour less than 4.5 cm in diameter or a multinodular tumour with a main tumour mass less than 3.5 cm) and "minute" (less than 3 cm in diameter) HCCs. Several centres in high incidence regions of the tumour are conducting programmes designed to detect tumours at a time when they will still be amenable to resection (2, 15, 19). These programmes involve long-term surveillance of individuals at high risk of developing this tumour, namely, chronic carriers of the hepatitis B virus and subjects with cirrhosis. AFP levels are measured at 3-, 4-, or 6-monthly intervals. A progressive rise in the serum AFP concentration or a sustained level above 200 ng/ml (some centres use 400 ng/ml) has proved to be a most reliable indicator of early tumour formation. Because many of the subjects being followed have liver disease and because various forms of benign liver may cause slight or unsustained increases in AFP values, slightly raised values or transient rises in concentration do not necessarily signify malignant transformation. Very early in the natural history of some "small" or "minute" HCCs a raised serum AFP value may be the only detectable abnormality and the concentration may be raised for as long as 2 years before the tumour becomes recognizable clinically.

Unfortunately, not all early HCCs cause an increase in serum AFP concentrations. Indeed, in most studies as many as 25 or 30% of the patients have not had a raised value and in a further approximately 20% the raised values do not reach a diagnostic level. AFP monitoring must therefore be undertaken in conjunction with the use of an imaging technique which is sufficiently sensitive to detect small hepatic tumours.

#### 2. Carcino-embryonic antigen (CEA)

Elevated serum concentrations of another onco-foetal protein, CEA are frequently present in patients with HCC, e.g., 39% of southern African Blacks (12) and 72% in a study in the United Kingdom (13). However, in the vast majority of these patients the rise is slight or moderate, with values similar to those encountered in various forms of benign hepatic parenchymal disease. In only about 4% of Black patients are the serum concentrations sufficiently high to be in the "tumour range," and an occasional patient only has a very high value. CEA is thus of limited value in the diagnosis of HCC. There is no correlation between serum CEA and AFP levels in individual patients (12).

#### 3. Tumour-associated isoenzymes of γ-glutamyl transferase (γ-GT)

Three novel or tumour-associated isoenzymes of γ-GT have recently been described in patients with hepatocellular carcinoma. One or more of these isoenzymes are present in the serum of approximately 60% of Japanese (8, 17) and southern African Black patients (7) with this tumour: 1′ isoenzyme is present in 54.5%, 1″ in 27.1%, and 11′ in 34% (7). The frequency with which these isoenzymes occur in populations with a low incidence of HCC has not yet been documented. They have not been detected in serum of healthy individuals and are only rarely found in association with other tumours or benign liver disease. Tumour-associated isoenzymes of γ-GT are not more useful than AFP in the diagnosis of HCC, but the two markers can profitably be used in conjunction. For example, 8% of southern African Blacks with HCC have normal serum AFP levels (less than 10 ng/ml); 40% of this group have one or more γ-GT isoenzymes, so that only 4% of Black patients have neither marker. Seventeen percent of Black patients have an AFP concentration which is in the non-diagnostic range (10–500 ng/ml): 50% of these have γ-GT isoenzymes. The production of tumour-associated γ-GT isoenzymes specifically by early HCCs has not been investigated to date.

### 4.  Tumour-specific isoferritins

Serum ferritin concentrations are elevated in the majority of patients with HCC (6). Tumour-specific acidic isoferritins have been demonstrated in HCC tissue (14), and it is conceivable that the high serum ferritin values could result from secretion of these onco-foetal isoenzymes by the tumour. If this were so, they may prove to be useful markers of HCC. Unfortunately, recent work has shown that the tumour-specific isoferritins appear to be immunologically indistinguishable from hepatic ferritin, and it has thus far not been possible to develop a specific immunoassay for their measurement.

### 5.  Tissue polypeptide antigen

A role for tissue polypeptide antigen, another recently described onco-foetal protein, in the recognition of HCC has been suggested (20). This membrane antigen is not specific for any particular type of tumour but rather is a marker for all types of malignant disease. The frequency with which raised values are found ranges from 100% in hypernephroma and leukaemia to 64% in testicular cancer. As an investigative tool in HCC tissue polypeptide antigen would therefore not be of value in differentiating between primary and metastatic hepatic malignancy. However, it might be useful in distinguishing HCC from benign space-occupying hepatic lesions, such as amoebic liver abscesses, and from cirrhosis or other forms of hepatic parenchymal disease which might be mistaken for HCC. Takahashi et al. recently reported finding high levels of this antigen in the serum of 15 of 18 Japanese patients with HCC (20). However, raised values were also recorded in 26% of patients with cirrhosis. We have found raised concentrations in 94% of our patients with HCC, but also in 53% of those with amoebic liver abscess and in 62% of those with hepatic parenchymal disease. In practise, therefore, this onco-foetal antigen is unlikely to be of value in differentiating between HCC and hepatic metastases, benign space-occupying lesions in the liver, or benign hepatic parenchymal disease.

### 6.  Des γ-carboxy prothrombin

This abnormal prothrombin was found in high concentration in the serum of 91% of Taiwanese and American patients with HCC (11). In two patients having a successful resection of the tumour the values returned to normal. Liebman et al. conclude that des-γ-carboxy prothrombin is synthesised by the tumour and may be an additional marker of HCC (11). The mean serum concentration in the tumour patients was 900ng/ml, whereas it was 10 ng/ml in patients with chronic active hepatitis and 42 ng/ml in those with hepatic metastases. This exciting new observation needs to be confirmed.

### 7. *Abnormal vitamin $B_{12}$ binders*

Abnormal vitamin $B_{12}$ binding proteins are found in a minority of patients with HCC, most of whom have been adolescents or young adults who do not have coexisting cirrhosis or raised serum AFP concentrations or show markers of hepatitis B virus infection. Moreover, these patients have a better prognosis than is usual in HCC. The ability to elaborate such a protein may define a sub-group of patients with this tumour, a suggestion reinforced by Paradinas *et al.* (16) who found that 7 of 10 patients with abnormal binders had the fibrolamellar variant of HCC. Indeed, they suggested that a high serum unsaturated vitamin $B_{12}$ binding capacity may be used as a marker for fibrolamellar HCC. A recent observation of ours lends indirect support to this possibility: we did not find either abnormal binders or an example of fibrolamellar HCC in any of 242 southern African Blacks with HCC.

### *Imaging Techniques*

While the various imaging techniques currently used in the diagnosis of advanced HCC have continued to be refined and a new method, nuclear magnetic resonance, has recently been introduced, the most meaningful new advances have been made in their use in the recognition of "small" and "minute" HCC (2, 15, 18, 19, 21). This has been accomplished as part of long-term surveillance programmes of populations at high risk of developing this tumour.

The most sensitive indicators of "minute" tumours are infusion hepatic angiography or dynamic computed tomography (also known as computed tomographic angiography). The former method is, however, obviously not suitable for routine use. Real-time ultrasonography or conventional computed tomography will almost always detect tumours between 2 and 3 cm in diameter and may detect those between 1 and 2 cm. Isotopic scintigraphy is the least sensitive technique in this type of surveillance with pick-up rates of as little as 20% and not more than 50%. In practice, to minimise expense and radiation exposure, real-time ultrasonography is used, in conjunction with AFP monitoring, as the initial screening technique.

Two-thirds of the patients with "small" or "minute" HCCs discovered in this way are asymptomatic, and the symptoms in the remainder are not suggestive of a tumour. Conventional tests of liver function are either normal or are mildly disturbed in a non-specific way.

High resolution real-time linear array or sector ultrasonography will demonstrate over 80% and as many as 94% of "small" HCCs. However, very small tumours may be missed. In current surveillance programmes, ultrasonography is being performed at 3-, 4-, or 6-monthly intervals. This method has the obvious advantages of minimal expense, safety and speed, and portability of the equipment. Moreover, the examination can be done repeatedly. An ultrasonographic biopsy probe allows small lesions to be biopsied either percutaneously or intraoperatively. Most (about 75%) " small" or "minute" HCC are hypoechoic. The majority of the remainder, like advanced tumours, are hyperechoic (echogenic); a small proportion are isoechoic and are recognised by a peripheral hypoechoic halo. The hypoechoic lesions have been shown to correlate histologically with solid tumour without necrosis; tumours with a mixed echogenicity have partial tumour necrosis; and hyperechoic tumours show fatty metamorphosis or marked sinusoidal dilatation (22).

One disadvantage of ultrasonography is the difficulty that may be experienced in detecting tumours located in the uppermost portions of the right hepatic lobe. Superficially located tumours may also be missed. "False-positive" results, i.e., the finding of lesions other than HCCs, including regenerating nodules in cirrhotic livers, are also a problem, and biopsy is required to ensure that unnecessary surgery is not performed.

Conventional computed tomography will detect 80 to 90% of "small" tumours. Most "small" or "minute" HCCs are less dense than the surrounding liver tissue and can readily be detected. However, isodense lesions may be missed. The recently introduced refinement of dynamic computed tomography, which makes use of rapid-sequence, bolus-enhanced tomograms which improve tumour detection by maximising differential contrast enhancement, will detect these isodense tumours, as well as those too small to be seen on conventional computed tomography (7 of 10 "minute" carcinomas in one study). This method will also demonstrate tumour thrombosis in the portal vessels and arteriovenous fistulae.

Although hepatic arteriography is not routinely used in the initial recognition of "small" HCCs, it provides essential information on the vascular supply of the tumour which is helpful in planning surgical treatment. Infusion hepatic angiography is capable of detecting very small tumours in the liver, and is used in selected cases.

Peritoneoscopy will only detect superficial lesions. It is, however, useful in assessing whether the non-neoplastic liver is cirrhotic.

*Acknowledgment*

This work was supported in part by the National Cancer Association of South Africa and the South African Chamber of Mines.

## REFERENCES

1. Chearanai, D., Plengvanit, U., Asavanich, C., Damrongsak, D., Sindhvananda, K., and Boonyapisit, S. Spontaneous rupture of primary hepatoma. *Cancer*, **51**, 1532–1536 (1983).
2. Chen, D. S., Shen, J. C., Sing, J. L., Lai, M. Y., Lee, C. S., Su, C. T., Tsang, Y. M., How, S. W., Wang, T. H., Yu, J. Y., Yang, T. H., Wang, C. Y., and Hsu, C. Y. Small hepatocellular carcinoma—a clinico-pathological study in thirteen patients. *Gastroenterology*, **83**, 1109–1119 (1982).
3. Kato, Y., Tanaka, N., Kobayashi, K., Ikeda, K., Hattori, N., and Nonomura, A. Growth of hepatocellular carcinoma into the right atrium. *Ann. Intern. Med.*, **99**, 472–474 (1983).
4. Kew, M. C. and Dusheiko, G. M. Paraneoplastic manifestations of hepatocellular carcinoma. *In* "Frontiers in Liver Disease," ed P. D. Berk and T. C. Chalmers, pp. 305–319 (1981). Thieme-Stratton Inc, New York.
5. Kew, M. C. and Paterson, A. C. Unusual clinical presentations of hepatocellular carcinoma *Tropical Gastroenterol.* (in press).
6. Kew, M. C., Torrance, J. D., Derman, D., Simon, M., Macnab, G. M., Charlton, R. W., and Bothwell, T. H. Serum and tumour ferritins in primary liver cancer. *Gut*, **19**, 294–299 (1978).
7. Kew, M. C., Wolf, P., Whittaker, D., and Rowe, P. Tumour-associated enzymes of γ-

glutamyl transferase in the serum of patients with hepatocellular carcinoma. *Br. J. Cancer*, **50**, 451–455 (1984).

8. Kojima, J., Kanatani, M., Nakamura, N., Kashiwagi, T., Tohjoh, F., and Akiyama, N. γ-Glutamyl transpeptidase in human hepatic cancer. *Clin. Chim. Acta*, **106**, 165–172 (1980).

9. Kojiro, M., Kawabata, K., Kawano, Y., Shirai, F., Takamoto, N., and Nakashima, T., Hepatocellular carcinoma presenting as intra-bile duct tumor growth. *Cancer*, **49**, 2144–2147 (1982).

10. Lai, C. L., Lam, K. C., Wong, K. P., Wu, P. C., and Todd, D. Clinical features of hepatocellular carcinoma: Review of 211 patients in Hong Kong. *Cancer*, **47**, 2746–2755 (1981).

11. Liebman, H. A., Furie, B. C., Tong, M. J., Blanchard, R. A., Lo, K. L., and Lee, S. D. Des-γ-carboxy (abnormal) prothrombin as a serum marker of primary hepatocellular carcinoma. *New Engl. J. Med.*, **310**, 1427–1431 (1984).

12. MacNab, G. M., Urbanowicz, J. M., and Kew, M. C. Carcinoembryonic antigen in hepatocellular carcinoma. *Br. J. Cancer*, **38**, 51–54 (1978).

13. Melia, W. M., Johnson, P. J., Carter, S., Munro-Neville, A., and Williams, R. Plasma carcinoembryonic antigen in the diagnosis and management of patients with hepatocellular carcinoma. *Cancer*, **48**, 1004–1008 (1981).

14. Niitsu, Y., Ohtsuka, S., Kohgo, Y., Watanabe, N., Koseki, J., and Urushizaki, J. Hepatoma ferritin in the tissue and serum. *Tumour Res.* **10**, 31–41 (1975).

15. Okuda, K., Kotoda, K., Obata, H., Hayashi, N., Hisamitsu, I., Tamiya, M., Kubo, Y., Yakushiji, F., Nagata, E., Jinnouchi, S., and Shimokawa, Y. Clinical observations during a relatively early stage of hepatocellular carcinoma, with special reference to serum α-fetoprotein levels. *Gastroenterology*, **69**, 226–234 (1975).

16. Paradinas, F. J., Melia, W. M., Wilkinson, M. C., Portmann, B., Johnson, P. J., Murray-Lyon, I. M., and Williams, R. High serum vitamin $B_{12}$ binding capacity as a marker of the fibrolamellar variant of hepatocellular carcinoma. *Br. Med. J.*, **285**, 840–842 (1982).

17. Sawabu, H., Nakagen, M., Ozaki, K., Wakabayashi, T., Toya, D., Hattori, N., and Ishii, M. Clinical evaluation of specific γ-GTP isoenzymes in patients with hepatocellular carcinoma. *Cancer*, **51**, 327–331 (1983).

18. Shen, J. C., Sung, J. L., Chen, D. S., Yu, L. Y., Wang, T. H., Su, C. T., and Tsang, Y. M. Ultrasonography of small hepatic tumours using high resolution linear-array real time instruments. *Radiology*, **150**, 797–802 (1984).

19. Shinagawa, T., Ohto, M., Kumura, K., Tsunetomi, S., Morito, M., Saisho, H., Tsuchiya, Y., Saotome, N., Karasawa, E., Miki, M., Neno, T., and Okuda, K. Diagnosis and clinical features of small hepatocellular carcinoma with emphasis on the utility of real-time ultrasonography. *Gastroenterology*, **86**, 495–502 (1984).

20. Takahashi, S., Utunomiya, K., Nakano, M., Saito, S., Abe, T., and Ayachi, T. Diagnostic value of tissue polypeptide antigen in hepatocellular carcinoma. *Hepatology*, **3**, 1045 (1983).

21. Takashima, T., Matsui, O., Suzuki, M., and Ida, M. Diagnosis and screening of small hepatocellular carcinomas. *Radiology*, **145**, 635–638 (1982).

22. Tanaka, S., Kitamura, T., Imaoka, S., Sasaki, Y., Taniguchi, H., and Ishiguro, S. Hepatocellular carcinoma. Sonographic and histologic correlation. *Am. J. Roentgenol.*, **140**, 701–707 (1983).

# HIGH RISK GROUP OF HEPATOCELLULAR CARCINOMA IN JAPAN: RISK SCORES TO PREDICT HEPATO-CELLULAR CARCINOMA DEVELOPMENT IN LIVER CIRRHOSIS

Nobu Hattori and Kenichi Kobayashi

*The First Department of Internal Medicine, School of Medicine, Kanazawa University**

It is of clinical importance to predict as precisely as possible what cases with liver cirrhosis (LC) might belong to the higher risk group of hepatocellular carcinoma (HCC) (the super high risk group). We calculated the score for each risk factor for the prediction of HCC development in LC by a computer generated statistical analysis. The material involved 375. Ten risk factors such as age ($\geq$60 years, 50–59 years, $\leq$49 years), ascites retention (during the past 3 years), sex difference, serum hepatitis B surface antigen (HBsAg) positivity, alcohol intake ($\geq$75 g/day, $\geq$10 years), familial clustering of chronic liver disease, the value of serum glutamic oxaloacetic transaminase (S-GOT) ($<$100), the level of $\alpha_1$-fetoprotein (AFP) ($>$21ng/ml), the type of cirrhosis (mixed type or other) and the retention rate of indocyanine green (ICG) (15 min) ($\leq$30%) or bromsulfophthalein (BSP) (45 min) ($\leq$25%) were selected when LC was diagnosed. Subsequently, each score of risk factors was calculated with the total possible being a maximum 10 points to a minimum of 0.

Retrospectively, 44 of 75 HCC-developed cases (58.5%) showed risk scores above 6 points, while only 7 out of 40 HCC non-developed autopsy cases showed risk scores above 6 points. The difference between the two groups was statistically significant ($p<0.05$). Accordingly, a case with a total risk score of above 6 points seemed to belong to the super high risk group. Thereafter, HCC developed in 9 cases with LC. In all but one case, the risk score was above 6 points at the time of LC diagnosis. The mean risk score of the 9 cases was 6.8 points. In 2 of these 9, HCC was radically resected. In contrast, the risk score was below 6 points in 4 autopsy cases which died of only LC with the mean being 4.4 points. These results suggest that risk score at the time of LC diagnosis may be useful in predicting HCC development in LC.

Hepatocellular carcinoma (HCC) is one of the most common malignancies in Japan. In 1982, approximately 14,000 people died of malignant neoplasms of the liver, primarily HCC, and this was respectively the third and fifth leading cause of death in men and women. Approximately 85% of the HCC cases have an underlying cirrhosis (4), and about 1/3 of the cirrhotic patients die of an associated HCC. Thus it seems clear that the presence of cirrhosis correlates with a high risk of HCC. Accordingly, it is clinically important to predict as precisely as possible what cases with liver cirrhosis might belong

---

* Takara-machi 13-1, Kanazawa, Ishikawa 920, Japan (服部　信，小林健一).

to the higher risk group (the super high risk group). We therefore aimed to identify the super high risk group of HCC in liver cirrhosis, using the scores for 10 readily available risk factors such as age, sex, ascites retention, and so on, according to multivariate computer analysis.

### Risk Factors for HCC Development

Three groups were concerned in our study: the first group is 75 HCC-developed and 300 HCC non-developed cases which were followed up more than one year after a diagnosis of liver cirrhosis (LC) by peritoneoscopic examination and/or biopsy. HCC development was detected by various imaging modalities including ultrasonography (US), computed tomography (CT) or hepatic angiography and was confirmed by operation or autopsy. The risk score was calculated according to the method described later.

The second group is 15 follow-up cases in our hospital. Ten of the 15 cases developed HCC, and the remaining 5 cases died of hepatic failure or rupture of esophageal varices. No HCC was found at autopsy.

The third group is 42 follow-up cases in two other large hospitals. Just half of these developed HCC; autopsy was done in all the remaining HCC non-developed cases.

Ten risk factors were selected: age ($\geqq 60$ years, 50–59 years, $\leqq 49$ years) absence of overt ascites retention during the past 3 years, sex difference, serum hepatitis B surface antigen (HBsAg) positivity, alcohol intake ($\geqq 75$ g/day, $\geqq 10$ years), familial clustering of chronic liver disease, the value of serum glutamic oxaloacetic transaminase (S-GOT) ($< 100$ I.U.), the level of $\alpha_1$-fetoprotein (AFP) (21 ng/ml), the type of cirrhosis (mixed type or other) and the retention rate of indocyanine green (ICG) (15 min) ($\leqq 30\%$) or bromsulfophtalein (BSP) (45 min) ($\leqq 25\%$).

Each score of these easily available 10 risk factors was calculated according to multivariate computer analysis. The figures initially obtained were complex, so they were changed to simple and easily countable ones, and the total score was made up of from a minimum of 0 to a maximum of 10 points.

### Super High Risk Group and Resected Cases

Table I shows each simple score of the 10 risk factors. Retrospectively, 44 of the 75 HCC-developed cases, approximately 60%, showed risk scores above 6 points. On the contrary, only 7 out of 40 HCC non-developed autopsy cases showed scores above 6 points. The difference between the groups was statistically significant ($p < 0.05$). Accordingly, a case with a total risk score above 6 points seemed to belong to a super high risk group.

Table II shows the risk score in the 11 radically resected cases, retrospectively and partially prospectively. All but one case, No. 7, showed a risk score above 6 points.

Figure 1 shows macroscopic and microscopic findings of case No. 1. His risk score at the diagnosis of LC was 8.0. Two years later HCC was detected angiographically. In Japan, there are many cases with a capsule like this case. This individual has survived for 4 years since the operation and he is still working well.

The size of the tumors of case Nos. 6, 9, and 10 was less than 2 cm in diameter. In this country, a so-called small liver cancer is defined as a tumor with a diameter of less than 2 cm.

TABLE I. Score of Parameters

| 1. | Age | ($\geqq 60$, $59\sim 50$, $\leqq 49$ yrs) | 2.2, 2.0, 0.0 |
|---|---|---|---|
| 2. | Ascites | $(-)$ | 1.5 |
| 3. | Sex | (male) | 1.4 |
| 4. | HBsAg | $(+)$ | 1.2 |
| 5. | Alcohol | $(+)$ | 0.9 |
| 6. | Familial clustering | | 0.9 |
| 7. | S-GOT | ($<100$ I.U.) | 0.6 |
| 8. | AFP | ($\geqq 21$ ng/ml) | 0.6 |
| 9. | Type of cirrhosis | | 0.4 |
| 10. | ICG (15′) ($\leqq 30\%$) or BSP (45′) ($\leqq 25\%$) | | 0.3 |
| | | | $+10.0$ |

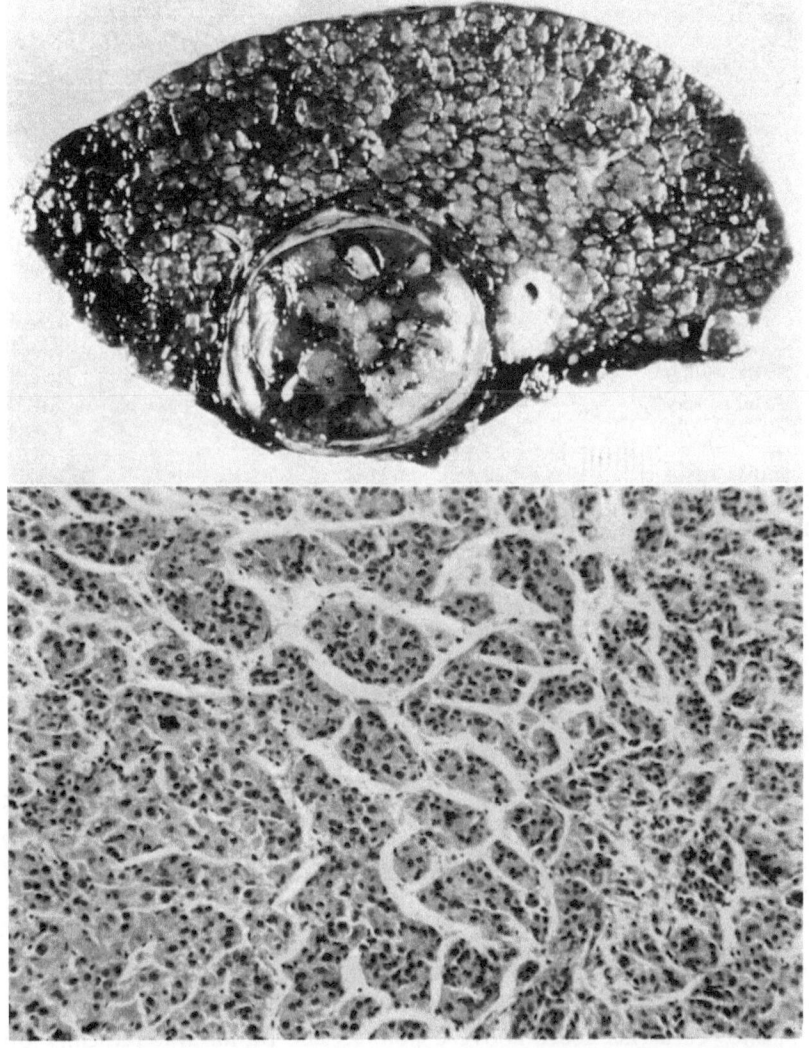

FIG. 1. Macroscopic and microscopic findings of a radically resected case.

TABLE II.  Risk Score in Radically Resected Cases (Sep. 1984)

| No. | Sex | Age | Risk score | Period to diag. | HBsAg | eAg or eAb | AFP (ng/ml) | Location and size | Capsule | Prognosis |
|---|---|---|---|---|---|---|---|---|---|---|
| 1 | M | 60 | 8.0 | 2 Y | + | both (−) | 105 | r. 3.5 cm | + | 48 M lived |
| 2 | F | 50 | 6.9 | 4 | + | eAb | — | r. 3.5 cm | + | 48 M lived |
| 3 | M | 62 | 6.4 | 2 | − | | 130 | r. 4.0 cm | + | 42 M died |
| 4 | M | 69 | 7.0 | 2 | + | eAg | 1124 | r. {2.5 cm / 1.2 cm} | + | 38 M lived |
| 5 | M | 62 | 8.3 | 3 | + | eAg | 121 | r. 2.5 cm | − | 37 M lived |
| 6 | F | 55 | 6.9 | 2 | + | eAb | 712 | r. 2 cm | − | 30 M died |
| 7 | M | 48 | 4.2 | 3 | − | | — | r. 3 cm | + | 19 M lived |
| 8 | M | 62 | 7.0 | 2 | − | | 724 | r. {2 cm / 0.7 cm} | + | 14 M died |
| 9 | M | 42 | 7.0 | 2 | + | eAg | 799 | r. 2 cm | − | 15 M lived |
| 10 | M | 28 | 6.9 | 2 | + | eAb | 151 | r. 1.6 cm | − | 13 M lived |
| 11 | M | 56 | 7.4 | 3 | + | both (−) | — | r. {2.5 cm / 1.2 cm} | − | 10 M lived |

TABLE III.  Risk Score for HCC (Super High Risk Group, Sep. 1984)

| No. | Sex | Age | Risk score | HBaAg | AFP (ng/ml) | "SOL" Local. and size | IHA | CT | US | Prognosis | Period to diag. |
|---|---|---|---|---|---|---|---|---|---|---|---|
| 1 | M | 42 | 7.0 | + | 799 | r. 2.0×2.0 cm | + | + | + | Rad. ope. | 2 Y |
| 2 | M | 28 | 6.9 | + | 151 | r. 1.6×1.0 cm | + | + | + | Rad. ope. | 2 |
| 3 | M | 43 | 6.9 | + | 39 | r. 1.4×1.4 cm | − | + | − | Lived | 3 |
| 4 | M | 51 | 9.2 | + | 100, 400 | diffuse | + | + | − | Died | 3 |
| 5 | M | 54 | 5.4 | + | 100 | r. multiple | + | + | − | Lived | 1 |
| 6 | M | 68 | 6.1 | − | 143 | r. multiple | N.D. | + | + | Lived | 3 |
| 7 | M | 76 | 6.1 | − | 129 | r. 1.5×1.5 cm | N.D. | + | + | Lived | 4 |
| 8 | M | 69 | 6.5 | − | 120 | r. 3.5×3.0 cm | N.D. | + | + | Lived | 3 |
| 9 | M | 60 | 6.9 | − | <20 | r. multiple | + | + | + | Lived | 5 |
| 10 | M | 72 | 7.9 | + | <20 | r. multiple | + | + | − | Lived | 2 |
| 11 | M | 63 | 4.4 | − | <20 | — | — | — | — | Died | |
| 12 | M | 46 | 5.8 | + | <20 | — | — | — | — | Died | |
| 13 | M | 40 | 1.5 | − | <20 | — | — | — | — | Died | |
| 14 | F | 69 | 5.7 | − | <20 | — | — | — | — | Died | |
| 15 | F | 53 | 3.0 | − | <20 | — | — | — | — | Died | |

No. 11–15: only LC.  IHA, infusion hepatic angiography.

TABLE IV.  Risk Score in Follow-up Cases (Groups II and III: 57 Cases)

| Risk score | HCC developed cases | Non-developed cases | Developed/ non-developed+developed |
|---|---|---|---|
| ≧6 | 21 | 9 | 21/30 (70.0%) |
| 4~5 | 9 | 12 | 9/21 (42.9%) |
| ≦3 | 1 | 5 | 1/6 (16.7%) |
| Total | 31 | 26 | |

Table III shows the risk score in the 15 follow-up cases in our hospital. Ten of the 15 developed HCC in from 2 to 5 years with a mean interval of 3.0 years. All but one case, No. 5, showed a risk score above 6 points. The tumor was radically operated in case Nos. 1 and 2.

Table IV shows correlation of the risk score with HCC development in the 57 follow-up cases, the 15 in our hospital and the 42 cases in the other two large hospitals. Twenty-one of 30 cases (70%) which had a risk score above 6 points developed HCC with a mean interval of 2.9 years after cirrhosis was diagnosed, although only 9 of 21 cases with risk scores of 4 or 5 points developed this disease. Fourteen of 16 cases (88%) with scores above 7 points developed HCC, while only one out of 6 cases with a score below 3 points did.

## Detection of Early HCC

It is clinically important to detect the association of HCC in cirrhosis as early as possible during the follow-up period (2, 3). However, it is difficult to predict which cases with cirrhosis may have a tendency to associate with HCC. The prognostic significance has been assessed in various diseases by statistical methods, using risk factors or variables (1, 5), but there is no report of a risk score predicting HCC development in LC. In the present study the risk score that we have proposed is simple and easily available and was useful in predicting the higher risk group, i.e., the super high risk group of HCC development in cirrhosis. For example, in a hypothetical case, the total risk score is calculated at the 10 point maximum. The patient is a 63-year-old male. No overt retention of ascites is observed. Serum HBsAg is positive; he has a history of alcohol intake and his uncle suffered from cirrhosis. S-GOT was 80 I.U. and serum AFP level 42 ng/ml. Peritoneoscopic examination revealed a mixed type of cirrhosis. Finally, ICG retention rate at 15 min was 25%.

On the contrary, in the case of a 37-year-old female with overt ascites, the type of cirrhosis is macronodular and there are no other risk factors; her risk score for HCC development is calculated as the 0 point minimum.

Table V demonstrates our strategy to detect early HCC, especially operable cases, based on the risk score. For the group having a risk score above 6 points in the top column, the super high risk group, stress is put on the follow-up intervals and methodologies, for example, the measurements of serum AFP level every two months, US every two or three months, and both angio-CT and infusion hepatic angiography (IHA) once a year.

TABLE V. Screening Methods for Detection of HCC

| | Group | AFP | US | CT | IHA |
|---|---|---|---|---|---|
| I | Risk score ≥6 | 1/2 M | 1/2–3 M | 1/Y (Angio-CT) | 1/Y |
| II | Risk score 4–5 | 1/2 M | 1/3 M | 1/Y | AFP ↑ or "SOL" ⊕ |
| III | Risk score ≤3 | 1/2 M | 1/3–4 M | 1/Y | AFP ↑ or "SOL" ⊕ |

## CONCLUSION

From the above described results, it is suggested that the prediction of HCC development in liver cirrhosis may be highly feasible, using the scores for 10 readily available factors that we have proposed.

## REFERENCES

1.  Hammermeister, K. E., Derouen, T. A., Dodge, H. T., and Zia, M. Prognostic and predictive value of exertional hypotension in suspected coronary heart disease. *Am. J. Cardiol.*, **51**, 1261–1266 (1983).
2.  Kobayashi, K., Kumagai, M., Kameda, S., Sugimoto, T., Suzuki, K., Nishimura, K., Kato, Y., Sugioka, G., and Hattori, N. Hepatoma development during long-term follow-up period of liver cirrhosis. *Acta Hepato-Gastroenterol.*, **25**, 344–349 (1978).
3.  Kobayashi, K., Sugimoto, T., Makino, H., Kumagai, M., Unoura, M., Tanaka, N., Kato, Y., and Hattori, N. Screening methods for early detection of hepatocellular carcinoma. *Hepatology* (1985), in press.
4.  Miyazi, T. Association of hepatocellular carcinoma with cirrhosis among autopsy cases in Japan during 14 years from 1958 to 1971. *GANN Monogr. Cancer Res.*, **18**, 129–149 (1976).
5.  Pike, M. C., Krailo, M. D., Henderson, B. E., Casagrande, J. T., and Hoel, D. G. Hormonal risk factors, breast tissue age and the age-incidence of breast cancer. *Nature*, **303**, 767–770 (1983).

# EARLY DIAGNOSIS OF PANCREATIC CANCER: FEASIBLE OR WORTHWHILE?

A. R. Moossa and Daniel M. Cohen

*Department of Surgery, University of California*[*1] *and*
*Department of Surgery, University of Illinois*[*2]

Our preliminary data and subsequent experience confirm our previous contention that the tests which are currently available can diagnose resectable cancer of the head of the pancreas in a symptomatic population. The most useful diagnostic tests are ultrasonography, computed tomography, endoscopic retrograde cholangiography, and cytology. About 1/3 of all diagnosed pancreatic cancers are resectable. About 1/3 of the resectable pancreatic (1/9 of the total number) are early. Early diagnosis of cancer of the body and tail of the pancreas cannot be achieved in a symptomatic population.

Either of the two currently popular procedures (Whipple operation or total pancreatectomy) can be performed with an acceptable operative mortality. The mean duration of survival is increasing when compared to previous reported experience. The long-term survival is still low because of delay in diagnosis leading to a high attrition rate from metastatic disease in the first 3 years after operation. Deaths occurring after 4 years are usually from unrelated disorders.

This review is based on our personal experience with diagnosis and surgical treatment of pancreatic cancer over the period 1970 to 1980 inclusive and on our evaluation of the current literature. We have attempted to answer three inter-related questions. 1) Is there delay in diagnosing pancreatic cancer? 2) Is diagnosis of early pancreatic cancer feasible? 3) Does resection of an early cancer prolong life?

## The Diagnosis of Early Pancreatic Cancer

To achieve this objective, the patient must present early with symptoms which are often vague and nonspecific. The physician must have a high index of suspicion that the symptoms are of pancreatic origin especially in the presence of a normal physical examination, normal hematologic and biochemical values, and normal contrast studies of the gastrointestinal tract. The diagnosis then will rest on the application of appropriate diagnostic tests and their relative sensitivity / specificity, predictive values, diagnostic accuracy, and technical failure rate in the particular institution.

Since any diagnostic program for pancreatic cancer can only involve a symptomatic population with a high clinical probability of pancreatic disease, multiple clinical subgroups will emerge when the eventual diagnoses are known. Thus, some patients will

---

[*1] San Diego, California 92103, U.S.A.

[*2] Chicago, Illinois 60612, U.S.A.

have no pancreatic disease, others will have chronic pancreatitis or nonresectable pancreatic cancer, while a minority will have a resectable pancreatic cancer.

Between July 1974 and January 1980, we evaluated prospectively 238 patients suspected, on clinical grounds, of potentially harboring a pancreatic cancer (12, 14, 15, 27). In order to qualify for this study, they had to be over 35 years old with an estimated life expectancy of more than 3 years. Their general health had to be adequate for extensive investigations and exploratory laparotomy. Pregnant women were excluded. The selected patients underwent the following investigations before a decision was made about laparotomy: 1) ultrasonography; 2) computed tomography; 3) radionuclide scan following injection of $^{75}$Se-selenomethionine. Longitudinal multiplane emission tomography was employed in the latter part of the study. Over the past 3 years, $^{11}$C-tryptophan has been substituted in place of selenomethionine; 4) duodenal drainage studies for pancreatic function tests and for cytologic examination of the juice collected after administration of secretin; 5) endoscopic retrograde cholangiopancreatography (ERCP) with cytology on the aspirated pancreatic juice; 6) celiac and superior mesenteric angiography; and 7) assay of various tumor markers in sera and plasma from systemic blood and, in patients undergoing laparotomy, from portal venous blood.

One hundred and ninety-one (80%) of the 238 patients underwent laparotomy. The eventual diagnoses were: pancreatic cancer—102 patients (43%); other cancers (including ampullary, duodenal, lower common bile duct, and islet cell)—33 patients (14%); chronic pancreatitis—39 patients (16%); other benign disorders with a normal pancreas—64 patients (27%). These data form the basis of our previous reports (12, 14, 15) that ultrasonography, computed tomography and ERCP with cytology are the best current methods of detecting pancreatic cancer with an individual diagnostic accuracy ranging from 85 to 95%. Pancreatic function tests, radionuclide scans with selenomethionine, assays of various tumor markers and angiography are not helpful in the diagnosis of pancreatic cancer since their diagnostic accuracy is below 75%. However, angiography may demonstrate major arterial and/or venous encasement which is usually a sign of unresectability. It also delineates variations in the foregut arterial vasculature and helps the surgeon in the planning of a major pancreatic resection. When ERCP fails technically, duodenal drainage is employed to obtain material for cytologic examination. The role of radionuclide scan, using $^{11}$C-tryptophan and the tomographic approach, remains uncertain.

Thirty-nine (38%) of the 102 pancreatic cancers were resectable. Thirty-eight were located in the head of the pancreas and the remaining one was located in the body and tail of the gland. Analysis of the relative sensitivities of the tests for the 39 resectable pancreatic cancers and the 63 unresectable ones shows that ultrasonography and ERCP with cytology are especially useful in diagnosing resectable tumors (12, 15).

In spite of the unusually high resectability rate in this population of patients with pancreatic cancer, delay in diagnosis from the onset of symptoms has been very conspicuous: the mean duration of symptoms was 4 months (range 2 to 18 months); the mean duration of jaundice was 5 weeks (range 3 weeks to 3 months); 40% of the pancreatic cancer patients had diabetes mellitus diagnosed within 2 years before presenting with the cancer; and 10% of the pancreatic cancer patients underwent a cholecystectomy within 2 years of presentation with the cancer. Factors responsible for the delay in diagnosis can be attributed to both the patient and his physician. The patient often tolerates vague, nonspecific, intermittent symptoms without reporting to a physician. The physician often relies on negative physical findings and takes reassurance in normal routine investigations such as contrast studies of the gastrointestinal and biliary tract.

Whether a tumor is "early" or not depends on the definition of "early" and this can only be determined by the pathologist after the tumor has been totally resected. We have arbitrarily defined an "early" pancreatic cancer as one that satisfies the following criteria: 1) tumor size not exceeding 2 cm in diameter; 2) no histological evidence of capsular invasion; 3) no histologic evidence of node involvement; and 4) the absence of distant metastases at laparotomy (15). Eleven of the 39 resected cancers satisfied these criteria and they were all located in the head of the gland.

## Does Resection of a Pancreatic Cancer Prolong Life?

Intense debate still persists among surgeons concerning the best operative procedure for patients with both resectable and unresectable pancreatic cancer. A proper evaluation of published series is difficult because of their retrospective nature, the lack of randomization, and inadequate histologic diagnosis and staging. Allocation to treatment groups has, quite rightly, been based on the age and fitness of the patient, on the extent of the disease and on the surgeon's personal preference. The small number of patients with early lesions that are included in the reported series makes any comprehensive data analysis impossible. The number of surgeons involved and their expertise or experience are virtually never mentioned.

Crile advocated, on the basis of his own experience during the period 1938–1966, bypass procedures over a pancreatoduodenectomy for carcinoma of the head of the pancreas. He concluded that the morbidity and mortality associated with pancreatic biopsy and radical surgery was offset by the remote possibility of cure. He added that the average patient lived longer and more comfortably following a bypass operation. We consider that analysis of the data from 1938–1966 is not valid in the modern clinical context. For patients operated upon between 1953–1966, the mean survival for bypass procedures was 12 months compared to 8.5 months following radical pancreatoduodenectomy. The number of patients in that group is small and the better mean survival in the bypass group leads us to question the types of carcinomas involved, considering Crile's reluctance to biopsy pancreatic lesions (3).

Shapiro found no statistically significant difference in the mean survival between patients who had a bypass procedure and those who underwent pancreatoduodenectomy (22). Since 66% of those patients who had bypass procedures did not have a histologic diagnosis established at laparotomy, we consider such a comparison spurious. In other reports, where histologic data on patients was obtained at laparotomy and the disease was apparently localized, the mean survival of bypassed patients was reduced when compared to resection (1, 5, 8, 13, 25). However, since about 50% of resected specimens have demonstrable extrapancreatic disease microscopically, understaging at the time of laparotomy is a frequent occurrence. Both the Brooks and Hermreck studies did not demonstrate an improved mean survival for resection over bypass procedures when metastases to regional lymph nodes were encountered (1, 8).

Our own early experience has been that the mean survival following resection was 23 months compared to less than 6 months for bypass operations. In those patients who underwent biopsy alone, the mean survival was 2.5 months. By pooling the data from major reports between 1964 and 1978, we found the mean survival following bypass surgery was 4.3 months compared to 16.5 months for resections of all types. Although the 5-year survival rate with resection remains discouragingly low (0–18%), no patient with histologically confirmed pancreatic cancer had survived 5 years after bypass alone (13).

We believe that the uncertainty of tissue diagnosis has been a frequent concomitant of "conservative" procedures. Pancreatic masses can be biopsied relatively safely with a low morbidity. Transduodenal biopsy using the Travenol Tru-Cut needle or fine needle aspiration for cytologic examination is recommended for lesions in the head of the pancreas. Once the diagnosis of pancreatic cancer has been established, a thorough examination of the peripancreatic tissues must be carried out to determine whether the disease is localized. From available data, we would conclude that only those with localized disease can potentially benefit from resection.

Surgeons once insisted on obtaining histologic proof of cancer before resecting a localized mass in the head of the pancreas. The smallest tumors (and probably those most amenable to cure by resection) may prove difficult to diagnose with any needle biopsy technique because of sampling error (7). Persistent efforts to biopsy a small mass in the head of the pancreas is unwarranted. Our decision to resect such lesions without a tissue diagnosis is based upon other factors, such as the overall clinical picture, the preoperative evaluation, and the intraoperative findings. The possibility of and the rationale for performing a pancreatoduodenal resection without a positive biopsy for cancer is always discussed in detail with the patient and his or her relatives prior to operation. Proper informed consent must be obtained to avoid medicolegal problems (16).

## What Type of Resection Should Be Undertaken in Patients Who Have Pancreatic Cancer?

Sommers and associates reported hyperplasia in the ducts of 41% of 141 cases of pancreatic carcinoma. In four cases, papillary hyperplasia, carcinoma *in situ*, and invasive cancer were identified in the same specimen, suggesting a transition from one to the other. Their findings were compared with 150 post-mortem specimens in which only 9% of cases demonstrated ductal hyperplasia (24). During the same year, Ross described two synchronous pancreatic tumors 13 cm apart and made a plea for total pancreatectomy (20). In 1966, Collins *et al.* examined their poor results with pancreatoduodenectomy of the Whipple type. In addition to multifocal tumor growth, they found residual cancer in the cut edge of the specimen. Since tumor often has spread into the peripancreatic tissues and could arise *de novo* in the pancreatic remnant, they suggested that extending the resection to include the remaining pancreas would offer a more realistic hope of improving the results with this disease (2). Lord Smith, while recognizing that tumor recurrence in the body and tail of the remaining pancreas remains a possibility following a Whipple procedure, noted that in his patients who died of recurrent cancer and in whom an autopsy was performed, metastatic disease rather than recurrence in the remaining gland was the prominent feature (23). Later reports also have recognized multifocal tumor growth in pancreatic cancer (10, 11, 18).

There are additional shortcomings associated with pancreatoduodenectomy of the Whipple type. Ross pointed out that viable malignant cells may be present in the obstructed pancreatic duct and following division of the gland, spillage with seeding of malignant cells could be a potential source of local tumor recurrence (20). Much of the morbidity and mortality following the Whipple procedure has been attributed to leakage from the pancreaticojejunal anastomosis; total pancreatectomy would obviate this. Many believe that an adequate cancer operation necessitates total pancreatectomy along with a splenectomy and *en bloc* regional lymphadenectomy (6, 9, 13, 19).

Arguments against total pancreatectomy are based on preserving the residual endocrine and exocrine function of the pancreatic remnant. We found that 34% of patients with pancreatic cancer were diabetic at the time of presentation and another 47% had abnormal glucose tolerance curves (21). There is some disagreement as to how brittle the diabetes actually is following total pancreatectomy. We believe that their diabetic state can be controlled safely and adequately provided that the patient and his or her immediate relatives are properly educated and good support and vigilance are available from the medical and nursing staff. The exocrine capacity of the residual gland following a Whipple procedure is variable. Some patients have little or no steatorrhea and require no enzyme replacement therapy; others have marked steatorrhea and need pancreatic enzymes.

Brooks and Culebras were among the first to report their experience with total pancreatectomy. They demonstrated an overall survival of 23 months and an operative mortality of 12.5%. In a similar group of patients following a Whipple procedure, overall survival was 7.6 months with a mortality of 21%. Patients who did not have positive lymph nodes at the time of resection had a mean survival for total pancreatectomy and Whipple procedures of 40 months and 12.7 months, respectively. The mean survival for total pancreatectomy and Whipple operations was 6.0 months in the group that demonstrated lymph node involvement. These latter figures were comparable to the bypass group (1). While this study was encouraging, suggesting considerable benefit from the *en bloc* resection in localized disease, patients with regional lymph node involvement have gained nothing from the more extensive procedure. Ihse *et al.* have recorded a 21% 5-year survival following total pancreatectomy with an overall operative mortality of 12% (10). However, their results are not comparable because a minority of their patients had other cancers besides pancreatic carcinoma. The Mayo Clinic has documented their operative experience with pancreatic carcinoma. Their overall operative mortality was 10% and the median survival was 13 months. Their 3- and 5-year survival rates were 9% and 2.3%, respectively (26). They have attributed their poor results, in part, to the high incidence of unsuspected regional lymph node metastases (49%) not detected intraoperatively. They could not demonstrate any difference in the overall mean survival between the Whipple operation and total pancreatectomy. It was concluded that total pancreatectomy did not provide any clear advantage over the Whipple operation in treating cancer of the head of the pancreas (4, 26).

We have examined our own data from a personal series of 64 patients operated on between 1970–1978 for pancreatic cancer. Nineteen patients had a Whipple procedure and 45 patients had a total pancreatectomy. All resectable cancers, except two, were **located in the head of the gland. Since it has been our bias that total pancreatectomy is** a superior operation for this disease, these two groups of patients are not strictly comparable. The Whipple operations were performed between 1970–1976 while the total pancreatecotomies were done from 1972–1978. The operative mortality for both groups was comparable (1 of 19 and 3 of 45) and was approximately 6%. The mean survival was 26.9 (±S.D.) months for the Whipple group and 33.2±23.1 (±S.D.) months for the total pancreatectomy group. The corresponding median survival after the two operations were 20 months and 37 months, respectively. The cumulative 3- and 5-year survivals were 37 and 16% for the Whipple group and 51 and 21% for total pancreatectomy. Eight of the 64 patients have survived 5 years, two following a Whipple operation and six following a total pancreatectomy. Six of the eight patients had "early" pancreatic cancer as defined previously. Four of the "early" cancers were "incidental" and were diagnosed histologically following total pancreatectomy for "chronic pancreatitis." Only three long-term survivors have been identified at the time of writing. Not all the patients died from pancreatic cancer metastases. Many succumbed from diseases such as primary lung cancer and cerebrovascular or cardiovascular catastrophes. These disorders are generally associated with cigarette smoking, which is believed to be a predisposing factor for pancreatic carcinoma. One patient died of an insulin overdose. None of the patients with cancer of the body and tail of the pancreas survived longer than one year. While we did not study the palliation provided by these two operations, we have not been able to demonstrate any clear statistical advantage of total pancreatectomy over Whipple procedure in this retrospective nonrandomized study. However, our clinical impression is that total pancreatectomy is the overall better operation (17).

## REFERENCES

1. Brooks, J. R. and Culebras, J. M. Cancer of the pancreas: palliative operation, Whipple procedure, or total pancreatectomy? *Am. J. Surg.*, **131**, 516 (1976).
2. Collins, J. J., Jr., Craighead, J. E., and Brooks, J. R. Rationale for total pancreatectomy for carcinoma of the pancreatic head. *New Engl. J. Med.*, **274**, 599 (1966).
3. Crile, G., Jr. The advantages of bypass operations over radical pancreatoduodenectomy in the treatment of pancreatic carcinoma. *Surg. Gynecol. Obstet.*, **130**, 1049 (1970).
4. Edis, A. J., Kiernan, P. D., and Taylor, W. F. Attempted curative resection of ductal carcinoma of the pancreas. Review of Mayo Clinic experience 1951–1975. *Mayo Clin. Proc.*, **55**, 531 (1980).
5. Forrest, J. F. and Longmire, W. P., Jr. Carcinoma of the pancreas and periampullary region: a study of 279 patients. *Ann. Surg.*, **189**, 129 (1979).
6. Fortner, J. G., Kim, D. K., Cubilla, A., Turnbull, A., Pahnke, L. D., and Shils, M. E. Regional pancreatectomy: *en bloc* pancreatic, portal vein and lymph node resection. *Ann. Surg.*, **186**, 42 (1977).
7. Hermann, R. E. and Cooperman, A. M. Current concepts in cancer. Cancer of the pancreas. *New Engl. J. Med.*, **301**, 482 (1979).
8. Hermreck, A. S., Thomas, C. Y. IV, and Friesen, S. R. Importance of pathologic staging in the surgical management of adenocarcinoma of the exocrine pancreas. *Am. J. Surg.*, **127**, 653 (1974).
9. Hicks, R. E. and Brooks, J. R. Total pancreatectomy for ductal carcinoma. *Surg. Gynecol. Obstet.*, **133**, 16 (1971).
10. Ihse, I., Lilja, P., Arnesjo, B., and Bengmak, S. Total pancreatectomy for cancer: an appraisal of 65 cases. *Ann. Surg.*, **186**, 675 (1976).
11. Levin, B., ReMine, W. M., Hermann, R. E., Schein, P. S., and Cohn, I., Jr. Panel: cancer of the pancreas. *Am. J. Surg.*, **135**, 185 (1978).
12. Mackie, C. R., Dhorajiwala, J., Blackstone, M. O., Bowie, J., and Moossa, A. R. Value of diagnostic aids in relation to the disease process in pancreatic cancer. *Lancet*, **ii**, 385 (1979).
13. Moossa, A. R., Lewis, M. H., and Mackie, C. R. Surgical treatment of pancreatic cancer. *Mayo Clin. Proc.*, **54**, 468 (1979).
14. Moossa, A. R. and Levin, B. Collaborative studies in the diagnosis of pancreatic cancer. *Semin. Oncol.*, **6**, 298 (1979).

15. Moossa, A. R. and Levin, B. The diagnosis of early pancreatic cancer. *Cancer*, **47**, 1688 (1981).

16. Moossa, A. R. and Altorki, N. Pancreatic biopsy. *Surg. Clin. North Am.*, **63** (6), 1205 (1983).

17. Moossa, A. R., Scott, M. H., and Lavelle-Jones, M. The place of total and extended total pancreatectomy in pancreatic cancer. *World J. Surg.*, **8**, 895 (1984).

18. Pliam, M. B. and ReMine, W. H. Further evaluation of total pancreatectomy. *Arch. Surg.*, **110**, 506 (1975).

19. ReMine, W. H., Priestly, J. T., Judd, E. S., and King, J. N. Total pancreatectomy. *Ann. Surg.*, **172**, 595 (1970).

20. Ross, D. E. Cancer of the pancreas: a plea for total pancreatectomy. *Am. J. Surg.*, **87**, 20 (1954).

21. Schwartz, S. S., Ziedler, A., Moossa, A. R., and Rubenstein, A. H. A prospective study of glucose tolerance, insulin, C-peptide and glucagon responses in patients with pancreatic carcinoma. *Am. J. Dig. Dis.*, **23**, 1107 (1978).

22. Shapiro, T. M. Adenocarcinoma of the pancreas: a statistical analysis of biliary bypass *vs.* Whipple resection in good risk patients. *Ann. Surg.*, **182**, 715 (1975).

23. Smith, R. Progress in the surgical treatment of pancreatic disease. *Am. J. Surg.*, **125**, 143 (1973).

24. Sommers, S. C., Murphy, S. A., and Warren, S. Pancreatic duct hyperplasia and cancer. *Gastroenterology*, **27**, 629 (1954).

25. van Heerden, J. A., Heath, P. M., and Alden, C. R. Biliary bypass for ductal adenocarcinoma of the pancreas. Mayo Clin Experience, 1970–1975. *Mayo Clin. Proc.*, **55**, 537 (1981).

26. van Heerden, J. A., ReMine, W. H., Weiland, L. H., McIlrath, D. C., and Ilstrup, D. M. Total pancreatectomy for ductal adenocarcinoma of the pancreas: Mayo Clinic experience. *Am. J. Surg.*, **142** (3), 308 (1981).

27. Wood, R.A.B., Hall, A. W., Moossa, A. R., Levin, B., and Skinner, D. B. Pancreatic cancer diagnosis: preliminary evaluation of a prospective study. *J. Surg. Res.*, **21**, 113 (1976).

# EARLY DETECTION OF SMALL PANCREATIC CARCINOMA

Itaru Oi

*Institute of Gastroenterology, Tokyo Women's Medical College\**

Sixty-five cases of small pancreatic cancer less than 2 cm in size, detected from 1981 to 1982 in a nationwide survey in Japan, were analyzed. The majority of lesions were clinically found by jaundice. Infiltration to the pancreatic capsule, intrapancreatic common duct, duodenum, or regional lymph nodes was often found. Although resection was done in 90% of the cases, the curative resection rate was only 38%. Clues-to discovery and method of diagnosis of small pancreatic cancer are described.

When we say "early diagnosis of pancreatic cancer," the word "early" would be expected to refer to the detection of pancreatic cancer in a curable stage, but this is far from true in the present situation. In this paper, we discuss only the clinical diagnosis of the small pancreatic carcinoma, because a small tumor has higher resectability and is expected to have a better prognosis. Diagnosis of a small tumor is one step in the detection of what may be a curable tumor. Mucous producing pancreatic cancer, cystadenocarcinoma, and islet cell tumor all behave differently, so our analysis is restricted to a usual ductal cell carcinoma. A small pancreatic carcinoma is defined herein as a tumor with a maximum diameter of 2 cm.

## Small Pancreatic Carcinomas in Japan

A survey by the Pancreatic Cancer Registration Committee of the Japanese Pancreatic Society (PCRC of JPS) (4) stated that there were 65 cases of small pancreatic cancer—which is a tumor with a maximum diameter of 2 cm—out of 2,005 total cases of pancreatic cancer registered from the period 1981–1982, or 3.2%. However, the data included all types of pancreatic cancers.

The resectability is 90% in small pancreatic carcinomas, and that of larger tumors is 25% (Table I). Curable resection, however, is only 38% even in small cancers. This means that half of the small pancreatic cancers are already in an incurable stage at the time of operation, though the value of 38% is extremely high compared with the 6% curable operation rate in larger tumors.

TABLE I. Small Pancreatic Cancer (1981–1982)

| | Cases | Resected | Curable resection | Jaundice |
|---|---|---|---|---|
| Small cancer | 65 | 59 (90%) | 25 (38%) | 25 (38%) |
| All cancer except small | 1,940 | [25%] | 109  (6%) | 434 (22%) |

[ ]: data in 1981. From PCRC of JPS.

\* 10 Kawada-cho, Shinjuku-ku, Tokyo 162, Japan (大井　至).

TABLE II.  Infiltration and Metastasis of Small Pancreatic Cancer (35 Cases, 1981)

| | Infiltration to | | | | | | | Metastasis to | |
|---|---|---|---|---|---|---|---|---|---|
| | Capsule | Retro. | CBD | Duode-num | Portal vein | Mesenteric artery | Perito-neum | Liver | Lymph nodes |
| Small cancer | 15% | 10% | 68% | 33% | 5% | 3% | 3% | 0% | 45% |
| All resected cancer except small (292 cases) | 60% | 47% | 59% | 36% | 47% | 26% | 3% | 5% | 64% |

From PCRC of JPS.

In small pancreatic carcinomas, infiltration to the portal vein or artery system, peritoneal dissemination and hepatic metastasis are very rare, but infiltration to the pancreatic capsule, retroperitoneum, intrapancreatic common bile duct, duodenum, and metastasis to the lymph nodes were found in about 15, 10, 68, 33, and 45% of the cases, respectively (Table II). Most of the small pancreatic cancers were found at the pancreatic head and were determined clinically by jaundice. A tumor of 2 cm in diameter may not be curable when it is located at the thin pancreatic body or tail. Because the cancer infiltrates the pancreatic capsule or retroperitoneum, it is not curable even though it is very small.

## Diagnosis of Small Pancreatic Cancer

Small pancreatic cancer can now be diagnosed by image-diagnoses which include ultrasonography (US) (3), computed tomography (CT) (5), endoscopic pancreatography (EPCG or ERCP) and superselective angiography (7); this latter is used only if pancreatic cancer is suspected. For small pancreatic carcinomas, US or CT is occasionally effective, and EPCG followed by superselective angiography is essential.

Most small pancreatic cancers show an obstruction or obvious stenosis of the main pancreatic duct, which is the same as those in advanced pancreatic cancer. Therefore, EPCG have an essential value in detecting a regional lesion of the pancreas; this may be a small pancreatic cancer, an advanced one or regional pancreatitis. Superselective angiography, which visualizes the intrapancreatic arteries and is used with information gained by EPCG, is essential in the diagnosis of small pancreatic carcinoma. Celiac angiography is not valuable in diagnosis of a small pancreatic cancer, but is useful to evaluate the extension of a larger tumor.

## How to Recognize a Patient

We can now diagnose small pancreatic cancer and determine its position, size, and extension. The problem is, however, how to select patients with this type of carcinoma. Jaundice is an important sign for both doctors and patients; in 25 cases, 38% of small pancreatic cancer sufferers developed jaundice, which is a higher percentage than the 22% with larger tumors.

The examination by which the small pancreatic tumors were firstly found varied (Table III). Percutaneous transhepatic cholangiography (PTC) and EPCG alone showed a higher detection rate of small cancers than larger ones, while US and CT proved more successful in detecting larger tumors.

TABLE III.  Type of Examination Effective for the First Detection

| | Clinical | Upper GI | US | CT | EPCG | PTC | Angio |
|---|---|---|---|---|---|---|---|
| Small cancer | 3% | 5% | 9% | 2% | 26% | 43% | 3% |
| All cancer except small (in 1981) | 6% | 6% | 25% | 12% | 16% | 21% | 3% |

From PCRC of JPS.

Epigastric pain is a main symptom even in small pancreatic cancer, but we cannot be certain that a small pancreatic tumor will develop any special symptoms except jaundice. The tumor-markers, CEA or CA19-9, are one of the potential detection methods (2), but their efficiency has not yet been confirmed for small pancreatic cancer. Hyperamylasemia and an attack of acute pancreatitis would be a clue to determining a small pancreatic cancer. The usefulness of mass survey, however, is not promising from a practical standpoint.

## DISCUSSION

The fear of gastric cancer is common in both doctors and patients in Japan, so that even mild epigastric trouble stimulate an individual to visit a hospital and a doctor will usually check for gastric cancer, even though the probability is not great. On such occasion, US might be utilized to check for pancreatic abnormalities, because US is a very easy examination even though its interpretation requires experience. We do not believe that small pancreatic cancer can be diagnosed only by US; this test is most useful to check for something on the pancreas and a patient would then be sent for further diagnosis. But, we must bear in mind that routine check methods like US cannot exclude the possibility of small pancreatic cancer.

Once a patient is suspected of having pancreatic cancer, almost all pancreatic tumors including small ones can be found and diagnosed by EPCG and superselective angiography. The essential problem is to suspect the patients. Tumor markers would be a possible method, and US is also a valuable procedure for checking something on the pancreas.

Up to now, clinical efforts against cancer have been directed toward earlier diagnosis and complete resection. But recent advances in oncogenesis and immunological techniques have changed this philosophy. We must now build a new symbiotic relationship between human life and cancer—it is no longer a medical problem but a social one.

## REFERENCES

1. Ariyama, J., Shirakabe, H., and Ikenobe, H. The diagnosis of the small resectable pancreatic carcinoma. *Clin. Radiol.*, **28**, 437–444 (1977).
2. Del Villano, B. C., Brennan, S., and Brock, P. Radioimmunometric assay for a monoclonal antibody-defined tumor marker, CA19-9. *Clin. Chem.*, **29**, 549–552 (1983).
3. Lawson, T. L. Sensitivity of pancreatic ultrasonography in the detection of pancreatic disease. *Radiology*, **128**, 733–736 (1978).
4. Pancreatic Cancer Registration Committee of the Japanese Pancreatic Society. Present state of treatment for pancreatic cancer (Japanese). *Tan to Sui*, **4**, 997–1025 (1983).
5. Stanley, R. J., Sagel, S. S., and Levitt, R. G. Computed tomographic evaluation of the pancreas. *Radiology*, **124**, 715–722 (1977).

# LONG-TERM SURVIVAL
# AND COMBINED MODALITY
# BY DIGESTIVE TRACT CANCER

# PRESENT STATUS OF CHEMOTHERAPY OF GASTROINTESTINAL TUMOURS

S. Eckhardt

*Department of Chemotherapy and Medical Oncology,*
*National Institute of Oncology\**

Chemotherapy of gastrointestinal malignancies is of major importance. Esophageal cancer in a multimodality treatment approach is sensitive to cytostatic agents. The role of chemotherapy of gastric cancer is well established; 5-fluorouracil (5-FU), adriamycin, mitomycin-C are active agents in adjuvant therapy and also in advanced disease. Some results can be expected in the treatment of pancreatic cancer with 5-FU, adriamycin, and mitomycin, while liver and gallbladder cancer are only marginally responding to antitumour agents. The chemotherapy of colorectal cancer is resulting in limited success and the value of adjuvant chemotherapy is under evaluation.

Gastrointestinal (GI) tract malignancies are frequent and account for 40–42% of cancer mortality; therefore chemotherapy plays a major role in the management of such patients. Nevertheless, GI tract malignancies are not very sensitive to cytostatic agents, and patients with advanced disease rarely respond to the treatment. It is therefore mandatory to explore the role of chemotherapy as an adjuvant treatment modality associated with surgery. This review enumerates in each major site of GI tract tumour the antitumour activity of cytostatic compounds as single agents and in combination and a critical analysis is made concerning their efficacy in an adjuvant setting.

*Esophageal Cancer*

Single agent activity varies between response rates from 17 to 33%. Adriamycin (ADM), bleomycin (BLM), 5-fluorouracil (5-FU), cisplatin, and the nitrosoureas seem to have well established antitumour effect which, however, is of short duration. These drugs in combination have synergistic action as is demonstrated in Table I.

As can be seen from Table I the response rate is increased. The median response duration, however, does not exceed 10.8 months. It is, therefore, important to combine chemotherapy with radiotherapy and surgery. Despite all multimodality therapy endeavours the median response duration increases only marginally (11.0 months), but the response rate is more frequent (52–62%).

*Gastric Cancer*

Antitumour activity of single agents (5-FU, ftorafur (FTF), mitomycin-C (MMC),

---

* 1525 Budapest, PF21 XII, Rath G Y. U. 7/9, Hungary.

TABLE I.   Esophageal Cancer Polychemotherapy

| Drugs | No. of patients | CR+PR (%) | Author |
|---|---|---|---|
| BLM+ADM | 16 | 19 ⎫ | Kelsen |
| BLM+CDDP | 38 | 19 ⎭ | |
| BLM+CDDP | 12 | 25 | Ogawa |
| BLM+CDDP+MTX | 10 | 50 | Hentek |
| BLM+CDDP+VDS | 53 | 55 | Ogawa |
| BLM+CDDP+ADM | 21 | 33 | Ogawa |
| BLM+VCR+MTX | 22 | 36 | Ogawa |
| 5-FU+MMC+ARA-C | 25 | 28 | Cocconi |
| 5-FU+ADM+BCNU | 35 | 52 | Ogawa |
| 5-FU+ADM+MeCCNU | 10 | 30 | GTSG |
| 5-FU+ADM+MeCCNU+MMC | 27 | 33 | Karlin |
| 5-FU+ADM+MMC | 62 | 42 | Ogawa |
| | 32 | 21 | Halm |
| | 45 | 44 | Beretta |
| | 12 | 25 | GTSG |

BLM, bleomycin; ADM, adriamycin; CDDP, cisplatin; MTX, methotrexate; VDS, vindesine sulfate; VCR, vincristine; ARA-C, cytosine arabinoside; BCNU, 1,3-bis(2-chloroethyl)-1-nitrosourea; 5-FU, 5-fluorouracil; MeCCNU, methyl cyclohexyl nitrosourea; MMC, mitomycin-C; GTSG, Gastrointestinal Tumour Study Group; CR, complete remission; PR, partial remission.

TABLE II.   Effect of Two Drug Combination in Gastric Cancer

| Drugs | No. of patients | CR+PR (%) | Author |
|---|---|---|---|
| 5-FU+BCNU | 34 | 41 ⎫ | |
| 5-FU | 28 | 29 ⎬ | Smith |
| BCNU | 23 | 17 ⎭ | |
| 5-FU+MeCCNU | 30 | 40 ⎫ | Smith |
| MeCCNU | 37 | 8 ⎭ | |
| ADM | 37 | 22 ⎫ | |
| 5-FU+MMC | 53 | 32 ⎬ | Moertel |
| 5-FU+MeCCNU | 49 | 24 ⎭ | |
| 5-FU+MMC | 43 | 14 ⎫ | Buroker |
| 5-FU+MeCCNU | 54 | 9 ⎭ | |
| ADM 40 mg/m² days 1, 22, 43, 64 | 18 | 38.8 | Eckhardt |
| FTF 800 mg/m² days 2–8, 23–29, 44–50, 65–71 | | | |

ADM) varies between 13.3–27.8%. A great number of investigational drugs have been also tested such as hexylcarbamoyl-5-FU, uracil+5-FU, neocarzinostatin aclacinomycin A, 2-nimustine·HCl (ACNU), amsacrin, Baker's antifol, etoposid, and cisplatin. It is, however, too early to judge their value in the chemotherapy of gastric cancer. Two drug combinations are more effective, as can be seen from Table II.

The most important three and four drug combinations are listed in Table III.

In Japan with two drug combinations on 195 patients a response rate of 23.6%, and with three drug combinations on 521 patients a 34.7% response rate was observed. Four drug combinations did not alter the number of responses (33.8%) and toxicity was considerable (3).

Adjuvant chemotherapy of gastric cancer resulted in controversial findings. More recently Kondo (2) was able to demonstrate on 1,670 patients treated postoperatively

TABLE III.  Effect of Three and Four Drug Combinations in Gastric Cancer

| Drugs | No. of patients | CR+PR (%) | Author |
|---|---|---|---|
| 5-FU+MMC+ARA-C | 18 | 17 ⎞ | |
| 5-FU+ADM+MeCCNU | 15 | 47 ⎬ | Gistg |
| ADM | 17 | 24 ⎠ | |
| 5-FU+MeCCNU | 22 | 9 ⎞ | |
| 5-FU+MeCCNU+ADM | 22 | 36 ⎠ | Lacave |
| 5-FU+ADM+MMC | 61 | 43 | Levi |
| | 11 | 55 | McDonald |
| | 62 | 40 | Bitran |
| | 63[a] | 28 | Panettiere |
| 5-FU+ADM+MeCCNU | 22 | 36 | Lacave |
| 5-FU+ADM+BCNU | 35 | 52 | Levi |
| 5-FU+ADM+MeCCNU+MMC | 18 | 11 | Bunn |
| 5-FU+ADM+BCNU+MMC | 16 | 50 | Bernath |

[a] Sequential therapy.

TABLE IV.  Pancreatic Cancer Results of Polychemotherapy

| Drugs | No. of patients | CR+PR (%) | Author |
|---|---|---|---|
| 5-FU+MeCCNU | 140 | 17 ⎞ | Buroker |
| 5-FU+MMC | | 30 ⎠ | |
| 5-FU+ADM+MMC | 23 | 40 | Smith |
| | 15 | 40 | Bitran |
| 5-FU+MMC+Stz | 23 | 43 | Wiggans |
| | 16 | 31 | Abderhalden |
| 5-FU+ADM+BCNU | 10 | 20 | Eckhardt |
| 5-FU+ADM+MMC+MeCCNU | 18 | 33 | Schachter |

Stz, streptozotocin.

with various doses of MMC and FTF that no statistically significant difference could be obtained in the 5-year survival rate. Other observations, however, showed benefit in favour of the treated group. At present, further investigations are needed for the establishment of the value of adjuvant chemotherapy with various dose schedules and different agents.

## Pancreatic Cancer

This malignancy is usually lethal within one year and the 5-year survival of patients is 0–2%. Results of chemotherapy with single agents are poor and their combination is only of a palliative value as is listed in Table IV.

## Primary Liver Cancer

Single agent activity is low and varies between 12 to 32%. Results of combination chemotherapy are no better. The most important data are presented in Table V.

Unfortunately, intraarterial administration of cytostatic agents results only in temporary palliation. The duration of response does not exceed 12 months by either

TABLE V.   Chemotherapy of Primary Liver Cancer

| Drugs | No. of patients | CR+PR (%) | Author |
|---|---|---|---|
| Single agents | | | |
| ADM   75 mg/m² | 41 | 16 | Vogel |
| 60 mg/m² | 44 | 32 | Johnson |
| 60 mg/m² | 36 | 8.3 | ECOG |
| m-AMSA | 23 | 13 | Bukowsky |
| Etoposid | 25 | 12 | Domingo |
| Cisplatin | 15 | 20 | Cheng |
| Neocarzinostatin | 15 | 40 | Sasaki |
| 5-FU   i.v., p.o. | 21 | — | Link |
| p.o. | 48 | — | ECOG |
| Combinations | | | |
| 5-FU+MeCCNU | | | |
| Malaysian | 20 | 20 | Joisky |
| African | 10 | — | Joisky |
| U.S. | 45 | 16 | Joisky |
| 5-FU+ADM | 38 | 3 | Domingo |
| 5-FU+ADM+VM26 | 36 | 44 | Bezwoda |
| 5-FU+AMSA+VM26 | 11 | 36 | Bezwoda |

AMSA, amsacrine; VM26, teniposide.

TABLE VI.   Polychemotherapy of Colorectal Cancer

| Drugs | No. of patients | No. of studies | CR+PR (%) | Med. resp. rate (%) |
|---|---|---|---|---|
| 5-FU+MTX | 133 | 6 | 6–53 | 32.3 |
| 5-FU+MeCCNU | 103 | 1 | 9 | — |
| 5-FU+HU | 85 | 1 | 18 | — |
| 5-FU+ADM+MMC | 28 | 1 | 21 | — |
| 5-FU+CCNU+VCR | 136 | 2 | 11 | 11 |
| 5-FU+CCNU+DTIC | 101 | 1 | 15 | — |
| 5-FU+CCNU+DTIC+VCR | 91 | 1 | 11 | — |
| FTF+ADM | 32 | 1 | 20 | — |

DTIC: dacarbazine.

type of therapy (1). Extrahepatic biliary cancer (bile duct, gall bladder) does not respond to any chemotherapy.

## Colorectal Cancer

Among single agents, fluorinated pyrimidines, ADM, MMC, and the nitrosoureas were found to be active. Polychemotherapy does not yield any better results than mono-therapy as is demonstrated in Table VI.

Adjuvant chemotherapy does not bring any benefit to the patient. A large series of randomised studies failed to prove their efficacy in preventing recurrency or metastases.

In conclusion, results of chemotherapy of GI tract malignancies are not satisfactory. New, more effective and less toxic agents are needed. Adjuvant chemotherapy has to be tested in a large number of patients with various dose schedules and different drugs.

Last but not least, early diagnosis, primary and secondary screening has to be prompted in order to be able to improve the prospects of therapy of GI tract neoplasms.

## REFERENCES

1. Falkson, G., Moertel, C. C., MacIntyre, J. M., Lavin, P., Engstrom, P. F., and Carbone, P. P. The value of cytostatic agents in the treatment of patients with primary liver cancer. *In* "Int. Congr. on Diagnosis and Treatment of Upper GI Tumors," Int. Congr. Ser. 542, pp. 455–459 (1981). Excerpta Medica, Amsterdam-Oxford-Princeton,
2. Kondo, T., Inokuchi, K., Hattori, T., Inoue, K., Taguchi, T., Akiyama, H., Abe, O., Ito, I., Nakajima, T., Muto, T., Kikuchi, K., Kasai, Y., Sugie, S., and Hayasaka A. Multi-hospital randomized study of the adjuvant chemotherapy with Mitomycin-C and futraful for gastric cancer. V. Estimation of five-year survival rate. *Japan. J. Cancer Chemother.*, **9**, 2016–2028 (1982).
3. Ogawa, M. An overview for advanced gastric cancer. *In* "Int. Congr. on Diagnosis and Treatment of Upper GI Tumors," Int. Congr. Ser. 542, pp. 357–366 (1981). Excerpta Medica, Amsterdam-Oxford-Princeton.

# EXPERIENCE WITH COMBINED PREOPERATIVE IRRADIATION AND SURGERY FOR CARCINOMA OF THE ESOPHAGUS

Guo-Jun HUANG, Xian-Zhi GU, Liang-Jun WANG, Wei-Bo YIN,
Ru-Gang ZHANG, Li-Jun ZHANG, Da-Wei ZHANG, Zhi-Xian ZHANG,
Zhen-Yan WANG, and Kan YANG

*Cancer Institute and Hospital, Chinese
Academy of Medical Sciences\**

Clinical studies with combined preoperative irradiation and surgery in the treatment of esophageal carcinoma were carried out in 408 selective cases (1959–1976) and in 83 randomized cases (1977–1982). In the first study the majority of patients had tumors of poor or questionable resectability as evaluated on clinical grounds before treatment. The primary tumors were located in the upper and middle thirds of the esophagus in 79.9% and were yp-TNM Stages III and IV in 81.6%. In this study the resectability rate was 81.9%, operative mortality 3.4%, and the 5-, 10-, and 15-year survival rates were 33.8, 23.0, and 17.9%, respectively. During the same time period 736 patients with tumors more distally located and of better resectability were treated by surgery alone. In 43.8% of these the tumor was located in the lower third of the esophagus. The operative mortality was 3.0% and the 5-year survival rate 29.8% in this group of cases.

In the randomized study 160 patients, all with midthoracic esophageal carcinoma averaging 5.2 cm in length, were eligible for analysis in which 83 were treated by combined therapy and 77 by surgery alone. The results, both early and late, as obtained by combined therapy *versus* those by surgery alone are as follows: resectability rate, 95.2 *vs.* 89.6%; 30 day resection mortality rate, 3.8 *vs.* 4.3%; incidence of intrathoracic anastomotic leakage, 0 *vs.* 1.7%; and 5-year survival rate, 45.5 *vs.* 25.0%.

Based on the results obtained in the two clinical studies, it was concluded that adjuvant preoperative irradiation with the dosage and methods recommended has the merits of enhancing surgical results for carcinoma of the esophagus.

Results of treatment of carcinoma of the esophagus by either radiotherapy or surgery alone have not been satisfactory. Reports on the combination of preoperative irradiation and surgery to improve treatment results for this malignancy have appeared more and more frequently in the literature during the past three decades. In 1960, Cliffton and associates (2) and Nakayama and associates (6) reported independently the experiences with this combined treatment modality in 20 cases and 114 cases respectively, both coming to the same conclusion that preoperative irradiation inhibited tumor growth and raised the resectability rate. Huang and associates (4) in 1962 reported 113 cases of eso-

---

\* Beijing, People's Republic of China.

phageal carcinoma treated by this combined therapy with a resectability rate of 70.8%, which was 12.4% higher than that of 161 cases treated at the same time period by surgery alone.

Subsequent reports by Akakura and associates in 1963 (1), Nakayama and associates in 1974 (7), Marks and associates in 1976 (5), Huang and associates in 1981 (3), and Parker and associates in 1982 (8) all indicated favorable results of this combined therapy in terms of resectability and long-term survivals over those of either radiotherapy or surgery alone.

The rationales for the combination of preoperative irradiation and surgery in the treatment of carcinoma of the esophagus are now widely accepted. Iatrogenic cancer cell dissemination at operation with the possibility of metastasis and cancer implantation is a well-known phenomenon. The cancer cells most easily disseminated during surgery are those in areas with a richer vascular supply which are better oxygenated and much more radiosensitive. Preoperative irradiation sterilizes or devitalizes the cancer cells in these areas and thus eliminates or reduces the risk of dissemination. The two common causes of surgical failure, namely, microscopic deposits of tumor cells not accessible to surgical resection and tumor invasion into adjacent vital organs, can be best controlled by preoperative irradiation. On the other hand, a bulky primary tumor usually contains large numbers of poorly oxygenated tumor cells which are radioresistant and are often the source of recurrence after radiotherapy. Surgery subsequent to radiotherapy removes the primary tumor not only eliminating the source of local recurrence but also rendering a high dose of preoperative irradiation unnecessary. It is therefore logical that by taking advantage of both preoperative irradiation and surgery in combination, better results can be achieved than by either modality alone.

The purpose of this report is to present our experiences with planned combined therapy of preoperative irradiation and surgery in two clinical studies, the first consisting of 408 selective patients treated from 1959 through 1976, preliminarily reported in 1981 (3), and the second of 83 randomized patients from 1977 through 1982. Patients who were primarily treated by radiotherapy but were later operated upon because of severe dysphagia, uncontrolled carcinoma, recurrences, etc., were excluded from both studies.

### Experience with 408 Selective Patients (1959–1976)

The majority of patients selected for combined therapy in this study were those with carcinoma of the midthoracic esophagus of poor or questionable resectability as evaluated on clinical grounds. As a result, there was a predominance of middle third esophageal carcinoma and Stage III cases in this series.

During the same time period most patients with carcinomas more distally located and of better resectability as assessed clinically were treated by surgery alone.

The tumor was located in the upper and middle thirds of the esophagus in 79.9% of the cases treated by combined therapy, as compared to 56.2% of those treated by surgery alone. This was the major difference of statistical significance between the two groups ($p < 0.001$).

### 1. yp-TNM staging

Postradiosurgical histopathologic staging of the 408 cases of the combined therapy group showed that 71.8% were Stage III with extra-esophageal invasion and/or regional lymph node involvement and 9.8% Stage IV with distant metastases. In only 2 cases, or 0.5%, was the carcinoma confined to only the mucosa and submucosa without lymph node involvement (Stage I). In 73 (17.9%), the lesion involved the muscular layer but was confined to the esophagus with no evidence of lymph node metastasis (Stage II). It is to be noted that preoperative irradiation probably had the effect of understaging some of the cases in which preexisting metastatic regional lymph nodes became cancer free after irradiation.

## 2. Preoperative irradiation

In this study telecobalt was used in 310 (76.0%) and betatron in 69 (16.9%), cases. In the remaining 29 (7.1%) cases either a combination of the two sources or deep X-ray, occasionally in the early years, was used.

Most patients were irradiated 5 days a week with a tumor dose of 200 rads each time through an anterior and a posterior portal of $6 \times 12$ or $6 \times 15$ cm depending on the tumor size. Table I shows the distribution of preoperative irradiation dosage in this study. In the later part of this study, the dosage was practically standardized to 4,000 rads in each case.

The interval between completion of preoperative irradiation and surgery ranged from 2–3 weeks, averaging 17.4 days.

## 3. Surgical intervention

Resection of the esophageal carcinoma was usually done through the left thoracotomy approach, in the vast majority of cases using the stomach as a substitute. The overall resectability rate was 81.9% for the 408 cases (Table II). It can be seen that carcinoma of the middle third of the esophagus has the lowest resectability rate of all three esophageal segments, as is true with surgery of esophageal carcinoma without preoperative irradiation.

At operation the lungs and pleura were found to be little affected by the preoperative irradiation. In some instances only mild congestion and edema were seen over the ir-

TABLE I. Distribution of Preoperative Irradiation Dosage in 408 Cases

| Dosage (rads) | Cases | % |
|---|---|---|
| <2,000 | 102 | 25.0 |
| 2,100–3,000 | 78 | 19.1 |
| 3,100–4,000 | 197 | 48.3 |
| >4,000 | 31 | 7.6 |
| Total | 408 | 100.0 |

TABLE II. Resectability Rates of 408 Cases Treated by Combined Therapy

| Site of lesion | Operations | Resections | Resectability (%) |
|---|---|---|---|
| Upper third | 27 | 26 | 96.3 |
| Middle third | 299 | 238 | 79.6 |
| Lower third | 82 | 70 | 85.4 |
| Entire group | 408 | 334 | 81.9 |

radiated mediastinal pleura. Usually there was some retraction and slight loss of luster of the mediastinal pleura overlying the tumor. Shrinkage of the tumor mass was noted in most cases. This was especially marked in cases in which the postradiation esophagram showed good radiation effects. Usually the tumor was much smaller in size and was softer in consistency with ill-defined boundaries. In some cases the tumor had so much regressed that it was indeed difficult for the exploring finger to exactly locate the lesion.

There were 15 deaths within 30 days of operation in the combined therapy group, an operative mortality of 3.4%. Thirteen of these deaths occurred in 334 resections, a resection mortality of 3.9%. In the 736 cases treated by surgery alone during the same time period, there were 22 (3.0%) operative deaths.

In the combined therapy group there were 15 postoperative anastomotic leaks among 334 resections, an incidence of 4.5%. The incidence of leakage of cervical anastomoses was 21% (5/24) and that of intrathoracic anastomoses was 3.2% (10/310).

There were 27 leaks among the 736 cases treated by surgery alone, an incidence of 3.7%.

It is estimated that in about 1/3 of the cases treated by combined therapy the esophagus at the site of anastomosis was within the field of preoperative irradiation.

## 4. Pathologic studies

Changes in esophageal cancer brought about by preoperative irradiation were classified as mild, moderate, or marked. Mild reaction included those with only minimal postradiation changes. The tumor showed no remarkable decrease in size and its cells showed slight regression with keratinization and necrosis. Moderate reaction included those with appreciable decrease in tumor size. Microscopically, there was more marked regression of the tumor cells which, however, were still distinguishable in discrete masses. Marked reaction included those in which the tumor mass had completely or nearly completely regressed. Microscopic findings consisted of either total disappearance of tumor cells or only remnants of degenerated tumor tissue.

Of the 279 cases who had complete records, mild reaction was found in 87 (31.2%), moderate reaction in 90 (32.2%), and marked reaction in 102 (36.6%).

Pathologic studies of the resected specimens showed evidence of extra-esophageal tumor invasion in 70.1% (230/328), and positive lymph node metastases in 34.3% (114/332), of the cases.

Of the 736 cases treated by surgery alone, lymph node involvement was found in 321, or 43.6%.

## 5. Long-term survivals

The 1- to 15-year survival rates of all 334 cases with tumor resection in the combined therapy group are shown in Table III. The 5-year survival of 33.8% in this group was, however, not statistically different from that of 29.8% (205/689) of those treated during the same time period by surgery alone ($\chi^2 = 1.75$, $p > 0.05$).

TABLE III.   Survival Rates of 334 Cases in the Combined Therapy Group

| Years postoperative | 1 | 3 | 5 | 10 | 15 |
|---|---|---|---|---|---|
| Resections | 334 | 334 | 334 | 248 | 179 |
| Survivors | 260 | 135 | 113 | 57 | 32 |
| Survival rate (%) | 77.8 | 40.4 | 33.8 | 23.0 | 17.9 |

It is to be noted that the criteria of case selection used in this study placed the group treated with combined therapy in an unfavorable prognostic situation as compared to the group treated by surgery alone. Taking this into consideration the gratifying results obtained in the group treated by combined therapy may well be attributed to the merits of adjuvant preoperative irradiation in improving the results of surgery.

### Experience with 83 Randomized Patients (1977–1982)

To further verify the value of preoperative irradiation a randomization study was started in 1977 of patients under 65 years of age with midthoracic esophageal carcinoma not exceeding 7 cm in length by roentgenography. In this study a linear accelerator was used almost exclusively with a total dose of 4,000 rads divided into 20 fractions over 4 weeks. Irradiation was given through an anterior and a posterior portal each 6 cm in width covering the whole mediastinum from the upper border of the manubrium sterni above to the xyphoid process below.

This study included 160 patients eligible for analysis up to the end of June, 1982. The combined therapy group consisted of 83 patients, 58 males and 25 females, with ages ranging from 28 to 65, and averaging 52.5 years. In the group treated by surgery alone there were 77 patients, 53 males and 24 females, with ages ranging from 34 to 65, and averaging 52.4 years. The average lengths of tumors in both groups were the same, 5.2cm.

The results, both early and late, as obtained by combined therapy *versus* those by surgery alone, are shown in Table IV, which further illustrates the advantages of the former over the latter treatment modality.

The fact that the incidence of anastomotic leak in the combined therapy group is no higher than that of the group treated by surgery alone serves to indicate that preoperative irradiation at the recommended dosage has no untoward effects on esophageal healing, as in about half of the cases of the combined therapy group the esophageal anastomotic site was within the field of preoperative irradiation. The absence of residual tumor at the esophageal stump in the cases treated by combined therapy, as compared to the incidence of 2.9% in the group treated by surgery alone, may also help to indicate the good tumoricidal effect of the preoperative irradiation.

The lower incidence of lymph node metastasis in the combined therapy groups of both the selective patients and the randomized patients can best be explained on the

TABLE IV.   Randomized Study of Combined Preoperative Irradiation and Surgery *versus* Surgery Alone for Carcinoma of the Esophagus:   Analysis of 160 Cases, 1977–1982

|  | Preop. irrad. and surgery | Surgery alone |
|---|---|---|
| Resectability rate (%) | 95.2 (79/83) | 89.6 (69/77) |
| 30-Day resection mortality (%) | 3.8 (3/79) | 4.3 (3/69) |
| Incidence of anastomotic leakage (%) | | |
|     Intrathoracic | 0 (0/77) | 1.7 (1/60) |
|     Cervical | 50 (1/2) | 44 (4/9) |
| Incidence of LN metastasis (%) | 21.5 (17/79) | 30.4 (21/69) |
| Residual tumor at esophageal stump (%) | 0 (0/79) | 2.9 (2/69) |
| 5-Year survival rate (%) | 45.5 (10/22) | 25.0 (4/16) |

Preop. irrad., preoperative irradiation; LN, lymph node.

basis of sterilization of cancer cells and inhibition of new lymph node metastasis by the preoperative irradiation.

## CONCLUSIONS

Based on our experiences with the two clinical studies, it may be concluded that the combination of preoperative irradiation and surgery in the treatment of carcinoma of the esophagus has merits in promoting resectability and long-term survivals over single modality by surgery alone. With the recommended dosage and rest intervals preoperative irradiation has no untoward effects on the healing power of the irradiated esophagus, and poses no additional difficulty on surgical manipulation. This combined modality is especially indicated in cases of midthoracic esophageal carcinoma with border-line resectability.

## REFERENCES

1. Akakura, I., Nakamura, Y., and Kakegawa, T. The combined treatment for carcinoma of the esophagus with the radical resection and the preoperative irradiation. *Keio. J. Med.*, **14**, 145 (1963).
2. Cliffton, E. E., Goodner, J. T., and Bronstein, E. Preoperative irradiation for cancer of the esophagus. *Cancer*, **13**, 37–45 (1960).
3. Huang, G. J., Gu, X. Z., Zhang, R. G., Zhang, L. J., Zhang, D. W., Miao, Y. J., Wang L. J., Lin, H., Wang, G. Q., and Xiao, Q. L. Combined preoperative irradiation and surgery in esophageal carcinoma: report of 408 cases. *Chin. Med. J.*, **94**, 73–76 (1981).
4. Huang, G. J., Wang, J. Z., Liu, Y. Q., and Wu, H. "Preoperative Irradiation for Carcinoma of the Esophagus: A Report on the Experiences in 113 Cases," pp. 1–10 (1962). Shanghai Sci. Tech. Publ., Shanghai.
5. Marks, R. D., Jr., Scruggs, H. J., and Wallace, K. M. Preoperative radiation therapy for carcinoma of the esophagus. *Cancer*, **38**, 84–89 (1976).
6. Nakayama, K. Combined surgical radiative treatment for cancerous lesions with particular interest in prevention of recurrence (Theoretical basis for the preoperative irradiation in the treatment of esophageal cancer), Proc. Japan, Cancer Assoc., 19th Gen. Meet, pp. 214–215 (1960).
7. Nakayama, K. and Kinoshita, Y. Surgical treatment combined with preoperative concentrated irradiation. *J. Am. Med. Assoc.*, **227**, 178–181 (1974).
8. Parker, E. F., Gregorie, H. B., Prioleau, W. H., Jr., Marks, R. D., and Barjles, D. M. Carcinoma of the esophagus: observation of 40 years. *Ann. Surg.*, **195**, 618–622 (1982).

# LONG-TERM SURVIVAL IN CASES OF EARLY AND ADVANCED GASTRIC CANCER IN CHILE

Roberto BURMEISTER

*Hospital Paula Jaraquemada**

The 5-year survival rate of 176 cases treated with curative resection at the Paula Jaraquemada Hospital during the years 1975–1979 was analyzed. In the resected group of patients the rate was 45.45% (80/176) and it was 27.49% (80/291) in relation to the laparotomied cases. No 5-year survival rate was available in patients submitted to palliative procedures. The prognosis is better when the lower portions of the stomach are involved than the upper stomach or when the lesion involves the entire organ. Ten to twenty percent of the patients with early gastric cancer had lymph node involvement, and those with serosa involvement presented more than 80% of lymph node dissemination up to the tertiary lymph node group in some cases. In the cases with no lymph node involvement there is an excellent prognosis which worsens as the cancer advances from lymph node level I to III. In relation to the depth of invasion and clinical stages, the 5-year survival rate was optimal in early lesions and stage I. There was a good survival rate in Borrmann types I, II, and V which at the same time showed a lower percentage of lymph node involvement. Concerning the survival rate according to histological type, the worst prognosis is observed in the mucocellular type. The surgical procedures are one of the most important factors influencing the prognosis. Survival is lower after total gastrectomy (37.25%) than with subtotal resection (63.51%).

The incidence of gastric cancer in Chile is very high and the overall death rate from this type of cancer is 32 per 100,000 individuals, according to Medina's 1970 statistics (4). Gastric cancer accounts for about 1/3 of all deaths caused by malignant tumors in Chile.

In recent years there has been marked progress in the surgery of gastric cancer, especially in Japan, with an improvement in long-term survival (3, 6). We began following the Japanese guidelines from the end of 1975.

In 1978 a diagnostic center for early gastric cancer detection was created at the Paula Jaraquemada Hospital, supported by the Japanese Government through its Japanese International Cooperative Agency. This paper represents our long-term results on a group of patients operated between 1975–1979 in this hospital.

## Number of Gastric Cancer Cases

During the 1975–1979 period, 291 patients with gastric cancer were operated. Among these, 176 underwent curative resection (60.48%) and 12 died within the operative

---

\* Santa Losa 1234, Santiago, Chile.

period (6.81%). All the resected cases were followed up and the removed specimens, which include 4,989 lymph nodes, were systematically examined. The guidelines established by "the general rules for gastric cancer study in surgery and pathology" were followed in this study (2).

## Factors Affecting Long-term Survival

Curative resection was carried out on 176 patients (60.48%) and the 5-year survival rate of this group was 45.45% (80/176); but from the total number of laparotomied cases those who survived represent only 27.49% (80/291). None of the patients with palliative resection survived 5 years. The survival rate was analyzed in relation to the site of the tumor, lymph node involvement, depth of invasion, clinical stage, gross classification, histological type, and surgical procedure.

### 1. Site of the tumor
The stomach was divided into the three parts suggested by the Japanese Society for Gastric Cancer. The 5-year survival rate is better in the lower portions than in the upper stomach or when the lesion involves the entire organ (Table I).

### 2. Lymph node involvement
The lymph node involvement constitutes one of the most important aspects to be considered in the prognosis of gastric cancer. In the 176 resected cases 4,989 lymph nodes were dissected with an average of 28.34 per patient. Of the total dissections, 17.54% showed an involvement. The incidence of lymph node metastases in resected patients was 70.46%, 10% in the mucosal type and over 80% in the transmural lesions (s2–s3), with dissemination to the tertiary group in some cases (Table II).

TABLE I.  Five-Year Survival Rate and Site of Cancer

| Tumor location | No. of cases | No. of survivors | Percentage |
|---|---|---|---|
| A | 57 | 34 | 59.64 |
| M | 46 | 25 | 54.34 |
| C | 47 | 16 | 34.04 |
| AMC-MC | 26 | 5 | 19.23 |
| Total | 176 | 80 | 45.45 |

TABLE II.  Relationship of Incidence of Lymph Node Metastases to Histologic Level of Invasion of Gastric Cancer in 176 Patients Who Underwent Curative Gastric Resection

| Level of invasion | No. of patients | Lymph node metastases (%) | | | |
|---|---|---|---|---|---|
| | | None | Primary | Secondary | Tertiary |
| Intramucosal | 10 | 90.00 | 5.00 | 5.00 | — |
| Summucosal | 13 | 84.61 | 7.69 | 7.69 | — |
| Intermediate | 20 | 45.00 | 50.00 | 5.00 | — |
| Subserosa | 11 | 36.36 | 45.55 | 18.18 | — |
| Transmural (s2) | 88 | 14.77 | 44.31 | 25.00 | 15.90 |
| To neighboring organs (s3) | 34 | 17.64 | 14.70 | 50.00 | 17.64 |
| Total | 176 | 29.54 | 34.09 | 25.00 | 11.36 |

TABLE III. Lymph Node Metastases and 5-Year Survival Rate

| Lymph node level | No. of cases | No. of survivors | Percentage |
|---|---|---|---|
| N 0 | 50 | 40 | 80.00 |
| N 1 | 62 | 29 | 46.77 |
| N 2 | 44 | 9 | 20.45 |
| N 3 | 20 | 2 | 10.00 |
| Total | 176 | 80 | 45.45 |

TABLE IV. Depth of Invasion of Gastric Cancer and 5-Year Survival Rate

| Depth of invasion | No. of cases | No. of survivors | Percentage |
|---|---|---|---|
| m | 10 | 9 | 90.00 |
| sm | 13 | 11 | 84.61 |
| mp | 20 | 15 | 75.00 |
| ss | 11 | 6 | 54.54 |
| s2 | 88 | 34 | 38.63 |
| s3 | 34 | 5 | 14.70 |
| Total | 176 | 80 | 45.45 |

TABLE V. Five-Year Survival Rate according to Clinical Stage

| Clinical stage | No. of cases | No. of survivors | Percentage |
|---|---|---|---|
| I | 30 | 27 | 90.00 |
| II | 19 | 15 | 78.94 |
| III | 79 | 32 | 40.50 |
| IV | 48 | 6 | 12.50 |
| Total | 176 | 80 | 45.45 |

In the cases with no lymph node involvement there is an excellent prognosis which worsens as the cancer advances from lymph node level I to level III (Table III).

### 3. Depth of invasion to gastric wall

This factor has a great influence on the prognosis of gastric cancer. In the lesions localized at the mucosa and submucosa the survival rate reaches nearly 90%. With serosal involvement the prognosis worsens (Table IV). Within the 176 resected cases there were 23 early cancers (13.08%), 20 intermediate (11.36%), and 133 with serosal involvement (75.56%).

### 4. Classification by stages

The prognosis in stage I is near 90%. The survival rate decreases as the disease advances (Table V).

### 5. Macroscopic classification

The survival rate was studied in relation to the macroscopic type of Borrmann's classification and according to the lymph node involvement in 153 advanced cases. Without lymph node involvement the survival rate was 56.25% and with lymph node

TABLE VI.   Five-Year Survival Rate according to Gross Classification and Incidence
of Lymph Node Metastases in 153 Advanced Gastric Cancer Cases

| 5-Year survivors (%) | Borrmann's classification of gastric cancer | | | | | |
|---|---|---|---|---|---|---|
| | I | II | III | IV | V | Total |
| Without node metastases | 66.66 | 66.66 | 28.57 | 50.00 | 60.00 | 56.25 |
| With node metastases | 50.00 | 40.90 | 28.57 | 21.42 | 33.33 | 33.38 |
| Total | 54.54 | 47.45 | 28.57 | 25.00 | 45.45 | 38.56 |
| | (8/11) | (28/59) | (16/56) | (4/16) | (5/11) | (59/153) |
| Incidence of lymph node | 72.00 | 74.57 | 87.00 | 87.50 | 54.54 | 79.08 |
| metastases | (8/11) | (44/59) | (49/56) | (14/16) | (6/11) | (121/153) |

TABLE VII.   Five-Year Survival Rate according to Histological Type of Gastric Cancer

| Histological type | No. of cases | No. of survivors | Percentage |
|---|---|---|---|
| Moderately to well differentiated | 50 | 27 | 54.00 |
| Poorly to undifferentiated | 32 | 17 | 53.12 |
| Signet-ring cell and gelatinous | 76 | 26 | 34.21 |
| Papillotubular | 18 | 10 | 55.55 |
| Total | 176 | 80 | 45.45 |

TABLE VIII.   Gastric Cancer Combined Resection Splenectomy
and or Distal Hemipancreatectomy

| Surgical procedures | No. of cases | With combined resection | Percentage |
|---|---|---|---|
| Total gastrectomy | 96 (10) | 86 (8) | 89.58 |
| Subtotal gastrectomy | 74 (2) | 7 (1) | 9.45 |
| Upper subtotal gastrectomy | 6 (0) | 4 (0) | 66.66 |
| Total | 176 (12) | 97 (9) | 55.11 |

( ): surg. death.

TABLE IX.   Five-Year Survival Rate according to Surgical Procedure

| Surgical procedures | No. of cases | No. of survivors | Percentage |
|---|---|---|---|
| Total gastrectomy | 96 | 30 | 31.25 |
| Subtotal gastrectomy | 74 | 47 | 63.51 |
| Upper subtotal gastrectomy | 6 | 3 | 50.00 |
| Total | 176 | 80 | 45.45 |

involvement it was only 33.38%. There was a good survival rate in types I, II, and V
that, at the same time, showed a lower percentage of lymph node involvement (Table VI).

### 6.   Histological type

Concerning the survival rate according to the histological type the worst prognosis
was observed in the mucocellular type (Table VII).

### 7.   Surgical procedure

In 54.54% of the cases total gastrectomy was performed, in 42.04% subtotal gastrectomy and in 3.40% upper subtotal gastrectomy. A combined resection was carried
out in 55% of the cases and in 89% of the total gastrectomies (Table VIII).

The surgical procedure is one of the most important factors influencing the prognosis. The survival is lower with total gastrectomy than with subtotal resection (Table IX).

## CONCLUSIONS

Our results have shown the enormous improvement experienced in the last 10 years, mainly due to better diagnostic methods and progress in surgical techniques. The new and better diagnostic procedures now available to our medical doctors in Japan have allowed us earlier gastric cancer detection, and today this represents 13.08% of our resected cases. Before 1972 this type of cancer was ignored in Chile. Using mass-survey methods even advanced lesions are detected sooner and thus are more amenable to resection. At present our percentage of resectability has reached 60.4% (Table X).

Routine lymph node dissection seems to be another of the important factors controlling long-term survival. Analysis of our material reveals a high percentage of lymph node involvement in advanced cancer; early lesions also show 10 to 20% lymph node involvement, in some cases up to the secondary lymph node group. For this reason we believe that it is necessary to perform a lymph node dissection to the secondary lymph node level in early lesions and to the tertiary lymph node group in advanced cases.

It is most important to choose the appropriate surgical procedure according to the site and extent of the tumor. In contrast to the opinions expressed in most scientific papers, total gastrectomy is the method we used most frequently in the cases reported on here (54.54%). This is due to the high percentage of advanced lesions localized in the middle and upper part of the stomach. In more than 80% of these cases a combined resection was added.

In spite of the extensive surgical procedures employed we have been able to lower the surgical mortality to 6.8% (Table XI).

TABLE X. Percentage of Operability and Resectability Cases in Chile

| Author (year) | | Resectability | Laparotomy | Not operated |
|---|---|---|---|---|
| Flores | (1964) | 39.0 | 50.0 | 11.0 |
| Flores | (1969) | 40.0 | 49.7 | 10.3 |
| Biel | (1960) | 48.0 | 13.0 | 39.0 |
| Vergara | (1961) | 39.0 | 39.0 | 22.0 |
| Otaiza | (1969) | 26.0 | 46.0 | 28.0 |
| De la Fuente | (1969) | 44.0 | 41.0 | 15.0 |
| Csendes | (1974) | 29.0 | 32.6 | 28.0 |
| Burmeister | (1984) | 60.4 | 33.6 | 6.0 |

TABLE XI. Operative Mortality in Chile

| Author (year) | | Resection | Laparotomy | Not operated |
|---|---|---|---|---|
| Flores | (1964) | 20.7 | 9.0 | 12.5 |
| Flores | (1969) | 16.4 | 16.4 | 10.5 |
| Biel | (1960) | 27.0 | 13.1 | 8.0 |
| Vergara | (1961) | 26.0 | 21.0 | — |
| Otaiza | (1969) | 25.0 | 12.7 | 18.4 |
| De la Fuente | (1969) | 12.7 | 6.2 | — |
| Csendes | (1974) | 19.0 | 9.3 | 20.0 |
| Burmeister | (1984) | 6.8 | — | — |

TABLE XII.    Comparative 5-Year Survival Rate in Chile

| Author (year) | % resected patients | % laparotomied patients |
|---|---|---|
| Otaiza       (1969) | 10.00 | 5.00 |
| Burmeister  (1984) | 45.45 | 27.49 |

Our survival rate of 45.45% constitutes a great improvement in our results compared with those published in 1969 by Otaiza *et al.* (5) (Table XII).

Our results, nevertheless, are still below the Japanese average, mainly due to a lower percentage of early gastric cancer and a higher operative mortality. However, we believe that the most important aspect to recognize is that using the same criteria and methods it is possible to reproduce anywhere the incredible results of the Japanese experience in gastric cancer.

## REFERENCES

1.  Csendes, A. Gastric cancer in Chile: a cooperative interhospital study. I. Clinical findings and diagnosis. II. Treatment and postoperative evolution. *Japan. J. Clin. Oncol.*, **5**(1), 41–52 (1975).
2.  Japanese Research Society for Gastric Cancer. The general rules for the gastric cancer study in surgery and pathology. *Japan. J. Surg.* **3**(1), 61–71. (1973).
3.  Kajitani, T. and Takagi, K. Cancer of the stomach at Cancer Institute Hospital, Tokyo. *Gann Monogr. Cancer Res.*, **22**, 77–87 (1979).
4.  Medina, E. Epidemiologia del cáncer gástrico en Chile. *Rev. Med. Chile*, **98**, 477–482 (1970).
5.  Otaiza, E., Lopetegui, G., and Csendes, A. Operabilidad y resecabilidad del cáncer gástrico. *Rev. Med. Valpo.*, **22**, 228–231 (1969).
6.  Soga, J. The role of lymphadenectomy in curative surgery for gastric cancer. *World J. Surg.*, **3**, 701–708 (1979).

# ADJUVANT CHEMOTHERAPY AFTER SURGERY FOR GASTRIC CANCER IN JAPAN

Takao Hattori, Minoru Niimoto, and Tetsuya Toge

*Department of Surgery, Research Institute for Nuclear Medicine and Biology, Hiroshima University**

The current of surgical adjuvant chemotherapy for gastric cancer in Japan can be divided into three periods. The first period was the 15 years from 1960 to 1975, in which the problem was to make clear the efficacy of mitomycin-C (MMC) as an adjunct to surgery, and the protocol was limited to (gastrectomy only) *vs.* (gastrectomy+MMC). The second period was the 5 years from 1975 to 1980, in which the focus of the study was confined to the use of long-term maintenance therapy with oral Tegafur (TG) after induction therapy with MMC. The protocol was (gastrectomy+ MMC) *vs.* (gastrectomy+MMC+oral TG). The third period was the years after 1980, in which the interest of the surgeons was directed to the combined use of immunopotentiators. The protocol was (gastrectomy+ MMC+oral TG) *vs.* (gastrectomy+MMC+oral TG+immunopotentiator). The representative studies in each period were reviewed. The 5-year survival rate in patients with stage III gastric cancer was increased from about 30–35% in the first period to about 55–60% in the third period.

Although surgical treatment for gastric cancer has improved the end results of gastrectomy in the last decade by extending operative procedures, the 5-year survival rate of curatively resected gastric cancer patients in Japan is still not satisfactory. Most Japanese surgeons now believe that the operative procedures cannot be further improved

TABLE I. History of Adjuvant Chemoimmunotherapy for Gastric Cancer in Japan

| 1960 The first period 1975 | The second period 1980 | The third period |
|---|---|---|
| Operation | Op.+MMC | Op.+MMC+Oral Tegafur |
| *vs.* | *vs.* | *vs.* |
| Op.+MMC | Op.+MMC+Oral Tegafur | Op.+MMC+Oral Tegafur+ Immunopotentiator |
| Study at National Cancer Center Hospital (*1–3*) (1963–65) | Cooperative Study Group of Surgical Adjuvant Chemotherapy for Gastric Cancer (SACGC) (Chairman: Prof. Inokuchi) | Cooperative Study Group organized by Japan Foundation for Multidisciplinary Treatment for Cancer (1981–83) |
| Cooperative Study Group cond. by Prof. Imanaga (*5*) (1965–68) | The first study (*6, 7*) (1975–76) The second study (*9*) (1977–79) | |
| | Pilot study at Hiroshima University Hospital (*4*) (1973–77) | |

Number in parenthesis indicates the references.

* Kasumi 1-2-3, Minami-ku, Hiroshima 734, Japan (服部孝雄, 新本 稔, 峠 哲哉).

to better the outcome of gastrectomized patients; they also believe that adjuvant chemotherapy after gastrectomy is absolutely necessary.

The development of surgical adjuvant chemotherapy for gastric cancer in Japan can be divided into three periods (Table I). In this paper the representative studies in each period are reviewed. The stages of gastric cancer are based on the directions for gastric cancer studies adopted by the Japanese Research Society for Gastric Cancer (8).

### The First Period (1960–1975)

The first period was the 15 years from 1960 to 1975, in which the problem was to make clear the efficacy of mitomycin-C (MMC) as an adjunct to surgery, and the protocol was limited to (gastrectomy only) vs. (gastrectomy+MMC). Various methods of administration of all possible sorts of MMC, including preoperative or postoperative, were examined by many surgeons. The study at the National Cancer Center Hospital was performed from 1963 to 1965. To our knowledge, it was the first prospective randomized controlled trial of adjuvant chemotherapy for gastric cancer in Japan done in one institution. The results were reported in 1964 (1), 1966 (2), and 1972 (3). Patients were randomly allocated into four groups.

Group 1 (278 cases): gastrectomy only (control group).

Group 2 (97 cases): gastrectomy plus large-dose MMC plus allogeneic bone marrow transplantation. Twenty mg (0.4 mg/kg) of MMC was given on the day of operation and an additional 10 mg (0.2 mg/kg) the next day. In patients more than 65 years old and with body weight of less than 40 kg, the additional 10 mg was not administered. Similar dose limitations were applied if total gastrectomy was associated with partial resection of the pancreas, liver or colon. On the 4th or 5th postoperative day, allogeneic bone marrow transplantation was performed.

Group 3 (146 cases): gastrectomy plus large-dose MMC. MMC was given in the same manner as in group 2.

Group 4 (100 cases): gastrectomy plus postoperative intermittent MMC. A dose of 10 mg (0.2 mg/kg) of MMC was given twice a week starting on the day of operation for a total of 40 mg (0.8 mg/kg).

The end results showed no differences in survival between groups in stages I or II. However, in stage III the 5-year survival rates were 13.7% in group 1, 36.4% in group 2, 30.3% in group 3, and 14.8% in group 4. Thus, groups 2 and 3 showed an excellent response as compared with the control group. As only one institution was involved in this trial, the number of cases in each group was relatively small and the differences were not significant.

A cooperative study on this same subject conducted by Prof. H. Imanaga is very famous in Japan (5). This cooperative group did their first study from 1965 to 1966. Patients were randomly allocated into two groups, a control group (gastrectomy only) and a MMC group. In the MMC group, MMC was administered in doses of 0.08 mg/kg ten times twice a week for a total of 0.8 mg/kg within 4 weeks after gastrectomy. Two hundred thirty-six cases in the control group and 269 cases in the MMC group were subjected to analysis. The MMC group showed superior results with a relative survival rate of 13.1% at 5 years and 8.7% at 10 years. The best results were observed in stage II cases with 37.5% at 5 years and 31.9% at 10 years in the relative survival rate.

Thus, many forms of induction chemotherapy using MMC after gastrectomy for gastric cancer were prescribed in this first period and all trials demonstrated the superiority of the MMC group as compared with the control.

### The Second Period (1975–1980)

In this period, the focus was directed on long-term maintenance chemotherapy combined with MMC induction therapy after gastrectomy. In this case, chemotherapy was performed on an out-patient basis. Therefore, a drug with sufficient anticancer activity and low toxicity on the one hand and convenient to use for out-patients on the other had to be selected. Fortunately, earlier trials in Japan with oral administration of Tegafur (TG) had provided a very compatible administration over a long period and had provoked a good response rate in recurrent or inoperable gastric cancer. The representative protocol was (gastrectomy+MMC) vs. (gastrectomy+MMC+oral TG). To promote the multihospital trial, the Cooperative Study Group of Surgical Adjuvant Chemotherapy for Gastric Cancer (SACGC) involving 297 major hospitals throughout Japan was established under the leadership of Prof. K. Inokuchi in 1975.

The first study of SACGC was performed in the period 1975 to 1976 and the results were reported in 1981 (6) and 1984 (7). Two protocols were offered and each hospital chose one of them. After gastrectomy patients, were assigned at random to either group A or B. In protocol I, patients received MMC intermittently with a single dose of 0.08 mg/kg twice a week for a total of 8–10 times. In protocol II, they received large-dose MMC, 20 mg on the day of gastrectomy and an additional 10 mg the next day in the same manner as in the study by the National Cancer Center Hospital described above. In group A of each protocol no further treatment was given and in group B TG was administered at a daily dose of 600–800 mg orally for 3 months.

Two thousand eight hundred and thirty-four patients were registered in total and 2,064 were analyzed (770 patients were excluded). The results are indicated in Table II. Generally, the survival rates of group B (MMC+TG) were superior to group A (MMC only) and a significant difference was observed in stage III patients and in n(+), ps(+) patients (positive lymphnode metastasis and positive serosal invasion) in protocol II. The advantage of TG addition was somewhat more pronounced in protocol II than in protocol I.

The second study of SACGC was performed from 1977 to 1979 and the preliminary results were reported in 1981 (9). In this study the patients were allocated at random into three groups after surgery. In group A, MMC was administered in the fashion of (20+ 10) mg as in protocol II of the first study. In group C, only TG was administered orally with a daily dose of 600 mg starting from 2 weeks after the operation for one year. In group C, both MMC and TG were given in the same manner as in group A or C. Four thousand seven hundred and seven patients were registered in total and 3,033 cases were analyzed for efficacy. As shown in Table III, group B had the best 5-year survival rates with significant differences in stage III patients and n(+), ps(+) patients compared to group A.

### The Third Period (after 1980)

The third period was the years after 1980, in which the interest of the surgeons was directed to the combined use of immunopotentiators. The protocol was (gastrectomy+

TABLE II.  Actuarial 5-Year Survival Rate of the First Study by the Cooperative
Study Group of Surgical Adjuvant Chemotherapy for Gastric Cancer
in Japan (SACGC) (1975–76)

|  | Protocol I | | Protocol II | |
|---|---|---|---|---|
|  | Group A | Group B | Group A | Group B |
| No. of cases | 698 | 550 | 416 | 400 |
| All cases | 46.7% | 47.3% | 54.6% | 56.1% |
| Stage I | 85.6 | 88.8 | 89.9 | 83.9 |
| Stage II | 52.4 | 65.8 | 66.0 | 71.5 |
| Stage III | 36.3 | 32.4 | 39.7 | 48.6* |
| Stage IV | 17.7 | 14.6 | 13.4 | 19.7 |
| n(−)ps(−)[a] | 84.4 | 89.5 | 89.1 | 82.2 |
| n(+)ps(−) | 49.7 | 61.8 | 66.2 | 67.6 |
| n(−)ps(+) | 54.7 | 46.1 | 61.7 | 70.4 |
| n(+)ps(+) | 22.8 | 21.3 | 27.1 | 35.8* |

[a] n, histological lymph node metastasis; ps, histological serosal invasion.
* Significant difference from group A ($p < 0.05$) by Generalized Wilcoxon test.

TABLE III.  Actuarial 5-Year Survival Rate of the Second Study by the Cooperative
Study Group of Surgical Adjuvant Chemotherapy for Gastric Cancer
in Japan (SACGC) (1977–79)

|  | Group A | Group B | Group C |
|---|---|---|---|
| No. of cases | 982 | 1,004 | 1,047 |
| All cases | 52.3% | 54.3% | 52.8% |
| Stage I | 87.9 | 89.9 | 90.1 |
| Stage II | 66.8 | 62.7 | 62.1 |
| Stage III | 33.8 | 50.9* | 40.6* |
| Stage IV | 13.1 | 18.0 | 17.8 |
| n(−)ps(−) | 86.4 | 88.1 | 89.6 |
| n(+)ps(−) | 63.7 | 64.9 | 62.7 |
| n(−)ps(+) | 57.5 | 59.4 | 56.3 |
| n(+)ps(+) | 23.5 | 32.7** | 25.4 |

See footnote for Table II.
*  Significant difference from group A ($p < 0.05$).
** Significant difference from groups A and C ($p < 0.05$).

MMC+oral TG) vs. (gastrectomy+MMC+oral TG+immunopotentiator). The curtain
raiser for this period was the pilot study performed at Hiroshima University from 1973
to 1977 (4). The protocol of this study is presented in Fig. 1. As an immunopotentiator,
PSK, extract from the mycelium of *Coriolus versicolor* (Fr.) Quel, was used. Patients
were allocated at random into three groups after MMC induction therapy: group P
(PSK only), group F (TG only), and group P+F (PSK+TG). The results are indicated
in Table IV. The best results were obtained in group P+F without significant differences compared to groups P and F. Some immunological parameters were investigated
during pre- and post-operative periods and an increased reaction to the PPD skin test
and lymphocyte blastogenesis induced by phytohemagglutinin (PHA) or pork weed

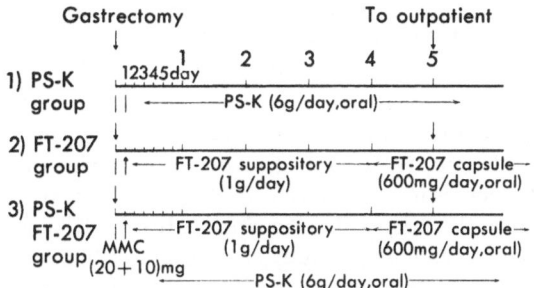

FIG. 1. Treatment schedules of adjuvant immunochemotherapy at Hiroshima University (1973–79) (the case of early cancer excluded).

TABLE IV. Actuarial 5-Year Survival Rate of Adjuvant Immunochemotherapy Performed at Hiroshima University (1973–79)

|  | Group P | Group F | Group P+F |
|---|---|---|---|
| No. of cases | 49 | 28 | 33 |
| All cases | 38.8% | 32.1% | 54.6% |
| Stage I+II | 91.0 | 40.0 | 81.8 |
| Stage III | 38.1 | 54.6 | 60.0 |
| Stage IV | 5.9 | 8.3 | 25.0 |
| n(−)ps(−) | 100.0 | 50.0 | 100.0 |
| n(+)ps(−) | 71.4 | 0 | 50.0 |
| n(−)ps(+) | 50.0 | 100.0 | 75.0 |
| n(+)ps(+) | 7.7 | 27.3 | 47.4* |

See footnote for Table II.
* Significant difference from group P ($p < 0.05$).

mitrogen (PWM) was found remarkable in group P+F at 3 and 6 months after gastrectomy compared to group P or F. Based on this pilot study a multicenter trial on the same problem was undertaken in 1980 by the Japanese Foundation for Multidisciplinary Treatment of Cancer.

Thus, adjuvant chemotherapy after surgery for gastric cancer in Japan has made solid progress in the past 20 years and the 5-year survival rate in patients with stage III gastric cancer has risen from 30–35% in the first period to about 55–60% in the third period.

## REFERENCES

1. Hattori, T., Ito, I., and Hirata, K. Large-dose administration of mitomycin-C during gastrectomy followed by homologous bone marrow transplantation. *Gann*, **55**, 211–224 (1964).
2. Hattori, T., Ito, I., Hirata, K., Iizuka, T., and Abe, K. Results of combined treatment in patients with cancer of the stomach; palliative gastrectomy, large-dose mitomycin-C and bone marrow transplantation. *Gann*, **57**, 441–451 (1966).
3. Hattori, T., Mori, A., Hirata, K., and Ito, I. Five year survival rate of gastric cancer pa-

tients treated with gastrectomy, large-dose mitomycin-C and/or allogeneic bone marrow transplantation. *Gann*, **63**, 517–522 (1972).

4. Hattori, T., Niimonto, M., Koh, T., Nakano, A., Oride, M., Takiyama, W., and Nishimawari, K. Postoperative long-term adjuvant immunochemotherapy with mitomycin-C, PSK and FT-207 in gastric cancer patients. *Japan. J. Surg.*, **9**, 110–117 (1979).

5. Imanaga, H. and Nakazato, H. Results of surgery for gastric cancer and effect of adjuvant mitomycin-C on cancer recurrence. *World J. Surg.*, **1**, 213–221 (1977).

6. Inokuchi, K., Hattori, T., Inoue, K., Kondo, T., Ito, I., Kikuchi, K., Sugie, S., and Taguchi, T. Multihospital randomized study on adjuvant chemotherapy with mitomycin-C ± futraful for gastric cancer; five year survival rate. 12th Int. Congr. Chemother., Florence (1981).

7. Inokuchi, K., Hattori, T., Taguchi, T., Abe, O., and Ogawa, N. Postoperative adjuvant chemotherapy for gastric cancer. Analysis of data on 1805 patients followed for 5 years. *Cancer*, **53**, 2393–2397 (1984).

8. Japanese Research Society for Gastric Cancer. The general rule for gastric cancer study in surgery and pathology in Japan. *Japan. J. Surg.*, **11**, 127–145 (1981).

9. Kasai, Y., Inokuchi, K., Hattori, T., Inoue, K., Taguchi, T., Kondo, T., Akiyama, H., Abe, O., Ito, I., Nakajima, T., Muto, T., Kikuchi, K., Sugie, S., and Hayasaka, A. Multihospital randomized study on adjuvant chemotherapy with mitomycin-C and futraful for gastric cancer; the second study. I. Two year survival rate. 18th Gen. Meet. Japan Soc. Gastroenterol. Surg., Hiroshima (1981).

# CONSIDERATIONS ON RECENT IMPROVEMENTS IN FIVE-YEAR SURVIVAL RATE OF COLON AND RECTAL CANCER

Takashi Takahashi and Tamaki Kajitani

*Department of Surgery, Cancer Institute Hospital\**

Five-year survival rates after radical surgery for colon and rectal cancer were calculated every decade since 1950. Definite improvements were seen for Dukes B and Dukes C cancer of both colon and rectum.

The technical improvements in regional lymph node dissection and identification of the separating plane around the tumor-bearing intestine which are supposed responsible for such improvements in 5-year survival rate, are discussed. The principles of procedure in a standard operation for advanced colon and rectal cancer are demonstrated, and the importance of anatomical understanding of regional lymphatic flow and fascial architecture of retroperitoneal space is stressed.

Colo-rectal cancer surgery has shown no sign of improvement for the last few decades. (*4–6*).

Thus it may be assumed that known surgical procedures have reached their maximum potential for improving the end-result of this cancer treatment. Despite this assumption, we have attempted since 1950 to develop a more radical operative procedure for colon and rectal cancer.

Determination of an anatomically reasonable method of the dissection of regional lymph nodes and of the separating plane around a tumor have been considered the most important aspects of research. Although the advances have not been rapid in the conduct of this research, they have been constant, and we can see a definite improvement in the results of surgical treatment of these types of cancer.

We will cite the impact of this improvement on the 5-year survival rate, and will then discuss details of our improved surgical procedures.

*Materials and 5-Year Survival Rates*

From 1950 through 1978, 341 colonic cancer cases and 701 rectal cancer cases were operated on with the intent to cure at the Cancer Institute Hospital in Tokyo. A few cases among them were given some kind of chemotherapy or radiotherapy, but in very small doses. (Rectosigmoid cancer is defined as a type of rectal cancer in this report.)

The 5-year survival rates which are calculated every decade, showed a definite improvement for colonic cancer for the 1970's: from 65.6% for the 1960's to 79.6% for the 1970's. There was also a clear improvement in cases of rectal cancer: from 56.7% for the 1960's to 73.2% for the 1970's (Table I).

---

\* Kami-Ikebukuro 1-37-1, Toshima-ku, Tokyo 170, Japan (高橋　孝, 梶谷　鐶).

TABLE I.   Five-Year Survival Rates of Colon and Rectal Cancer
Cases Operated on for Cure

|            | 1950–1959          | 1960–1969          | 1970–1978            |
|------------|--------------------|--------------------|----------------------|
| Colon ca.  | 77.8% (42/54)      | 65.6% (63/96)      | 79.6% (152/191)      |
| Rectal ca. | 54.8% (102/186)    | 56.7% (127/224)    | 73.2% (213/291)      |

TABLE II.   Five-Year Survival Rates on Each Stage of Dukes' Classification

|            |         | 1950–1959        | 1960–1969        | 1970–1978        |
|------------|---------|------------------|------------------|------------------|
| Colon ca.  | Dukes A | 100% (10/10)     | 100% (11/11)     | 93.9% (31/33)    |
|            | B       | 77.8 (21/27)     | 70.8 (34/48)     | 84.7 (78/92)     |
|            | C       | 64.7 (11/17)     | 48.6 (18/37)     | 65.1 (43/66)     |
| Rectal ca. | Dukes A | 100% (5/5)       | 100% (9/9)       | 88.0% (37/42)    |
|            | B       | 72.5 (63/87)     | 74.8 (77/103)    | 82.3 (98/119)    |
|            | C       | 36.2 (34/94)     | 36.6 (41/112)    | 65.5 (78/130)    |

These differences in survival rates between the two decades are significant when statistically analyzed, though further analysis is required to determine the particular aspect of the surgical procedures which has led to such improvement.

The survival rates are calculated separately for each stage of Dukes' classification. In both colonic and rectal cancer there is a remarkable improvement in the Dukes B and C cases. The 5-year survival rate for Dukes B colonic cancer was 70.8% for the 1960's and 84.7% for the 1970's; for Dukes C, it was respectively 48.6 and 65.1%. For Dukes B rectal cancer, the survival rate was 74.8% for the 1960's and 82.3% for the 1970's, and for Dukes C, it was 36.8 and 65.5% (Table II). The improvement in Dukes B cases indicates a better anatomical understanding of the fascial arrangement around the tumor, and a definite advance in the idea of separating the plane around the tumor-bearing intestine. Improvement in the 5-year survival rate for Dukes C cases suggests progress in the topographical understanding of the regional lymphatic way from the intestine, and technical improvement in the nodal dissection of the tumor.

## The Principles of Surgery for Colo-Rectal Cancer, and Operative Technique

There follows a summary of the results of our clinical research program to determine the reasonable separating plane and to clarify the idea of complete dissection of the regional lymph nodes. This was done by dissecting several cadavers, operative specimens, and analyzing operative materials.

### 1.   The principle of separation

The principle of separation is to insure the removal of the tissues surrounding the tumor widely enough to get a safety margin. There are two different dimensions: these are how to define the separating line of the intestine distal to and proximal to the tumor, and how to maintain a sufficient safety margin at the top of the depth of invasion of the tumor. In either right or left side colonic cancer, the fusion fascia of Toldt (7) just beneath the colon and mesocolon must be separated from the retroperitoneal space. Sometimes, in advanced cancer, the sub-peritoneal fascia which is deeper in the retroperitoneal space is separated. In right side colonic cancer, full exposure of the duodenum and the head

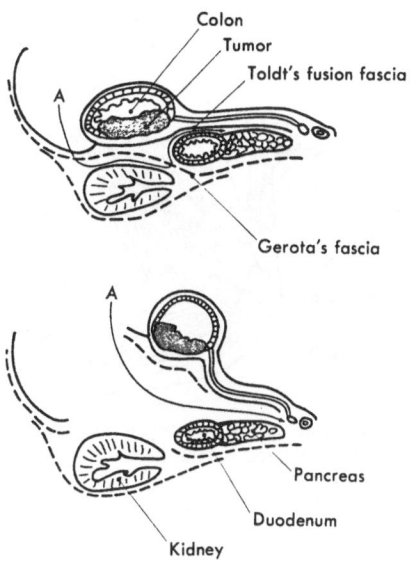

FIG. 1.  Transverse section at the site of hepatic flexure of the colon.

Line A indicates the separating plane in an advanced colonic cancer. Toldt's fusion fascia and a part of Gerota's fascia are separated, exposing the 2nd part of the duodenum and pancreas.

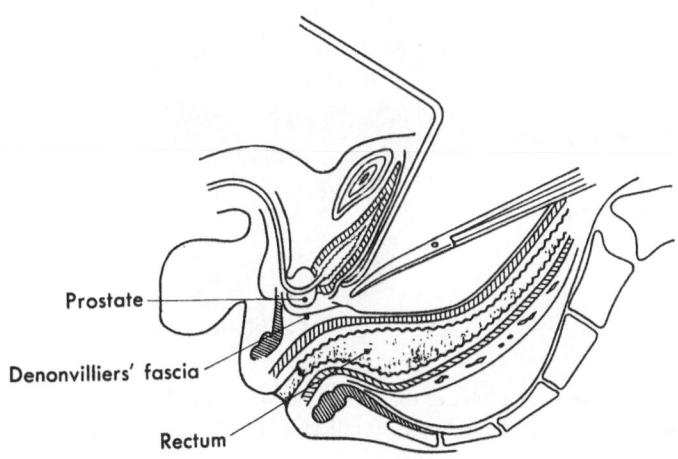

FIG. 2.  On the anterior side of the rectum, scissors must be inserted just above Denonvilliers' fascia, peeling it off from the posterior surface of the prostate.

of the pancreas are required to obtain a safety margin from the tumor (Fig. 1). Two separating lines of the intestine, either **distal to or proximal** to the tumor, are made 10 cm from the tumor margin. It is also important to clear the lymph nodes along **the** marginal vessels so as to keep a distance of 10 cm on both sides.

The principle of separation plays an important role in rectal cancer surgery. Separation must be made outside the Denonvilliers' fascia anteriorly, so that the seminal vesicle and prostate in the male, or vaginal muscle layer in the female can be clearly seen (Fig. 2). Posteriorly, the separation must be made from the visceral pelvic fascia, and the

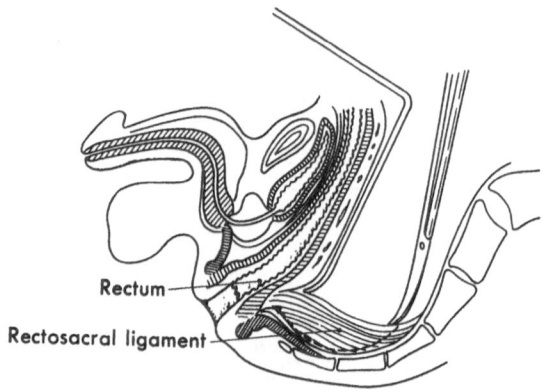

FIG. 3. On the posterior side of the rectum, scissors must be inserted along the curve of the sacral bone as indicated by the dotted line, so that the rectosacral ligament is completely separated.

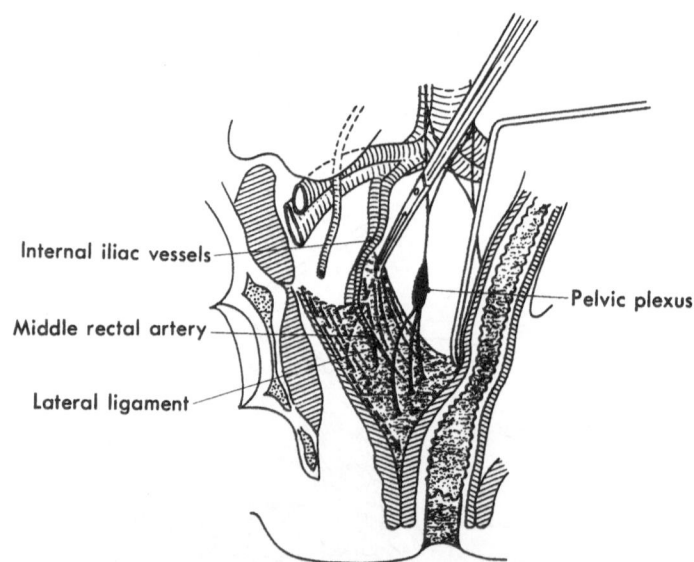

FIG. 4. On both lateral sides of the rectum, scissors must be used closely along the internal iliac vessels as the dotted line indicates. The lateral ligaments are separated from their bases.

dense fiber of the recto-sacral ligament is then completely removed from the surface of the sacral bone (Fig. 3). On both lateral sides of the rectum, the separation must be made closely along the internal iliac artery and vein, down to the base of the levator ani muscles. The lateral ligaments on both sides are completely separated, with the middle rectal arteries inside them (Fig. 4). In the case of rectal amputation, the levator ani muscles are naturally separated from their origins. The most important factor in separation is that we do not hesitate to remove a part or all of the neighboring organs when there is doubt of whether cancer cells might remain in the operating field. The proximal separating line of the intestine is put on a level more than 10 cm from the tumor edge, and then the tumor-bearing rectum is removed leaving a healthy intestine 3.0 cm distal to the lower margin of the tumor in the case of Dukes A, and 4.0 to 5.0 cm in Dukes B and C. When the distal separating line is located just above the anal canal or far from its upper limit, one of the sphincter-saving operations is carried out as a radical procedure.

When length of the normal intestine between the lower margin of the tumor and the anal canal is insufficient, rectal amputation is the procedure of choice.

### 2. The principle of lymph node dissection

For right side colonic cancer, lymph node dissection up to the root of the superior mesenteric vein must be done, and the trunk of this vein exposed to its full length. To complete this, the ileocolic artery and right colic artery are separated at their origins and corresponding veins are also clamped at the pouring sites to the superior mesenteric vein, so that the outer layer of that vein trunk itself is fully exposed up to the lower border of the pancreas body (Figs. 5, 6).

In left side colonic cancer, the dissecting process must reach the root of the inferior mesenteric artery, and for this full exposure of the origin of this artery is required. When the dissection is completed, a part of the abdominal aorta is visible at the site of the origin of the inferior mesenteric artery which is then fully exposed. This artery is then cut off at the origin and the inferior mesenteric vein is separated at the same level (Fig. 7.)

Although the lymphatic system of the rectum is thought to be rather complex, we can recognize two main lymphatic flows with their topographic situations: the upward lymphatic flow along the course of the inferior mesenteric vessel, and the lateral lymphatic flow along the internal iliac vessels and their tributaries. Even in a rectal cancer, the lymph node dissection along the inferior mesenteric vessel is required up to the origin of the inferior mesenteric artery. The operative technique of the dissection is the same as that for left side colonic cancer. Also in a rectal cancer, especially that which is low lying, the meticulous dissection of lymph nodes along the internal iliac artery and vein

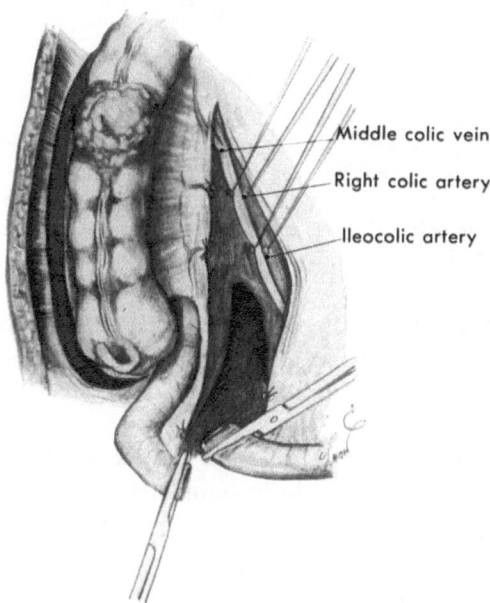

FIG. 5.   In right side colonic cancer, to complete the nodal dissection the mesocolon is separated and the ileocolic and right colic vessels are separated at their origins.

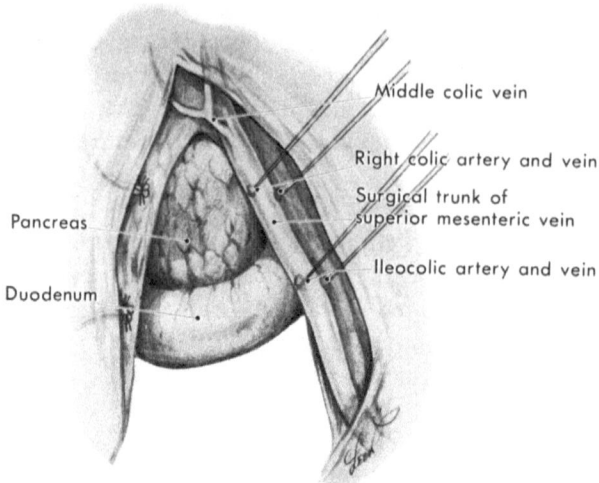

FIG. 6. We can see that the surgical trunk of the superior mesenteric vein is fully exposed and the 3rd portion of the duodenum and pancreas are also exposed.

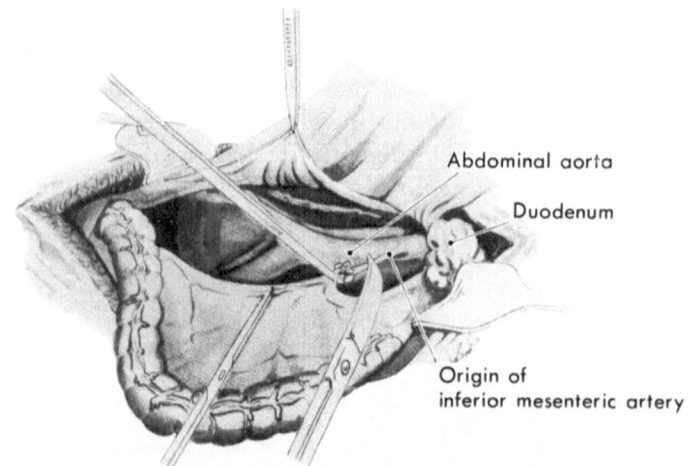

FIG. 7. In left side colonic cancer, to complete the nodal dissection the origin of the inferior mesenteric artery from the abdominal aorta is exposed.

on both sides is required. For this to be done completely, the paravesical space, the space between the course of the internal iliac artery and the true pelvic wall must be dilated; this is composed of fat tissues containing lymph nodes which are scheduled to be removed (Fig. 8).

The full exposure of the obturator nerve in the center of the paravesical space is a sign that the lateral node dissection has been completed.

## COMMENTS

Wide removal of the tissues surrounding the tumor is one of several principles for colo-rectal cancer surgery which has been generally accepted. We would like to stress

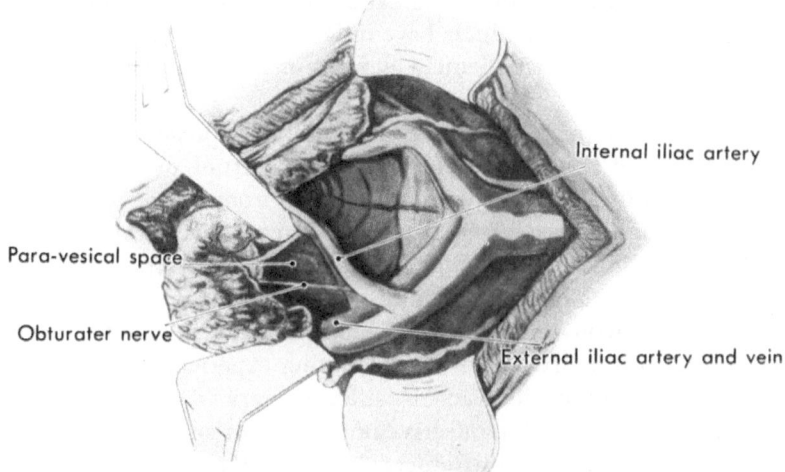

Internal iliac artery

Para-vesical space

Obturater nerve

External iliac artery and vein

FIG. 8.   For lateral node dissection, the paravesical space is widened with a retractor placed on the superior vesical artery. The full exposure of the obturator nerve at the center of the space is an indication of complete lateral node dissection.

that this type of procedure must be done under direct viewing, and should be undertaken with a full understanding of the architecture of the retroperitoneal space; this has already been done by several enthusiastic anatomists like Curtis (1) and Tobin (10).

The separating procedure has become more effective in cancer cure because the fascial arrangment in the retroperitoneal space acts as a kind of barrier against the spread of the disease. In the process of separation of colonic cancer, especially right side and left side, it is important to recognize Toldt's fusion fascia and sub-peritoneal fascia during an operation not only to maintain the radicability of cancer cure but also for safety of the operation. These fascias retain a constant relationship with the retroperitoneal elements such as ureter, vesical or ovarian vessels. Goligher's textbook (3) is, in our opinion, the only book which appropriately acknowledges the importance of Toldt's fusion fascia in the separating process for colonic cancer. We would like to go a step further and recommend cutting off the sub-peritoneal fascia situated in the deeper layer for an advanced colonic cancer. In the course of the separating process around the rectum, the connection of the pelvic fascia around the rectum to the sub-peritoneal fascia which is no more than the lower part of Gerota's renal fascia should be realized. Almost all textbooks concerning rectal surgery indicate the importance of peeling off the pelvic fascia at the posterior side of the rectum. In addition, another critical point is that the peeling off of the pelvic fascia is the first step in the complete separation of the rectosacral ligament which is located at the bottom of the pelvis.

Many operative drawings for rectal cancer recommend that the lateral ligament be **separated at its origin.** After searching for the best way to reach the base of the lateral ligament, we have concluded that the separating **process at the lateral** side of the rectum is best done closely along the internal iliac artery and vein to the base of the lateral ligament. This process is easier and more radical. As to the area which is removed in order to clear the course of the regional lymphatic flow, various drawings indicate it as having different sizes. Stearns' drawing (9) indicates a rather large area extending beyond the course of the inferior mesenteric vessels. Turnbull's operative sketch (11) shows a little smaller area limited to the leaf of mesocolon and the drawing of Goligher (3) suggests an area of medium size. These individuals have different ideas of regional lymphatic nodes and do not indicate any concrete element defined anatomically as the limit of the area of regional lymphatic flow.

We tried to define the regional area of the lymphatic spread by anatomical elements from the point of view of clinical practice. The surgical trunk of the superior mesenteric vein is the upper limit of the regional lymphatic flow from the right side colon, and the origin of the inferior mesenteric artery is the uppermost point from the left side colon and rectum. In our definition, the lymph nodes along the internal iliac vessels, that is, the lateral lymph nodes, are included within the area of the regional nodes.

Deddish (2) and Bacon (8) have investigated the clinical significance of dissection of the lateral nodes and reported their disappointing experiences, suggesting that these lateral nodes are already out of the reach of radical surgery. We have made an anatomical analysis of the lateral lymph nodes and have improved our surgical dissection technique. We believe the advances we have introduced partly account for the improvement of the 5-year survival rate of rectal cancer in our hospital, especially of Dukes C cancer.

## REFERENCES

1.   Curtis, A. H., Anson, B. J., and Beaton, L. E. The anatomy of the subperitoneal tissues and ligamentous structures in relation to surgery of the female pelvic viscera. *Surg. Gyne col. Obstet.*, **70**, 643-656 (1940).
2.   Deddish, M. R. Discussion on the treatment of advanced cancer of the rectum. *Proc. R. Soc. Med.*, **43**, 1075-1081 (1950).
3.   Goligher, J. C. *In* "Surgery of the Anus, Rectum and Colon," 5th ed., ed. J. C. Goligher, p. 496 (1984). Bailliere Tindal, London.
4.   Hawley, P. R. *In* "Surgery of the Anus, Rectum and Colon," 5th ed., ed. J. C. Goligher, p. 549 (1984). Bailliere Tindal, London.
5.   Lockhart-Mummery, H. E., Ritchie, J. K., and Hawley, P. R. The results of surgical treatment for carcinoma of the rectum at St. Mark's Hospital from 1948 to 1972. *Br. J. Surg.*, **63**, 673-677 (1976).
6.   McDermott, F. T., Hughes, E.S.R., Pihl, E. A., and Milne, B. J. Changing survival prospects in carcinoma of the rectum. *Br. J. Surg.*, **67**, 775-780 (1980).
7.   Perlemuter, L. and Waligora, J. "Cahiers d'Anatomie, Abdomen, II," 4th ed. (1976). Masson, Paris.
8.   Sauer, I. and Bacon, H. E. A new approach for excision of carcinoma of the lower portion of the rectum and anal canal. *Surg. Gynecol Obstet.*, **95**, 229-242 (1952).
9.   Stearns, M. W., Jr. Adenocarcinoma. *In* "Neoplasma of the Colon, Rectum and Anus," pp. 84-85 (1980). John Wiley and Sons, New York.
10.   Tobin, C. E. and Benjamin, J. A. Anatomical and surgical restudy of Denonvilliers' fascia. *Surg. Gynecol. Obstet.*, **80**, 373-388 (1945).
11.   Turnbull, R. B., Jr., Kyle, K., Watson, F. R., and Spratt, J. Cancer of colon: the influence of no-touch isolation technic on survival rate. *Ann. Surg.*, **166**, 420-427 (1967).

# LONG-TERM SURVIVAL OF HEPATOCELLULAR CARCINOMA WITH REFERENCE TO THE ROLE OF EARLY RESECTION, MULTIOPERATION AND MULTIMODALITY TREATMENT

Zhao-You TANG and Ye-Qin YU

*Liver Cancer Research Unit, Zhong Shan Hospital,*
*Shanghai First Medical College\**

Despite the tremendous efforts made in the past decades, the dismal long-term survival rate of hepatocellular carcinoma (HCC) has changed little. Nevertheless, encouraging results have appeared in the authors' hospital. A comparative study of pathologically proven HCC between 258 cases in 1964–1973 and 539 cases in 1974–1983 showed remarkable improvement in overall rates of 1-year (14.6 *vs.* 36.0%), 3-year 5.3 *vs.* 20.6%), and 5-year survival (3.7 *vs.* 15.2%). Analyses revealed: a) the increasing number (3 cases *vs.* 63 cases) of small HCC ($\leq 5$ cm) resection played a major role, 5-year survival increased to 71.2% after resection of small HCC. b) The increasing number of patients (0 *vs.* 30 cases) receiving multioperations (24 reoperations for subclinical recurrence or solitary lung metastasis after radical resection, 6 second step resections after palliative surgery) was the second factor improving 5-year survival. c) Multimodality treatment such as hepatic artery cannulation or occlusion, cryosurgery, laser vaporization, and their combination also added to improvement of 1- and 3-year survival. Thus, multioperation and multimodality treatment might be effective approaches to improving long-term survival of HCC in those institutions which have not yet started an early detection program.

In China, primary liver cancer (PLC) causes 100,000 deaths every year, amounting to about 40% of the liver cancer deaths in the world. The standarized mortality rate has been reported to be as high as 14.52/100,000 in males and 5.61/100,000 in females and it ranks third in male and fourth in female malignancies (*9*). The peak age affected is in the years 40–49, with the average 43.7 (*18*). The geographic distribution showed a narrow belt of high endemicity along the southeastern seacoast, which is the country's most populated area (*9*). Hepatocellular carcinoma (HCC) has attracted the most attention; first because it accounted for 89.9% of PLC in China; secondly, strong evidence of liver disease background has been noted, in a survey of 500 HCC autopsied cases 80.2 and 56.2% of nontumorous hepatocytes contained HBsAg and HBcAg, respectively, and 84.6% of HCC patients had cirrhosis (*11*); thirdly, 89.6% of HCC patients had elevated serum $\alpha$-fetoprotein (AFP) higher than 20 ng/m*l* (*20*). This offers the possibility of primary and secondary prevention particularly in HCC.

Unfortunately, the dismal long-term survival rate of HCC has been recorded for decades, with 5-year survival around 3% (*1, 13*). However, encouraging results have been

---

\* Shanghai 200032, People's Republic of China.

TABLE I. Long-Term Survival of Pathologically Proven HCC—a Comparison
between 1964–1973(A) and 1974–1983(B) of Patients Treated in Zhong
Shan Hospital, Shanghai First Medical College

| Treatment modality | | No. of cases | Survival % (life table method) | | | | |
|---|---|---|---|---|---|---|---|
| | | | 1-year | 2-year | 3-year | 4-year | 5-year |
| Radical resection | (A) | 29 | 79.3 | 55.2 | 37.9 | 31.0 | 31.0 |
| | (B)[a] | 116 | 95.3 | 79.6 | 72.1 | 68.5 | 61.0 |
| Hepatic artery cannulation | (A) | 0 | — | — | — | — | — |
| +occlusion+2nd step op. | (B)[b] | 39 | 48.9 | 25.4 | 19.0 | 19.0 | — |
| Cryosurgery+cannulation | (A) | 0 | — | — | — | — | — |
| and/or occlusion | (B) | 18 | 37.4 | 22.5 | — | — | — |
| Cryosurgery or laser | (A) | 0 | — | — | — | — | — |
| | (B) | 22 | 40.9 | 13.6 | 9.1 | 4.6 | — |
| Hepatic artery cannulation | (A) | 43 | 9.3 | 0 | 0 | 0 | 0 |
| | (B) | 49 | 26.7 | 9.7 | 9.7 | 6.5 | — |
| Hepatic artery occlusion | (A) | 0 | — | — | — | — | — |
| | (B) | 38 | 14.3 | 5.4 | 0 | 0 | 0 |
| Palliative resection | (A) | 46 | 4.4 | 0 | 0 | 0 | 0 |
| | (B) | 74 | 23.5 | 2.4 | 0 | 0 | 0 |
| Conservative treatment | (A) | 140 | 4.3 | 2.2 | 0.7 | 0 | 0 |
| | (B) | 183 | 5.4 | 1.8 | 0.6 | 0 | 0 |
| Total | (A) | 258 | 14.6 | 8.1 | 5.3 | 3.7 | 3.7 |
| | (B) | 539 | 36.0 | 23.9 | 20.6 | 17.2 | 15.2 |

[a] With reoperation in 24 cases.
[b] With second step operation in 6 cases.

obtained in recent years, particularly in the field of early detection of subclinical HCC
(4, 7, 12, 17) as well as subclinical recurrence or metastasis (23, 30) using AFP serosurvey
and early resection (8, 10, 19, 22, 26). Early detection and early resection is doubtlessly
of prime importance to prolong overall long-term survival. Presently clinical rather than
subclinical HCC still accounts for the majority of HCC in our clinical work, particularly
in those institutions which have not yet introduced an early detection program, and thus
endeavors should also be made to prolong the overall survival of symptomatic clinical
HCC patients. Based on a comparative study of long-term survival of pathologically
proven HCC in Zhong Shan Hospital of Shanghai First Medical College between 258
cases in 1964–1973 and 539 cases in 1974–1983, factors influencing long-term survival
with respect to treatment modality were analyzed. Results demonstrated that multioperation and multimodality treatment might be effective approaches.

*Evolution of Long-Term Survival of HCC and the Role of Early Detection and Early
Resection*

Recently, as a result of earlier diagnosis, higher resectability and postoperative
adjuvant therapy, more favorable results were observed (2). In a study of 600 cases of
HCC, the median survival of resection ($n=98$) was reported to be 19.6 months, 2.8
months in those with nonsurgical treatment and only 1.6 months in patients without
treatment (14). However, the 5-year survival rate of overall PLC or HCC has rarely
been recorded in the literature. In the United States, the PLC 5-year survival rate was

2% in the period 1940–1949 (371 cases), 1% in 1950–1959 (724 cases), and 4% in 1960–1964 (505 cases) (*1*). In Japan, a 5-year survival rate of 2.4% in 1968–1977 (1,424 cases of HCC) was reported (*13*). In the authors' hospital, it was 2.6% in 1961–1970 (387 cases) (*28*). In the present study, however, as shown in Table I, the overall 5-year survival rate increased from 3.7% in 1964–1973 to 15.2% in 1974–1983. The only factor that might be involved in this improvement is radical resection, because no 5-year survival could be observed when other treatment modalities were used. Of course, the increase in proportion of radical resection in the whole series from 11.2% (29/258) to 21.4% (116/539) played an important role; however, the remarkable increase in 5-year survival from 31.0 to 61.0% after the same radical resection deserves particular attention. Further analysis revealed that early detection of small HCC (≦5 cm) contributed to both aspects mentioned above. As a result of AFP screening either in a natural population or recently in a high risk population, the proportion of small HCC in the resection group (radical and palliative) increased from 4.0% (3/75) to 33.2% (63/190), thus markedly improving the radical resection rate in overall resection cases from 38.7% (29/75) to 61.1% (116/190). The exciting thing was that 5-year survival as high as 71.2% was obtained after resection of small HCC. Similar data were also reported in Chinese literature: 49.3% in 42 cases (*8*), 53.8% in 38 cases (*26*), and 59.6% in 15 cases (*10*). Clearly, early detection and early resection of small HCC played a major role in the improvement of the overall 5-year survival in the whole series.

*Evaluation of Multioperation for the Improvement of Long-Term Survival of HCC*

Multioperation includes: a) reoperation for liver recurrence or metastatic lesions after a radical resection; b) second step resection of liver cancer after a palliative surgery. Wilson reported a case with 13 repeated resections of metastases in the abdomen with 15-year survival (*25*). Foster collected 10 cases with reoperation from the literature, one of them had received three reoperations (left lung metastasis, left liver recurrence, right lung metastasis) and was still alive 172 months after the initial operation (*6*). However, Chen *et al.* reported 8 cases with re-resection in symptomatic recurrence, the average survival being only 11.4 months and no significant comparative difference being observed from the group without re-resection (*5*). Recently, the sequence of regional chemotherapy and second step resection of a tumor either in PLC (*30*) or in secondary liver cancer (*24*) has been reported of value in improving the salvage rate.

The present study showed that multioperation may be of importance in improving overall long-term survival. During 1964–1973, no patient received more than one operation, but 30 cases underwent more than one operation in the period 1974–1983. Of these 30 cases, 24 underwent reoperation, which was performed twice in 3 cases and thrice in 2 cases for either liver recurrence or solitary lung metastasis after an initial radical resection; 6 underwent second step resection after an initial palliative surgical treatment with hepatic artery ligation plus cannulation. According to our data, the 1-, 3-, and 5-year recurrent rates after radical resection in a series of 76 cases of AFP positive HCC were 17.1, 32.5, and 61.5%, respectively. The median survival from the onset of recurrence was only 11 months in patients without reoperation. If reoperation had not been performed in this series, the survival time of the 24 cases would have had to be revised by adding 11 months after the onset of recurrence, and then the 5-year survival rate of radical resection would have been 41.2%, showing only a 10% increase as compared with that of 1964–1973 (31.0%). However, it was 61.0% according to the present data, indicating that reoperation had resulted in a 20% increase in 5-year survival in the radical resection group and played an important role in the overall improvement of that statistic. As shown in Table I, the 2- and 4-year survival rates were 25.4 and 19.0% respectively in the 39 cases that underwent hepatic artery cannulation and occlusion; in 6 of these second step resection was performed. If second step resection had not been performed in this series, the survival time of the 6 cases would have had to be revised by the median survival of cannulation plus occlusion—9 months, and then the 2- and 4-year survival rates of this group would have been 14.2 and 0%. Therefore, second step resection played a certain role in the improvement of the overall 2- and 4-year survival.

### The Importance of Multimodality Treatment in Prolonging 1-, 2-, and 3-Year Survival of HCC

Considering that the majority of clinical HCC patients had an unresectable tumor, multimodality treatment might prove to be of importance. Based on the new concept of surgical oncology, the more the tumor is eradicated, the better the recovery of the host status. Therefore, numerous modes of palliative surgery have been developed and employed. Cryosurgery (31) and high power YAG laser beam vaporization (29) have been of demonstrable value in treating superficially confined HCC. A 1-year survival of 44% has been reported in 120 patients with unresectable hepatoma in which hepatic artery embolization was used (27). Hepatic artery ligation or cannulation with chemotherapeutic perfusion provided acceptable results (16). It is particularly worthy of mention that combined multimodality treatment using hepatic arterial infusion plus occlusion seems to be the latest trend in the treatment of unresectable HCC (3, 15, 21). This combination treatment provided hope for sequence removal of HCC in patients with marked regression (by 50%) of well encapsulated tumors.

As shown in Table I, the overall 1-, 2-, and 3-year survival rates were also markedly increased as compared with the previous 10 years, 14.6 vs. 36.0%, 8.1 vs. 23.9%, and 5.3 vs. 20.6%, respectively. Of course, the above two factors were of importance; however, multimodality treatment also remained an important factor because it was clear that no remarkable improvement could be observed in the fields of palliative resection and conservative treatment (see Table I). On the other hand, the marked improvement of the ultimate outcome of hepatic artery cannulation and chemotherapeutic perfusion by more accurate positioning of the catheter and longer perfusion period was observed (9.3 vs. 26.7% in 1-year, 0 vs. 9.7% in 2-years). In addition, a combination of 2 or 3 modalities (hepatic artery occlusion, cryosurgery, and laser) and second step resection had been employed, and all these had contributed to the improvement of 1–3-year survival rates. The combination of multimodality treatment was better than each of the modalities used alone.

It may be concluded that early detection, early resection, and multioperation remain the major factors in the improvement of the overall 4- and 5-year survival rates and that multimodality treatment plays an important role in the improvement of overall 1-, 2-, and 3-year survival. Early resection is doubtlessly the modality of choice in the treatment of subclinical HCC with compensated liver function. Multioperation and multimodality treatment are of significant value in prolonging survival of clinical HCC.

## REFERENCES

1. Axtell, I. M., Cutler, S. J., and Mayers, M. H. "End Results in Cancer—Report No. 4," pp. 72–76 (1972). U.S. Department of Health, Education and Welfare, Public Health Service, NIH, NCI, Bethesda.

2. Bengmark, S., Hafstrom, L., Jeppsson, B., and Sundqvist, K. Primary carcinoma of the liver—improvement in sight? *World J. Surg.*, 6, 54–60 (1982).

3. Berjian, R. A., Douglass, H. O., Nava, H. R., and Karakousis, C. The role of hepatic artery ligation and dearterialization with infusion chemotherapy in advanced malignancies in the liver. *J. Surg. Oncol.*, 14, 379–387 (1980).

4. Chen, D. S., Sheu, J. C., Sung, J. L., Lai, M. Y., Lee, C. S., Su, C. T., Tsang, Y. M., How, S. W., Wang, T. H., Yu, J. Y., Yang, T. H., Wang, C. Y., and Hsu, C. Y. Small hepatocellular carcinoma—a clinicopathological study in thirteen patients. *Gastroenterology*, 83, 1109–1119 (1982).

5. Chen, H., Wu, M. C., and Zhang, X. H. Reoperation of primary liver cancer (in Chinese) *Shanghai Med. J.*, 2, 794–796 (1979).

6. Foster, J. H. and Berman, M. M. "Solid Liver Tumors," pp. 62–104 (1977). Saunders, Philadelphia.

7. Heyward, W. L., Lanier, A. P., Bender, T. R., McMahon, B. J., Kilkenny, S., Paprocki, T. R., Kline, K. T., Silimperi, D. R., and Maynard, J. E. Early detection of primary hepatocellular carcinoma by screening for alpha-fetoprotein in high-risk families—a case report. *Lancet*, ii, 1161–1162 (1983).

8. Huang, X. Y. and Zhang, Q. M. Results of surgical treatment of carcinoma of liver—report of 181 cases (in Chinese). *Chin. J. Surg.*, 20, 68–70 (1982).

9. Li, B. and Li, J. Y. National survey of cancer mortality in China (in Chinese). *Chin. J. Oncol.*, 2, 1–10 (1980).

10. Li, G. C., Li, G. H., and Liu, G. S. Resection of small hepatocellular carcinoma—analysis of 15 cases (in Chinese). *Cancer Control (Guangdong, China)*, 4, 24–29 (1980).

11. National Coordination Group of Pathology of Liver Cancer. Relationship between hepatocellular carcinoma, liver cirrhosis and hepatitis B—a pathological study (in Chinese). *Natl. Med. J. China*, 62, 257–261 (1982).

12. Okuda, K., Kotoda, K., Obata, H., Hayashi, N., Hisamitsu, T., Tamiya, M., Kubo, Y., Yakushui, F., Nagata, E., Jinnouchi, S., and Shimokawa, Y. Clinical observations during a relatively early stage of hepatocellular carcinoma, with special reference to serum alpha fetoprotein levels. *Gastroenterology*, 69, 226–234 (1975).

13. Okuda, K. (The Liver Cancer Study Group of Japan). Primary liver cancer in Japan. *Cancer*, 45, 2663–2669 (1980).

14. Okuda, K., Obata, H., Nakajima, Y., Ohtsuki, T. Okazaki, N., and Ohnishi, K. Prognosis of primary hepatocellular carcinoma. *Hepatology*, 4, 3s–6s (1984).

15. Patt, Y. Z., Chuang, V. P., Wallace, S., Benjamin, R. S., Fuqua, R., and Mavligit, G. M. Hepatic arterial chemotherapy and occlusion for palliation of primary hepatocellular carcinoma and unknown primary neoplasms in the liver. *Cancer*, 51, 1359–1363 (1983).

16. Reed, M. L., Vaitkevicius, V. K., Al-Sarraf, M., Vaughn, C., Singhakowinta, A., Sexonporte, M., Izbicki, R., Baker, L., and Straatsma, G. W. The practicality of chronic hepatic artery infusion therapy of primary and metastatic hepatic malignancies—ten year results of 124 patients in a prospective protocol. *Cancer*, 47, 402–409 (1981).

17. Shanghai Coordinating Group for Research on Liver Cancer. AFP serosurvey in diagnosis and screening of hepatocellular carcinoma (in Chinese). *Natl. Med. J. China*, 53, 455–457 (1973).

18. Shanghai Coordinating Group for Research on Liver Cancer. Primary liver cancer—clini-

cal analysis of 3,254 cases (from 11 provinces 21 hospitals in China) (in Chinese). *Tumor Prevent. Treat. Study*, **2**, 207–215 (1974).

19. Shanghai Coordinating Group for Research on Liver Cancer. Diagnosis and treatment of primary hepatocellular carcinoma in early stage—report of 134 cases. *Chin. Med. J.* **92**, 801–806 (1979).

20. Tang, Z. Y. and Yang, B. H. Clinical evaluation of alpha fetoprotein as tumor marker for hepatocellular carcinoma (in Chinese). *Chin. J. Oncol.*, **3**, 205–209 (1981).

21. Tang, Z. Y., Yu, Y. Q., Lin, Z. Y., Yang, B. H., Zhou, X. D., and Cao, Y. Z. Clinical research of primary liver cancer—a 10 year (1970–1979) survey. *Chin. Med. J.*, **96**, 247–250 (1983).

22. Tang, Z. Y., Yu, Y. Q., Zhou, X. D., and Zhou, N. Q. Surgical treatment of subclinical hepatocellular carcinoma (HCC) and its ultimate outcome—a comparative study of 74 cases of subclinical HCC and 229 cases of clinical HCC undergone surgery. *J. Exp. Clin. Cancer Res.*, **2**, 261–268 (1983).

23. Tang, Z. Y., Yu, Y. Q., and Zhou, X. D. An important approach to prolonging survival further after radical resection of AFP positive hepatocellular carcinoma. *J. Exp. Clin. Cancer Res.*, **3**, 359–366 (1984).

24. Tilchen, E., Patt, Y. Z., Mcbride, C. M., Wallace, S., Chuang, V., and Mavligit, C. M. Sequence of regional chemotherapy and surgery—management of colorectal adenocarcinoma confined to the liver. *Arch. Surg.*, **116**, 959–960 (1981).

25. Wilson, E. Malignant hepatoma—repeated resection of metastases with survival for 15 years. *Med. J. Aust.*, **2**, 889–893 (1966).

26. Wu, M. C., Zhang, X. H., Chen, H., and Wu, B. W. Experiences in hepatectomies of 467 cases (in Chinese). *Chin. J. Digest.*, **2**, 190–193 (1982).

27. Yamada, R., Sato, M., Kawabata, M., Nakatsuka, H., Nakamura, K., and Takashima, S. Hepatic artery embolization in 120 patients with unresectable hepatoma. *Radiology*, **148**, 397–401 (1983).

28. Yang, B. H. and Tang, Z. Y. Improvement in diagnosis and treatment of primary liver cancer—an analysis of 1,045 cases (in Chinese). *Chin. J. Oncol.*, **4**, 279–282 (1982).

29. Yu, Y. Q., Tang, Z. Y., Zhou, X. D., Lin, Z. Y., Yang, B. H., Lu, J. Z., Zhou, N. Q., Lu, J. M., and Lu, H. X. Treatment of primary hepatic cancer by YAG laser, a preliminary report (in Chinese). *Acta Acad. Med. Primae Shanghai*, **8**, 29–31 (1981).

30. Yu, Y. Q., Tang, Z. Y., Zhou, X. D., Lu, J. Z., Zhou, N. Q., and Yang, B. H. Treatment of huge primary liver cancer in stages (in Chinese). *Chin. J. Surg.*, **21**, 92–93 (1983).

31. Zhou, X. D., Tang, Z. Y., Yu, Y. Q., Lu, H. X., Chen, C. G., Jiang, Y. M., and Xu, Y. D. Cryosurgery for liver cancer—experimental and clinical study (in Chinese). *Chin. J. Surg.*, **17**, 480–483 (1979).

# CURRENT STATUS OF SURGICAL THERAPY FOR PRIMARY LIVER CANCER IN JAPAN

Takayoshi TOBE

*First Department of Surgery, Faculty of
Medicine, Kyoto University**

The follow-up study of primary liver cancer analyzed by the Liver Cancer Study Group in Japan revealed that this malignant tumor was prevalent in men in the sixth decade of life, and that about 83.2% of these patients were cirrhotic. Periodic surveillance of serum $\alpha$-fetoprotein together with ultrasound and computed tomography in this high risk group appeared to be most important for detection of primary liver cancer at the early stage.

When surgical intervention is being contemplated, serious consideration should be given to not only anatomical condition but also hepatocellular reserve, particularly in cases with cirrhosis. Standard major resection can be done only when hepatocellular function is well preserved. Small hepatic resection should be a procedure of choice in cases of impaired liver function since this can lead to decreased postoperative morbidity and mortality. Subsegmental hepatectomy combined with intraoperative ultrasound examination, which was developed in Japan, appears one of the most suitable approaches in such patients.

Comparing results achieved by various types of medical treatment, the survival is extended in patients undergoing hepatectomy.

## Characteristics of Primary Liver Cancer in Japan

The Liver Cancer Study Group in Japan has been analyzing a follow-up study of primary liver cancer since 1965. Based on 4,658 patients treated in 1980 and 1981, primary liver cancer in this country has the following characteristics:

1.  Hepatocellular carcinoma is quite common, accounting for 89.2% of all cases of microscopically proved liver cancer.
2.  It is more prevalent in men: the male/female ratio is 5.2/1.
3.  The incidence is higher in the sixth decade of life.
4.  Many patients have a history of hepatitis B from an earlier blood transfusion and are carriers of HBs antigen; they frequently have hepatic cirrhosis (83.2%).

## Important Points in Diagnosis

On the basis of the above characteristics, the following three points are important in diagnosing primary liver cancer.

1.  Follow-up study of high risk groups: high risk patients are men in the sixth

---

\* Kawara-cho 54, Shogoin, Sakyo-ku, Kyoto 606, Japan (戸部隆吉).

decade of life with a past history of blood transfusion or hepatitis B, patients with hepatic cirrhosis, and HBs antigen carriers.

2. Regular screening for $\alpha$-fetoprotein (AFP).

3. Greater use of ultrasonography (US) or computerized tomography (CT) for lesions suspected of being malignant.

## Indications for Surgical Therapy

In the normal liver there is such a large functional reserve capacity that hepatic function remains normal even when 40 to 50% of the liver is removed. The remnant liver can regenerate to regain its original size in 4 to 6 months even after 75% hepatectomy. However, in hepatic cirrhosis even minimal surgical intervention may induce hepatic failure after operation.

My associates and I routinely analyze the grade of hepatic cirrhosis not only by inspection of the hepatic surface but also by measuring the amount of cytochrome $a$ ($+a_3$) in the mitochondria of the hepatic cells after performing a liver biopsy. Serum albumin and bilirubin levels, ICG tests and the oral glucose tolerance test are useful routine laboratory procedures.

Child's criteria were first used to select patients with esophageal varices for shunt operations. If a patient is classified as grade C, it is recommended that operation be avoided.

Recent advances of CT or US in the diagnosis of liver cancer have made it possible to determine preoperatively not only the anatomic location and size of the tumor but also the degree of infiltration. Cirrhosis of the liver can be demonstrated.

Enhanced contrast study can reveal hepatocellular carcinoma more clearly.

Obstruction of the portal vein by tumor emboli is a contraindication for surgery.

Tumor invasion of the inferior vena cava indicates that surgery will be very difficult or impossible.

Selective angiography is one of the essential preoperative examinations to determine the area to be resected and is more effective in determining the presence of daughter nodules or intrahepatic small metastases.

If intrahepatic metastases are demonstrated in the opposite lobe, surgery is contraindicated.

## Selection of the Appropriate Surgical Approach (3)

When hepatic cirrhosis is minimum and a good functional reserve of the liver can be predicated, established hepatectomy can be performed: left lateral segmentectomy, left lobectomy, right lobectomy, or trisegmentectomy (Fig. 1).

When a high degree of hepatic cirrhosis is detected, resection of the liver should be only partial.

However, it is well known that hepatocellular carcinomas metastasize easily through the portal vein to form multiple daughter nodules in other portions of the liver. Therefore, segmental resection of the liver is much better than enucleation of the tumor. This procedure was developed in our country by Makuuchi and others (1) (Fig. 2).

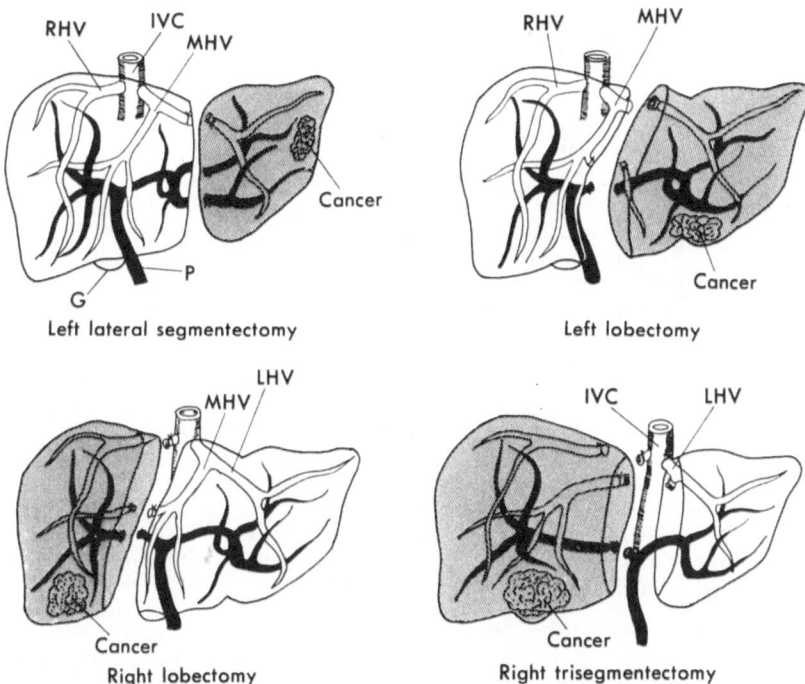

FIG. 1. Selection of appropriate surgical procedure—minimum degree of hepatic cirrhosis.

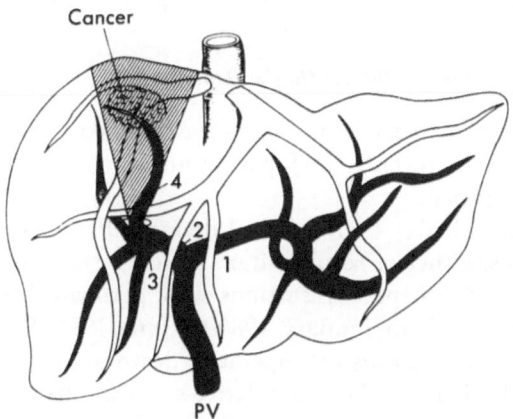

FIG. 2. Selection of appropriate surgical procedure—liver cancer associated with hepatic cirrhosis.

PV, portal vein; 1, left branch; 2, right branch; 3, right anterior portal vein; 4, right anterior superior portal vein.

## Subsegmental Hepatectomy

After mobilization of the liver, the probe of the ultrasonograph is placed on the liver surface. The location of the tumor and its relationship to the portal vein, hepatic veins and bile duct are identified. Using US, a 22-gauge percutaneous transhepatic cholangiography (PTC) needle is inserted into the liver. The tip is placed in the portal vein which

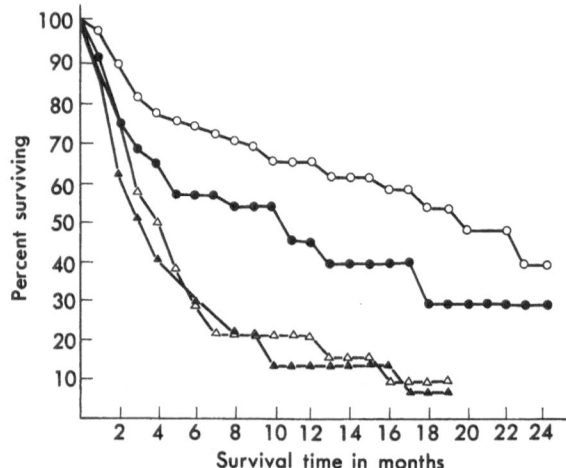

FIG. 3.  Surgical results for primary cancer in Japan.
○ non-cirrhotic, laparotomy with tumor resection (N=135); △ non-cirrhotic, without tumor resection (N=91); ● cirrhotic, laparotomy with tumor resection (N=67); ▲ cirrhotic, without tumor resection (N=39).

supplies the hepatic tumor. After ascertaining the location of the needle, indigocarmine or ICG is injected through the PTC needle until the surface of the liver is clearly stained. On the ultrasonogram the flow of the staining solution can be demonstrated clearly as an echogenic tiny spot in the portal vein. When the subsegmental region is clearly visible with this technique, subsegmental resection can be performed.

*Surgical Results in Japan and in the Author's Department*

The use of this limited resection has greatly decreased intraoperative mortality and postoperative complications recently in Japan. Figure 3 shows the results of therapy for primary liver cancer in Japan.

Surgical treatment is better than medical therapy. Patients with either cirrhotic or non-cirrhotic livers showed better results after surgical resection.

In our department, 127 hepatic resections were performed for primary liver cancer during the 4.5 year period from January 1980 to June 1984. Since January of 1980 in the past 4 years, there has been only one operative death per year; each of these occurred in a patient with a cirrhotic liver. The cumulative survival rate for patients with cirrhosis over the last 4 years in our department is 33.5%, while that of non-cirrhotic patients is 56.2%.

We have demonstrated that the cytochrome *a* content is closely related to the functional reserve and the regenerating capacity of the cirrhotic liver (2). It appears that the measurement of the cytochrome *a* content of the remnant liver is important in determining the extent to which hepatic resection can be safely performed and also in determining the prognosis and survival rate.

## REFERENCES

1.  Makuuchi, M., Hasegawa, H., Yamazaki, S., Mandai, Y., Ito, T., Watanabe, G., Abe, H., and Muroi, T. Intraoperative ultrasonic examination for liver surgery and new concept in partial hepatectomy (in Japanese). *Geka Chiryo*, **44**, 579 (1981).
2.  Ozawa, K., Yamaoka, Y., Kitamura, O., Nambu, H., Kamiyama, Y., Takeda, H., Takasan, H., and Honjo, I. Clinical application of cytochrome $a$ $(+a_3)$ of mitochondria from liver specimens: an aid in determining metabolic tolerance of liver remnant for hepatic resection. *Ann. Surg.*, **180**, 868 (1974).
3.  Tobe, T. Hepatectomy in patients with cirrhotic liver. *In* " Surgery Annual 1984," Vol. 16, ed. L. M. Nyhus, pp. 177–202 (1984). Appleton-Century-Crofts, Norwalk, Connecticut.

# RESULTS OF SURGERY AND COMBINED MODALITY THERAPY FOR CARCINOMA OF THE PANCREAS

Toshio Sato, Hidemi Yamauchi, and Seiki Matsuno

*First Department of Surgery, Tohoku University
School of Medicine\**

Extended operations for carcinoma of the pancreas may not greatly influence 5-year survival rate although they may contribute slightly to increasing survival periods. The time now seems ripe for surgeons to define the most promising type of operation for each stage of the disease. Intensive investigative efforts should proceed for the diagnosis and treatment of small pancreatic cancer as well as for the combined modality treatment of advanced pancreatic cancer.

The incidence of carcinoma of the pancreas arising from ductal cells has steadily increased recently. Despite the various newly developed examinations and diagnostic tools available, a high percentage of lesions are still unresectable and the survival rate following the operation is truly disappointing. The present status of the treatment of pancreatic carcinoma including combined modality therapy is summarized in this report.

*Radical Resection of Carcinoma of the Pancreas*

### 1. Resectability rate

Resectability rates of carcinoma of the head of the pancreas range from 19 to 26% (*2, 10*). Carcinoma of the body and tail of the pancreas is rarely resectable and rates reported are less than 10%. Of the 295 patients of periampullary carcinoma who were operated on at our clinic of Tohoku University Hospital, 116 were subjected to radical resection. For 171 patients with carcinoma of the head of the pancreas, Whipple operation was performed on 28 patients and total pancreatectomy on 10, and for 92 patients with carcinoma of the body and tail of the pancreas, caudal pancreatectomy on 7 and total pancreatectomy on one. Resectability rates were 22.2 and 8.7%, respectively. The operative mortality rate of the Whipple operation has decreased to less than 10% in the 1970's, while that of a total pancreatectomy for pancreatic carcinoma ranged from 7 to 17% (*2, 6*).

### 2. Late results after resection of the pancreas

In a survey of late results for 1,005 pancreaticoduodenectomies summarized by Levin and ReMine (*5*) in 1978, only 39 patients (4%) survived more than 5 years. The various reported 5-year survival rates varied from 0 to 10%, and many of them fell in the less than 5% category. Survival period after pancreaticoduodenectomy ranged from 9 to 18 months in most reported series except that Moossa *et al.* (*6*) reported that of 23 months. In our series, 5-year survival rates after pancreaticoduodenectomy were 8.7% for patients

---

* Seiryo-cho 2-1, Sendai 980, Japan (佐藤寿雄, 山内英生, 松野正紀).

TABLE I.   Survival by Months and Stage of Carcinoma of the Head
of the Pancreas (146 Patients) (1984. 8)

| Stage | Survival (months) of patients | | | Average months |
|:---:|:---:|:---:|:---:|:---:|
|  | Resection | Palliative operation | Exploratory laparotomy |  |
| I | 34.8  (9) | 1.5  (1) |  | 31.6  (10) |
| II | 26.9  (16) | 4.7  (9) |  | 17.3  (26) |
| III | 7.1  (8) | 5.9  (30) | 3.5  (2) | 6.0  (39) |
| IV |  | 4.9  (63) | 3.3  (8) | 4.6  (71) |
| Average months | 25.1  (33) | 5.2  (103) | 3.4  (10) | 9.3  (146) |

( ): No. of patients.

with carcinoma of the head of the pancreas, 28.5% for those with carcinoma of the bile
duct, and 38.1% for those with carcinoma of the papilla of Vater.

In recent years, total pancreatectomy has been attempted by many surgeons in
different parts of the world. In 51 patients who underwent this operation for carcinoma
of the pancreas in Mayo Clinic, the 5-year survival rate was as low as 2.3% (9). Although
some reported somewhat superior survival periods after total pancreatectomy to pancreaticoduodenectomy, little benefit could be seen with total pancreatectomy (2, 9, 10).

Average survival and stage of carcinoma of the head of the pancreas (7) with reference
to the type of operation performed in our series are listed in Table I. Survival periods
became shorter in accordance with the advancement of stages. Mean survival periods
were 25.1 months for patients who underwent resection, 5.2 months who underwent
palliative operation, and 3.4 months who underwent exploratory laparotomy. In patients
who underwent resection, those with stage III disease had a survival period of 7.1 months
which was markedly shorter than those with stage I or stage II disease. Difference between stage II and stage III is mainly related to the existence either of cancer invasion
to the capsule or of the involvement of group I or II lymph nodes. From the point of
view of possibly eradicating the cancer spread in the pancreatic duct as well as in the
lymphatic network behind the pancreas, extended pancreatic resection combined with
thorough dissection of the regional lymph nodes has been attempted by many surgeons
(1, 6, 9).

### 3.   Problems with extended pancreatectomy

Among the problems concerned with the radicality of pancreaticoduodenectomy
for carcinoma of the pancreas are residual cancer at the cut edge of the pancreas, multi-
centricity, residual cancer in the distal pancreatic duct, and incomplete dissection of
lymph nodes along the distal pancreas. These problems are always associated with patients
who are not subjected to total pancreatectomy. To overcome them, regional pancreatectomy has been proposed by Fortner (3). There have been some reports on this procedure giving higher resectability, curativity, and consequent better prognosis. Several
surgeons have reported that there were no significant differences in late operative results
between conventional pancreatectomy and regional pancreatectomy in advanced stages
of carcinoma of the pancreas. This suggests that regional pancreatectomy has limited
indication and cannot be recommended in an advanced stage of disease which presents
a cancer invasion to the pancreatic capsule.

#### 4. Surgical treatment of small pancreatic cancer

Small pancreatic cancer less than 2 cm in size accounts for only 3% of carcinoma of the pancreas. Most tumors are located in the head of the pancreas and are diagnosed by manifestation of jaundice.

In the treatment of small pancreatic cancer, great controversy continues as to the extent of lymph node dissection and the operative procedures selected: partial or total resection of the pancreas.

According to our study on 32 patients resected, pancreatic cancer without invasion to the pancreatic capsule appears to have metastasis limited to group I lymph nodes; in contrast, those with capsular invasion have metastasis to group II or III lymph nodes.

Wider dissection of lymph nodes, therefore, would be recommended when cancer invasion to the capsule is highly suspected, even in patients with small pancreatic cancer. Curative operation can be reasonably expected by the standard lymph node dissection procedure in patients without invasion to the pancreatic capsule. The authors have been performing the conventional Whipple operation in patients whose tumors are located within the capsule and bear a clear boundary, and total pancreatectomy in those whose tumors are not.

### Combined Modality Treatment for Carcinoma of the Pancreas

#### 1. Radiation therapy

In patients with carcinoma of the pancreas, definitive radiation in high doses cannot be applied because of its close proximity to radiosensitive structures such as the intestine and other important organs manifesting significant side effects. Therefore, the use of intraoperative radiation therapy directed into the open abdomen aimed specifically at the tumor is being investigated. Intraoperative radiation may result in either the prevention of local recurrence after resection of the tumor, or antitumor effectiveness of the tumor residue in non-curatively resected or unresected cases.

We have employed intraoperative radiation in high doses on 37 patients with stage IV unresectable carcinoma of the pancreas since August, 1974. Several studies have shown that relief of pain was achieved in about 70% of these individuals. In the 37 patients treated by the authors, pain palliation including excellent and good results was achieved in 40% in cancer of the head, in 55% in that of the body and the tail of the pancreas and in 49% overall (Table II). Our studies revealed that 5 out of 15 patients (33.3%) who underwent clipping by radio-opaque markers around the tumor margin manifested reduced tumor size after the radiation. The authors believe that intraoperative radiation may result in reducing tumor size to some extent and in contributing to a patient's longer survival.

TABLE II. Effect of Intraoperative Irradiation on Abdominal Pain (1974. 8–1984. 8)

| | Response | | | | Total |
|---|---|---|---|---|---|
| | Excellent | Good | Poor | Uncertain | |
| Cancer of the head | 3 (1) | 3 (1) | 4 (1) | 5 (2) | 15 (5) |
| Cancer of the body and tail | 7 (5) | 5 (4) | 7 (5) | 3 (2) | 22 (16) |
| Total | 10 (6) | 8 (5) | 11 (6) | 8 (4) | 37 (21) |

( ): No. of patients with chemical splanchnicectomy.

Palliative bypass procedures seemed to have poor prognosis showing overall mean survival time of 3 to 6 months, and an even more unfavorable survival of 3 to 4 months could be seen in carcinoma of the body and tail of the pancreas. The mean survival of patients treated with intraoperative radiation in our series was 7.2 months, which was double the time of survival of patients who did not undergo radiation therapy. Goldson (4) reported a median survival time of 5.5 months after intraoperative radiation.

In addition to ordinary radiation therapy, radiation using high-performance neutron beam, heavy charge particle or high linear energy transfer system has recently been introduced. Shipley et al. (8) reviewed the effectiveness of $^{125}$I implantation into tumor tissues to prolong the survival of the patients.

## 2. Cancer chemotherapy

Chemotherapy of pancreatic carcinoma, most of which arises from ductal cells, has not met with much success due to poor blood supply to the tumor. The authors have been performing extensive studies on combined chemotherapeutic agents of 5-fluorouracil, neocarzinostatin, and acracinomycin (or mitomycin) associated with the adjuvant agent of OK-432. The survival up to 8 months after the operations was considerably better in patients with chemotherapy than in those without.

The authors have been applying chemotherapeutic agents not only for systemic use but also for regional use to the lesions. Slow releasing agents which were molded to needle-shape were directly injected into the tumor under the open abdomen in 12 patients. The slow releasing anticancer drug injected into the tumor can maintain a high concentration of agent in the tissue for a certain period and can, therefore, intensify the anticancer effects with little adverse side-effect. A few cases in our series evidenced a stabilization of their disease after this treatment.

## REFERENCES

1.  Brooks, J. R. Cancer of the pancreas. *In* "Surgery of the Pancreas," ed. J. R. Brooks, pp. 263–298 (1983). W. B. Saunders Co., Philadelphia.
2.  Forrest, J. F. and Longmire, W. P. Carcinoma of the pancreas and periampullary region. A study of 279 patients. *Ann. Surg.*, **189**, 128–138 (1979)
3.  Fortner, J. E. Regional resection of cancer of the pancreas. A new surgical approach. *Surgery*, **73**, 307–320 (1973).
4.  Goldson, A. L. Techniques and indications for intraoperative radiotherapy of pancreatic carcinoma. *In* "Pancreatic Cancer. New Directions in Therapeutic Management," ed. I. Cohn, pp. 23–29 (1980). Masson Publ. U.S.A., Inc., New York.
5.  Levin, B., ReMine, W. H., Hermann, R. E., Schein, P. S., and Cohn, I., Jr. Panel: Cancer of the pancreas. *Am. J. Surg.*, **135**, 185–191 (1978).
6.  Moossa, A. R., Levis, M. H., and Mackie, C. R. Surgical treatment of pancreatic cancer. *Mayo Clin. Proc.*, **54**, 468–474 (1979).
7.  Sato, T., Saitoh, Y., Noto, N., and Matsuno, S. Factors influencing the late results of operation for carcinoma of the pancreas. *Am. J. Surg.*, **136**, 582–586 (1978).
8.  Shipley, W. U., Nardi, G. L., Cohen, A. M., and Clifton Ling, C. Iodine-125 implant and external beam irradiation in patients with localized pancreatic carcinoma. *Cancer*, **45**, 709–714 (1980).
9.  Van Heerden, J. A. and ReMine, W. H. Total pancreatectomy for ductal adenocarcinoma of the pancreas. *Am. J. Surg.*, **142**, 308–311 (1981).
10. Warren, K. W., Christophi, C., Armendariz, R., and Basu, S. Current trends in the diagnosis and treatment of carcinoma of the pancreas. *Am. J. Surg.*, **145**, 813–818 (1983).

# RISK OF CARCINOMA AFTER
# PARTIAL GASTRECTOMY

# INTRODUCTORY REMARKS

Tomio HIROHATA

*Department of Public Health, School of Medicine, Kurume University**

The risk of carcinoma in the remnant stomach after partial gastrectomy has been the subject of controversy for the past 2–3 decades. This issue has been of great interest not only from an academic but also from a practical point of view, because the choice of surgical procedures may be affected if risk increase in the remnant stomach is real. Therefore, I believe the present panel discussion was very timely, and may shed new light on the subject with its current information from Japan and abroad. The first two reports of the panel were on human population studies and the remaining three were on laboratory investigations.

Dr. Domellöf from Sweden reported that ulcer patients with partial gastrectomy in Umeå had a high risk of developing carcinoma in the remnant stomach, and this was in concert with some other reports of Scandinavian countries. In contrast, Dr. Kuratsune of Japan reported that his series of partial gastrectomy patients showed no risk increase and, in fact, had a much lower risk than the general population. It is of course up to the readers to study the reports of these two distinguished investigators and draw their own conclusions. However, I may state my own views as additional reference information.

Some of the discrepancies between these two studies may appear to be more factual than they really are. Scandinavian countries are known to provide very favorable environments for long-term, say 20–30 years, follow-up studies because of the completeness of various registration systems. If risk increase is limited to those patients followed up for more than 17 years after surgery, as claimed by Dr. Domellöf, then his very long-term study would tend to show a higher risk on that account. Further, the patients were subjected to intensive endoscopic examinations and multiple biopsies, which must have inflated the observed number of gastric carcinoma cases. He was aware of this bias and tried to accommodate this in his analysis. In so doing, a large risk increase ($p=0.0002$) of male patients for the follow-up period of 17 or more years was greatly reduced and was barely statistically significant ($p=0.05$).

In contrast, Dr. Kuratsune and his associates found no increase but actually a decrease in mortality from gastric carcinoma among patients who had undergone a partial gastrectomy in Japan. Even those with Billroth II type gastrectomy, who were likely to be exposed to a more duodenogastric reflux, did not show a risk increase. One problem is that their study appears to be the first on this issue reported from Japan and further investigations among Japanese are needed to confirm their results. As is well known, gastric carcinoma is unusually prevalent in Japan. Mortality from this cause has decreased greatly among Japanese who immigrated to the United States and dietary habits are very suspect for the noted decline of this condition. Could it be possible that an inevitable change of dietary habits among patients after partial gastrectomy might have actually been beneficial and led to a decreased risk of gastric carcinoma? The points

* Asahi-machi 67, Kurume, Fukuoka 830, Japan (廣畑富雄).

described are only a few that must be considered. As proposed by Dr. Kuratsune, it may be desirable for a multidisciplinary group of experts to make a critical review of the issue utilizing studies available throughout the world.

In contrast to these two studies, laboratory investigations resulted in good agreement and only a few comments are needed. Drs. Kaibara and Koga from Japan presented the results of laboratory animal experiments on the relationship between operative procedures and the incidence of gastric carcinoma. The surgical procedures with greater duodenogastric reflux led to a higher incidence of gastric carcinoma in rats, and this finding was supported by *in vitro* test systems where bile acids clearly affected cell transformation. Dr. Kondo and his associates from Japan also presented results of animal experiments where surgical procedures led to a complete reflux of duodenal contents into the stomach of rats. It was clear that the development of gastric carcinoma was greatly related to exposure to the duodenal contents. Drs. Drasar and Cook from England reported colonization of bacteria in the stomach after surgical procedures, which might be associated with later development of gastric carcinoma. It may be emphasized that results of laboratory animal experiments, although very clear and impressive, did not necessarily indicate that human patients with partial gastrectomy sustained increased risk of gastric carcinoma, because of the difference in susceptibility and far less exposure to duodenal contents in humans.

In conclusion, I believe that this panel, with active participation from the audience, was very informative in exploring the issue of risk of carcinoma after partial gastrectomy.

# RISK OF CARCINOMA AFTER PARTIAL GASTRECTOMY

Lennart DOMELLÖF

*Division of Surgical Oncology, Department of*
*Surgery, University Hospital**

To learn whether gastric resection implies a greater risk for gastric carcinoma than is expected in non-operated ulcer patients, we performed a follow-up of 1,095 patients who underwent gastric resection and of 527 radiologically verified non-operated ulcer patients. The highest proportion of gastric cancer was found in operated males compared to non-operated males, however, the difference was not statistically different. Relative risk for carcinoma in males with and without risk-adjustment for the size of gastric resection was significantly increased after a 50% resection. When the male confidence limits corresponding to the observed *versus* the expected number of carcinomas (O/E ratio) was determined by time, a significant increase was found after 17 years. When analyzing the risk ratio compared to municipality controls, a significantly increased risk was present in males with duodenal ulcer operated before age 40γ. The risk was also increased in this group of younger males operated according to the Billroth II-principle. Younger males operated for gastric or duodenal ulcer should be offered screening starting 15–20 years postoperatively.

Carcinoma of the gastric remnant after an operation for benign ulcer disease was first described by Balfour in 1922 (*1*). During the following decades several case reports were published. From autopsy and retrospective clinical studies, an increased cancer incidence was claimed late after ulcer surgery (*11*, *12*). In 1972 Morgenstern and co-workers compiled 1,100 cases from the medical literature including several cases of their own (*16*). Even though they stressed that different opinions existed with regard to the risk of cancer development, they agreed to a slightly increased risk, when considering the general decline in stomach cancer. Over the following years endoscopical studies and work with experimental stomach cancer models added to our knowledge of pathophysiological events. Stump cancer was commonly regarded as a clinical entity and as an operation-sequel carcinoma (*5*, *16*). The prevalent view is that an interval of 5 years from the operation has to pass in order to rule out cancer not diagnosed at the time of ulcer surgery (*5*).

Recent studies with endoscopy have notified intestinogastric reflux, fecal bacterial flora, the concentration of nitrite and carcinogenic *N*-nitroso-compounds (*7*, *18*), or **postoperative mucosal changes such as atrophic gastritis with intestinal metaplasia** (*13*). These probably sequential alterations have in several cases been accompanied by inflammatory and neoplastic polyps, dysplasia, or cancer. Accordingly, many authors regard the resected stomach as a precancerous state and partially gastrectomized patients as a high risk group (*19*). However, others have not been able to confirm an increased

---

* S-901 85 Umeå, Sweden.

risk for cancer development (see Refs. *9, 17, 21*). The reason for this enduring discrepancy may be selection bias, dietary or geographical differences, and lack of proper controls such as non-operated ulcer patients. It is easy to be critical of follow-up studies after ulcer surgery, especially when we require well controlled long-term prospective studies. A decreased risk of cancer during the first 10 years may balance an increased risk during the next decades, indicating that clinical follow-up studies must be conducted during a sufficiently long time. Keeping this in mind, we have systematically followed up all patients partially gastrectomized for ulcer in Umeå. The cancer incidence in non-operated ulcer patients and the expected incidence from municipality based data have been used for the risk evaluation.

Based upon results achieved early during our follow-up we voiced concern that partial gastrectomy in male patients would result in an increased risk for later cancer in the retained stump (*6*). Accordingly, we feel obliged to report on our current experience of the prospective study, including endoscopic surveillance, in a 10 year perspective.

## Prospective Study Design

Starting in 1973 we performed a follow-up of all patients operated during the period 1952–1969 for benign peptic ulcer at the Department of Surgery in Umeå. Patients with less common benign disorders such as gastric polyps or patients submitted to gastro-enterostomy with or without vagotomy, have been excluded. The total number of patients with a follow-up time of 6 years or more was 1095.

Histological diagnosis of the resected stomach was available in 97.8% and was compared with the operation records. All operation records were thoroughly checked. Partial gastrectomy always implied that at least 50% and in males often 75% of the stomach was resected. Billroth I-operation (BI) was performed in 318 patients (193 males, 125 females). In this group the mean follow-up time was 16.8 years and the person years at risk 5,332. Gastric ulcer was present in 146 patients (49.5%), duodenal ulcer in 140 (44%), combined or pyloric ulcer in 27, and not distinctly stated diagnosis in 5. The mean age at surgery was 52.5 years (range 19–78). Endoscopies with multiple biopsies were performed in 179 cases (56%).

Billroth II-operation with Braun's enteroanastomosis (BII) was performed in 777 patients (599 males, 178 females). The mean follow-up time was 22 years and the person years at risk 17,126. Gastric ulcer was the cause of the operation in 214 cases (27.5%), duodenal ulcer in 486 (62.5%), pyloric or combined ulcers in 55, gastritis in 3, and not distinctly stated disease in 19. The mean age at surgery was 47.7 years (range 18–76). Endoscopies with biopsies were performed in 354 patients (45.6%).

The observed number of stomach cancers after partial gastrectomy was compared with the expected number, estimated from municipality based age specific incidence data in the regional cancer registry.

Radiologically verified, non-operated ulcer patients from the period 1960–1966 surviving 6 years or more, were also used as controls: 267 with gastric ulcer (131 males, 136 females) and 260 duodenal ulcer patients (175 males, 85 females). The mean follow-up time was 17.9 and 19 years, respectively. The total person years at risk were 4,773 and 4,945, respectively. All patients were checked with the National Cancer Registry in order to obtain information of possible cancers in the individuals who relocated to other regions.

## Statistical Evaluation

Confidence limits corresponding to the observed *versus* the expected number of carcinomas (O/E ratio) were obtained using the procedure based on Fisher's exact test.

At the estimation of relative risk for developing cancer, operated and non-operated individuals were compared in subgroups according to operation method and ulcer disease. The occurrence of carcinomas can be considered as Poisson-distributed over time. The probability that an operated patient will get a stump carcinoma was estimated as a function of age. A maximum likelihood estimation was performed under the restriction of non-decreasing probability with increasing age (2).

## Present Occurrence of Gastric Cancer

Gastric stump cancer was observed in 21 cases, 5 after BI and 16 after B II-operation. The male: female ratio was 20: 1. Ten males and 1 female had gastric ulcer as primary disease. Four cancers were diagnosed in the non-operated gastric ulcer controls (2 males, 2 females), and 1 male stomach cancer was found in the duodenal ulcer group. The time interval between operation or ulcer diagnosis to cancer was 10–26 years. As of this writing 424 of all patients (40%) have been followed until death and nearly half of these have been examined at routine autopsy. The evaluation and vital status are as of June 15, 1984. Totally 533 patients (48.7%) have been checked with endoscopy, 110 (21%) once, 423 (79%) two times or more, 268 (50%) three times or more, and 162 (30%) with four or more examinations. Stump cancer was found in 9 of these patients (5 early carcinomas). The highest proportion of gastric cancer, 10/240 (4.2%) was found in males operated for gastric ulcer compared to non-operated males 2/131 (1.5%). In males operated for duodenal ulcer, cancer was present in 9/474 cases (1.9%) compared to 1/ 175 (0.6%) in non-operated males. The risk in the operated *versus* non-operated patients was not significantly different. However, this estimation was performed under the assumption of a constant risk over time.

Assuming that ulcer surgery might reduce the risk for later cancer development, proportional to the area of resection, this hypothesis was tested after 50 and 75% resections (Table I). When compared with non-operated ulcer patients it was shown that the

TABLE I. Estimation of Relative Risk for Carcinoma in Males with and without Risk-Adjustment for the Size of Gastric Resection[a]

| All operated *vs.* non-operated | Relative risk | | | 95% confidence limits | | | *p*-value | | |
|---|---|---|---|---|---|---|---|---|---|
| | 100% risk | 50% risk | 25% risk | 100% risk | 50% risk | 25% risk | 100% risk | 50% risk | 25% risk |
| Gastric ulcer | 2.5 | 5.0 | 10.0 | 0.53, 11.7 | 1.1, 23.5 | 2.1, 47.0 | N.S. | 0.04 | 0.003 |
| Duodenal ulcer | 2.9 | 5.8 | 11.6 | 0.35, 23.9 | 0.7, 47.8 | 1.4, 95.6 | N.S. | N.S. | 0.02 |
| Gastric and duodenal ulcer | 2.4 | 4.8 | 9.5 | 0.69, 8.3 | 1.4, 16.6 | 2.8, 33.2 | N.S. | 0.01 | 0.0004 |

[a] Testing of the hypothesis of a reduced risk proportional to a 50% and a three-quarter resection.

TABLE II.   Observed and Expected Number of Patients with
Carcinoma after Partial Gastrectomy

| Years post-operatively O/E | Results in 1977 (Ref. 6) | | | | Years post-operatively O/E | Present results (June 1984) | | | |
|---|---|---|---|---|---|---|---|---|---|
| | Male | Female | Total | p | | Male | Female | Total | p |
| 0–8 years | 0/2.5 | 0/0.8 | 0/3.3 | N.S. | 0–9 years | 0/4.3 (p=0.03) | 0/1.2 | 0/5.5 | 0.008 |
| 9–11 years[a] | 1.7/2 | 0/0.4 | 2/2.1 | N.S. | 10–16 years[a] | 4/4.7 | 0/1.1 | 4/5.8 | N.S. |
| ≧12 years | 11/4 (p=0.006) | 1/0.7 | 12/4.7 | 0.007 | ≧17 years | 16/5.2 (p=0.0002) | 1/1 | 17/6.2 | 0.0006 |

[a] Time interval in which the risk ratio became less than 1.

relative risk was significantly increased in male patients after a 50% resection and BI or BII anastomoses (p=0.01 and 0.02).

When the male O/E was determined by time, a significant increase was found after 17 years (p=0.0002) (Table II). As 5 early gastric cancers were found at the endoscopical follow-up, this O/E ratio was calculated with the assumption that these carcinomas were detected 5 years earlier, the p-value being 0.05.

When analyzing the risk ratio compared to municipality controls, a significantly increased risk (p=0.02) was present in males with duodenal ulcer operated before the age of 40. The O/E ratio was 4/0.78 (1.397–13.130, 95% confidence limits). The risk was also increased (borderline) in males of this age group operated for gastric ulcer, the O/E ratio being 2/0.24 (1.009–30.103, 95% confidence limits). Furthermore, the risk ratio was significantly increased (p=0.01) in males operated according to BII before the age of 40. The O/E ratio was 5/0.96 (1.692–12.154, 95% confidence limits).

*Risk Evaluation*

It has been claimed that "gastric cancer is no more common among patients with prior gastric surgery for peptic ulcer disease than among members of the population at large" (17) and that the size of an increased risk is only one argument against screening after gastric surgery (14). It is noteworthy that neither the fact that partial gastrectomy conceivably reduces the target area for cancer development, nor the lower cancer risk in non-operated duodenal ulcer patients have been taken into consideration. Our results from a prospective cohort study show a significantly increased proportion of cancer in males younger than 40 years when operated for gastric or duodenal ulcer or when operated according to the BII principle when compared to municipality controls. This may reflect an increased risk, most likely mediated through promotion by bile reflux. Moreover, when compared with non-operated gastric or duodenal ulcer patients a 5- to 10-fold increase in relative risk was found under the assumption that surgery might exert a protective effect by removing the most cancer-prone distal part of the stomach.

The estimated annual incidence of carcinoma was 10 times higher in operated males aged 50 to 55 years compared to the general male population in the region (Fig. 1). This finding is in accordance with our previous results (4) and supported by Eriksson and coworkers from the south of Sweden (8).

Age is difinitely of crucial importance in the risk evaluation. We have to consider the well-known fact that duodenal ulcer occurs at an earlier age than gastric ulcer. Ac-

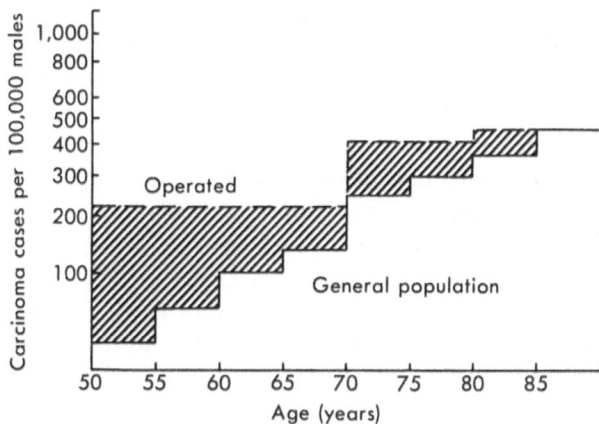

FIG. 1. Estimated annual probability for gastric carcinoma in operated males and in the general male population in the county of Väterbotten.

cordingly, we have found that duodenal ulcer patients are about 7 years younger at partial gastrectomy. Furthermore, the difference in sex ratio has been reconfirmed. Thus the male predominance in our stump cancer material is about 4 times the estimated. This may be surprising as males with duodenal ulcer frequently were submitted to three-quarter resections leaving a very small gastric residue. Consequently, we feel strongly that subgroups at risk can be identified by age, sex, and ulcer disease.

It should be emphasized that the final risk in the cohort remains to be established as most of the patients are still alive. Moreover, the effects of the present annual decline in stomach cancer in Sweden of about 3% have to be accounted for.

Our previous and present results are very similar. Thus, we found an early protective effect during the first 8–9 years after partial gastrectomy (Table II). However, this was balanced by a significant increase in the O/E ratio after 17 years or more. The increase by time from gastrectomy was pointed out by Stalsberg and Taksdal in 1971 (20) and has been confirmed by several studies. It is of interest to note that the time from operation to development of stump cancer is similar to the time lag suggested by Fujita (10) for a single neoplastic cell to grow into manifest cancer. The process of initiation may have occurred prior to or after partial gastrectomy. However, the operation is inevitably followed by a reduction in mucosal height and a number of degenerative histological alterations. Thus, provided that the initiation has taken place, the surrounding cells may not be capable of restraining a neoplastic cell from proliferating in the presence of sufficient stimuli (3).

The relevance of our findings might be restricted to certain geographical areas. However, in Scandinavia cancer of the resected stomach has become an increasing problem. The National Cancer Registry in Norway is probably unique in having a special code for previous gastric surgery. Thus it is important to note that Lund of Norway (15) has shown increased rates of gastric cancer in all age groups of operated males and females and decreased rates in non-operated individuals.

Partial gastrectomy still is the most common operation procedure for ulcer disease (4). Being so, and stimulated by the relatively high proportion of early gastric carcinomas diagnosed at endoscopy in these patients, we find careful endoscopic surveillance justified in certain high risk groups and areas. Needless to say, patients with symptoms should be examined by endoscopy. Furthermore, younger males operated for duodenal or gastric ulcer should be offered screening starting from 15–20 years postoperatively.

Many questions concerning cancer development in the operated stomach are not yet resolved. Key factors such as genetically determined mucosal protection and differences in diet or abuse have to be studied. Thus, by analyzing the geographical differences in risk ratio, these factors could be further elucidated, adding to a better understanding of the pathophysiology and hopefully the prevention of stomach cancer.

*Acknowledgments*

This work has been performed in collaboration with K. G. Janunger, M. D., Ph.D., K. Edin, M. D., S. Eriksson, M. D., and R. Stenling, M. D., Ph.D. It was supported by grants from the Swedish Cancer Society, project numbers 797-10XC and 797-11X.

## REFERENCES

1.  Balfour, D. C. Factors influencing the life expectancy of patients operated for gastric ulcer. *Ann. Surg.*, **76**, 405–408 (1922).
2.  Barlow, R. E., Bartholomew, D. J., Bremner, J. M., and Brunk, H. D. "Statistical Inference under Order Restriction" (1972). John Wiley, New York.
3.  Berenblum I. "Carcinogenesis as a Biological Problem" (1974). North Holland-American Elsevier, New York.
4.  Chan, M. and Kay, C. S. A prospective study of proximal gastric vagotomy and Polya gastrectomy for the treatment of duodenal ulcer in Chinese: an interim report. *Southeast Asian J. Surg.*, **5**, 52 (1982).
5.  Dahm, K. and Rehner, M. "Das Karzinoms im Operierten Magen" (1975). Georg Thieme Verlag, Stuttgart.
6.  Domellöf, L. and Janunger, K. G. The risk for gastric carcinoma after partial gastrectomy. *Am. J. Surg.*, **134**, 581–584 (1977).
7.  Domellöf, L., Reddy, B. S., and Weisburger, J. H. Microflora and deconjugation of bile acids in alkaline reflux after gastrectomy. *Am. J. Surg.*, **140**, 291–295 (1980).
8.  Eriksson, S.B.S. The operated stomach. Thesis. Bulletin No. 36 from the Department of Surgery, University of Lund (1983).
9.  Fischer, A. B., Graem, N., and Jensen, O. M. Risk of gastric cancer after Billroth II-resection for duodenal ulcer. *Br. J. Surg.*, **70**, 552–554 (1983).
10. Fujita, S. Kinetics of cellular proliferation and growth of human cancers. *In* "Cancer", ed. T. Sugimura and Y. Yamamura (1976). Iwanami Publ. Co., Tokyo.
11. Griesser, G. and Schmidt, H. Statistische Erhebungen über die Häufigkeit des Karzinoms nach Magenoperationen wegen eines Geschwürsleidens. *Med. Welt.*, **35**, 1836–1840 (1964).
12. Helsingen, N. and Hillestad, L. Cancer development in the gastric stump after partial gastrectomy for ulcer. *Ann. Surg.*, **143**, 173–179 (1956).
13. Janunger, K. G., Domellöf, L., and Eriksson, S. The development of mucosal changes after gastric surgery for ulcer disease. *Scand. J. Gastroenterol.*, **13**, 217–223 (1978).
14. Logan, R.F.A. and Langman, M.J.S. Screening for gastric cancer after gastric surgery. *Lancet*, **ii**, 667–670 (1984).
15. Lund, E. Gastric cancer after gastric surgery; an increasing problem in Norway. *Lancet*, **ii**, 973 (1983); personal communication (1984).
16. Morgenstern, L., Yamakawa, T., and Seltzer D. Carcinoma of the gastric stump. *Am. J. Surg.*, **125**, 29–37 (1973).
17. Schafter, L. W., Larson, D. E., Melton, L. J., Higgins, J. A., and Ilstrup, D. M. The risk

of gastric carcinoma after surgical treatment for benign ulcer disease. *New Engl. J. Med.*, **309**, 1210–1213 (1983).

18. Schlag, P., Böcklar, R., Ulrich, H., Peter M., Merkle, P., and Herfarth, C. Are nitrite and N-nitroso compounds in gastric juice risk factors for carcinoma in the operated stomach? *Lancet*, **i**, 727–729 (1980).

19. Siurala, M., Lawson, H. H., Morson, B. C., and Dahm, K. The resected stomach—its dynamics and premalignant properties. Symposium. 7th World Congr. Gastroenterol., *OMGE Bull.*, **18**, 15–16 (1983).

20. Stalsberg, H. and Taksdal, S. Stomach cancer following gastric surgery for benign conditions. *Lancet*, **ii**, 1175–1177 (1971).

21. Tokudome, S., Kono, S., Ikeda, M., Kuratsune, M., Sano, C., Inokuchi, K., Kodama, Y., Ischimiya, H., Kanayama, F., Kaibara, N., Koga, S., Yamada, H., Ikejiri, T., Oka, N., and Tsurumaru, H. A prospective study on primary gastric stump cancer following partial gastrectomy for benign gastroduodenal diseases. *Cancer Res.*, **44**, 2208–2212 (1984).

# MORTALITY FROM CANCER AFTER PARTIAL GASTRECTOMY IN JAPAN

Masanori Kuratsune,[*1] Kiyoshi Inokuchi,[*2] Ryunosuke Kumashiro,[*2] and Shinkan Tokudome[*3]

*Department of Food and Nutrition, Nakamura Gakuen College,[*1] Department of Surgery II, Faculty of Medicine, Kyushu University,[*2] and Department of Community Health Science, Saga Medical School[*3]*

A cohort analysis was made on the cancer deaths seen among 3,827 patients partially gastrectomized for benign gastroduodenal diseases. The patients were followed up from the time of surgery (from 1948 to 1970) to June 30, 1981, the average follow-up period being 16.3 years. Of 3,701 patients (96.7%), the vital status at the end of observation was determined, the total person-years at risk being 62,286. The observed deaths were compared with the expected deaths calculated from the mortality rates of Japan. The observed and expected deaths from primary gastric stump cancer which were calculated for the patients surviving 10 years or more after gastrectomy were 11 and 52.85, respectively, an O/E ratio of 0.21 ($p < 0.01$). Thus, contrary to some other authors, we observed a much reduced mortality from cancer of the remnant stomach. Possible biases which might be involved in our study were carefully considered, and hardly any serious ones found. A need for examining possible difference in operation procedures used by various authors was then suggested. A proposal was made to UICC and IARC to set up a workshop to critically examine and evaluate all the published papers dealing with the risk of remnant stomach cancer. A significantly elevated mortality from cancer of the lung and liver and from liver cirrhosis was also observed among our cases. A similar significantly elevated mortality from cancer of the colon and the rectum was observed among those operated on by Billroth II with retrocolic anastomosis but without Braun's anastomosis. Thus, not only the remnant stomach but also other organs must be considered for possible excess risk of cancer after partial gastrectomy.

The risk of cancer in the remnant stomach following partial gastrectomy has been reported to have increased by some European authors (*2, 5, 8, 14*), but others could not confirm this (*1, 3, 4, 6, 10, 12, 13, 15, 16*). Since only a few studies (*16*) have been made on this important issue in Japan where gastrectomy is commonly practiced, we analyzed the mortality from cancer of the remnant stomach as well as cancer at other sites among patients who had undergone partial gastrectomy for benign gastroduodenal diseases. Our findings (*15*) were quite different from those reported by others. They will be outlined here again and discussed from several relevant points of view.

---

[*1] Befu 5-7-1, Jyonan-ku, Fukuoka 814, Japan (倉恒国徳).
[*2] Maidashi 3-1-1, Higashi-ku, Fukuoka 812, Japan (井口　潔, 神代龍之介).
[*3] Nabeshima-cho, Saga 840-01, Japan (徳留信寛).

*Our Study*

Altogether 3,827 patients who had been partially gastrectomized from 1948 to 1970 were followed from the time of gastrectomy to the date of death or to the end of June, 1981. The average observation period was 16.3 years and the total person-years at risk 62,286. The patients were predominantly males (83%) and 53% of them had been operated on by Billroth II without Braun's anastomosis, about 39% by Billroth I, and about 8% by Billroth II with Braun's anastomosis. They had been operated on for gastric and/or duodenal ulcer (84%) and for polyp, gastritis, and other conditions (16%). Histological examination of the resected stomach had been done for 63% of them.

The vital status of all the subjects was determined by referring to the city, town, or village office of their *honseki*, that is, permanent address. For the deceased, death certificates were requested from the District Legal Affairs Bureau. Patients lost to follow-up were observed up to the date last known alive. When this date was unknown, they were assumed to be alive up to the end of observation. The observed number of deaths from cancer at a specific site was compared with the expected number of deaths which was calculated by multiplying the patients' age-, sex-, calendar year-, and operative procedure specific person-years at risk by sex- and age-specific mortality rates for the specific cancer in 1955, 1960, 1965, 1970, and 1975 in Japan. The O/E ratio was calculated and the difference was statistically tested by Poisson distribution.

Sixty-eight percent of the subjects were confirmed to be alive and 28% to be dead, with the status of 3% unknown as of June 30, 1981; thus the follow-up loss was reasonably small. The observed and expected deaths from all causes numbered respectively 938 and 930.97 for males and 146 and 156.29 for females. The O/E ratios were close to unity. O/E ratio for cancer at all sites was 0.95 for both males and females. Neither excess nor reduced mortality was seen with any statistical significance.

The observed and expected number of deaths from stomach cancer for both sexes was 34 and 100.63, the difference being very statistically significant. Patients operated on by Billroth I or by Billroth II without Braun's anastomosis showed similar small O/E ratios, 0.31 and 0.29, respectively. The O/E ratio for those operated on by Billroth II with Braun's anastomosis was also smaller than unity but not significantly so. Similar facts were seen for males and females but were statistically significant only for males.

To select primary gastric stump cancer cases, a postoperative time interval of 10

TABLE I.   Observed and Expected Number of Deaths from Primary Gastric Stump Cancer by Operation Type for Patients Surviving 10 Years or More after Partial Gastrectomy

| Operation type | Male | | | Female | | | Total | | |
|---|---|---|---|---|---|---|---|---|---|
| | Observed No. of deaths | Expected No. of deaths | O/E ratio | Observed No. of deaths | Expected No. of deaths | O/E ratio | Observed No. of deaths | Expected No. of deaths | O/E ratio |
| BI | 3 | 18.80 | 0.16** | 2 | 2.15 | 0.93 | 5 | 20.95 | 0.24** |
| BII, B(+)[a] | 2 | 3.13 | 0.64 | 0 | 0.42 | 0 | 2 | 3.55 | 0.56 |
| BII, B(−)[a] | 4 | 25.54 | 0.16** | 0 | 2.81 | 0 | 4 | 28.35 | 0.14** |
| Total | 9 | 47.47 | 0.19** | 2 | 5.38 | 0.37 | 11 | 52.85 | 0.21** |

[a]   With or without Braun's anastomosis.
**   Significant at $p < 0.01$ (2-tailed).
From Ref. *15*.

TABLE II. Observed and Expected Number of Deaths from Cancer at Various Sites

| Organ involved | Deaths | Male | Female | Total |
|---|---|---|---|---|
| Esophagus | Observed | 7 | 0 | 7 |
| | Expected | 10.97 | 0.70 | 11.67 |
| | O/E | 0.64 | 0 | 0.60 |
| Intestine and colon | Observed | 11 | 2 | 13 |
| | Expected | 6.09 | 1.44 | 7.53 |
| | O/E | 1.81 | 1.39 | 1.73 |
| Rectum | Observed | 13 | 2 | 15 |
| | Expected | 7.48 | 1.36 | 8.84 |
| | O/E | 1.74 | 1.47 | 1.70 |
| Liver | Observed | 46 | 1 | 47 |
| | Expected | 18.22 | 2.30 | 20.52 |
| | O/E | 2.52** | 0.43 | 2.29** |
| Lung | Observed | 36 | 5 | 41 |
| | Expected | 26.30 | 2.11 | 28.41 |
| | O/E | 1.37 | 2.37 | 1.44* |
| Pancreas | Observed | 3 | 1 | 4 |
| | Expected | 7.95 | 1.32 | 9.27 |
| | O/E | 0.38 | 0.75 | 0.43 |

\* Significant at 5% level (two-tailed).
\*\* Significant at 1% level (two-tailed).
From Ref. 7.

years was arbitrarily set not only to exclude recurrent, remaining, or multiple cancer but also to allow a latency period for development of a new cancer. For comparison, the expected number of deaths from stomach cancer was calculated based upon the population at risk who survived 10 years or more after the operation. As shown in Table I, the observed number of deaths from primary gastric stump cancer for both sexes was 11, which was only one fifth the expected number of deaths. Similarly, very small O/E ratios were observed for those operated on by Billroth I or Billroth II without Braun's anastomosis. The ratio was also smaller than unity for those operated on by Billroth II with Braun's anastomosis but statistically not significant. When the subjects were divided by sex, male patients again showed very similar O/E ratios but the females showed no definite trend probably due to the limited number of deaths. All these facts indicate that mortality from gastric stump cancer was not elevated but rather much reduced among our series of partially gastrectomized patients. This is quite contrary to the findings reported by some Scandinavian authors (2, 5, 8, 14).

A significantly increased mortality from liver cancer was observed among patients, O/E ratio being 2.29 for the combined sexes and 2.52 for males (Table II). Both ratios significantly differ from unity. For females, however, no excess mortality was indicated. It is also interesting to note that the O/E ratio for liver cirrhosis was also significantly increased for the combined sexes and for males, being 1.79 and 1.76, respectively. An elevated O/E ratio was also seen for females but was statistically not significant. At present, we suspect that these excess mortalities from liver diseases might be connected with hepatitis from which patients tended to suffer after gastrectomy. A slight but significantly increased mortality from lung cancer was also observed among the patients. For cancer of the intestine and colon, an excess mortality was observed for both sexes, males, and females, but without statistical significance (Table II). When the patients

TABLE III.   Observed and Expected Number of Deaths from Colon and
Rectal Cancer and O/E Ratios by Operation Type

| Operation procedure | Deaths | Colon cancer | | | Rectal cancer | | |
|---|---|---|---|---|---|---|---|
| | | Male | Female | Total | Male | Female | Total |
| Billroth I | Observed | 2 | 0 | 2 | 4 | 2 | 6 |
| | Expected | 2.53 | 0.66 | 3.19 | 3.10 | 0.62 | 3.72 |
| | O/E | 0.79 | 0 | 0.63 | 1.29 | 3.21 | 1.61 |
| Billroth II | Observed | 9 | 2 | 11 | 9 | 0 | 9 |
| | Expected | 3.57 | 0.78 | 4.35 | 4.38 | 0.74 | 5.12 |
| | O/E | 2.52* | 2.56 | 2.53* | 2.05 | 0 | 1.76 |
| Retro, Braun (−) | Observed | 5 | 2 | 7 | 8 | 0 | 8 |
| | Expected | 2.24 | 0.51 | 2.75 | 2.72 | 0.48 | 3.20 |
| | O/E | 2.23 | 3.95 | 2.55* | 2.94* | 0 | 2.50* |
| Ante, Braun (−) | Observed | 2 | 0 | 2 | 0 | 0 | 0 |
| | Expected | 0.93 | 0.18 | 1.11 | 1.17 | 0.17 | 1.34 |
| | O/E | 2.15 | 0 | 1.80 | 0 | 0 | 0 |
| Ante, Braun (+) | Observed | 2 | 0 | 2 | 1 | 0 | 1 |
| | Expected | 0.40 | 0.09 | 0.49 | 0.49 | 0.09 | 0.58 |
| | O/E | 5.05 | 0 | 4.08 | 2.05 | 0 | 1.72 |
| Total | Observed | 11 | 2 | 13 | 13 | 2 | 15 |
| | Expected | 6.09 | 1.44 | 7.53 | 7.48 | 1.36 | 8.84 |
| | O/E | 1.81 | 1.39 | 1.73 | 1.74 | 1.47 | 1.70 |

* Significant at $p < 0.05$.
From Ref. 7.

were divided according to operation type, no excess mortality was seen for those operated on by Billroth I, but a significantly higher mortality was observed for those operated on by Billroth II (Table III). Such excess mortality was seen for both males and females, but only the excess for the former was statistically significant. Furthermore, those undergoing Billroth II gastrectomy were divided by anastomosis type. Most of the O/E ratios calculated for the combined sexes and for males were larger than unity but only the ratio for those operated on with retrocolic anastomosis but without Braun's anastomosis was significantly larger than unity. For rectal cancer, O/E ratios for the combined sexes, males, and females were all larger than unity but none of them significantly so. When the patients were divided according to operation type, O/E ratios were all larger than unity for the combined sexes and for males but only the ratio for those gastrectomized with retrocolic anastomosis but without Braun's anastomosis was significantly elevated. Thus, an increased mortality from cancer of the intestine and colon and the rectum was seen for patients operated on by a specific gastrectomy procedure but no conclusive remarks can be made because the observed number of deaths from these cancers was fairly small. However, these facts suggest that not only the risk of cancer of the remnant stomach but also that of cancer at other sites must be adequately examined to evaluate the possible risk after partial gastrectomy.

## DISCUSSION

Why did our study observe a greatly reduced mortality from cancer of the remnant stomach among partially gastrectomized Japanese patients, quite in contrast to other studies so far reported (2, 5, 8, 14)? The following aspects must be considered.

## 1. Possible biases

Observational epidemiologic studies are often liable to various kinds of bias and our study may be no exception. Since neither reduced nor increased overall mortality or overall cancer mortality was observed in these studies, although significantly increased mortality was observed for cancer at certain sites, systematic biases cannot really be suspected in our study, particularly in the detection of deaths and the collection of information. However, a slight bias may be involved in our sampling of cases, because 77% of our series of patients were those operated on at university hospitals which very poor patients known to be more prone to gastric cancer usually are not able to visit. Therefore, the gastric cancer risk among our cases might be lower than the national average. However, such possible selection bias can hardly explain our finding of markedly reduced mortality from gastric stump cancer, because the socioeconomic gradient of gastric cancer is not so large (11) and extremely poor patients who are unable to visit university hospitals are very limited in number. Thus, we could find no serious biases in our study which could explain the present findings.

It is interesting to note that most of the studies designed and undertaken with adequate epidemiologic caution have shown hardly any excess risk of gastric stump cancer (3, 6, 12, 13, 15). They describe the technical details of their studies so that they can be well understood. Unfortunately, however, most of those reporting increased risk are difficult to understand mainly due to their lack of detailed methodology explanation. Explanation of the comparability of the gastrectomized group and the control group, observation period, calculation of expected cancer risk, type of risk (mortality, incidence, or prevalence), uniformity in detection of cancer cases or cancer deaths between the patient group and the control group, sampling of cases and controls, or collection of information from cases and controls, is often lacking making it very hard to compare their findings with ours.

## 2. Better health care of patients

Partially gastrectomized patients are probably more concerned about their own health than are most other persons. They must be more careful about diet and nutrition in particular. This greater health consciousness decreases the risk of stomach cancer after the operation. They probably visit a good hospital whenever they feel something wrong with their stomach just as they did when they had benign gastroduodenal disease. This, of course, leads to early detection of gastric stump cancer. Since stomach cancer is so prevalent in Japan and the medical profession and related institutions including public health centers throughout the country are so concerned about its early detection, even gastrectomized patients who live in remote areas can enjoy such medical care. Furthermore, particular caution is exercised in checking for gastric stump cancer by doctors whenever they examine the remnant stomach. All these aspects lower the mortality from cancer of the remnant stomach among partially gastrectomized patients, at least in part contributing to our present findings.

## 3. Extent of partial gastrectomy

The fact that even among the studies reported by Scandinavian authors there is a distinct discrepancy in regard to the risk of gastric stump cancer (2–5, 8, 10, 14) strongly suggests a possible technical difference in the gastrectomy they practice, for instance, in the extent of the stomach resection. This has already been expressed by two of us (9) and by Professor Shigemasa Koga, Faculty of Medicine, Tottori University (S. Koga, personal communication). A mutual exchange of expert gastroenterologists between our hospitals and those where an excess risk of gastric stump cancer has been observed might well help to resolve this question.

*Proposal*

Partial gastrectomy is widely practiced throughout the world. The question whether or not the operation increases the cancer risk of the remnant stomach is crucially important and urgently requires solution. Since quite a few reports on this issue have already been published and their findings are unfortunately quite diverse, we would like to propose that the International Union Against Cancer and the International Agency for Research on Cancer set up a workshop which will critically examine and evaluate all these reports. It is recommended that such workshop be composed of experienced epidemiologists, biostatisticians, surgeons, internists, and other specialists who have not been involved in the present controversial issue.

## REFERENCES

1.  Denck, H. and Salzer, G. 21 Yahre Ulcuschirurgie an der Klinik Denk in Wien. 1933–1954. *Gastroenterologia*, **83**, 94–109 (1957).
2.  Domellöf, L. and Janunger, K.-G. The risk for gastric carcinoma after partial gastrectomy. *Am. J. Surg.*, **134**, 581–584 (1977).
3.  Fischer, A. B., Graem, N., and Jensen, O. M. Risk of gastric cancer after Billroth II resection for duodenal ulcer. *Br. J. Surg.*, **70**, 552–554 (1983).
4.  Hakkiluoto, A. Long-term follow-up study of patients operated on for benign peptic ulcer. *Ann. Chir. Gynaecol.*, **65**, 361–368 (1976).
5.  Helsingen, N. and Hillestad, L. Cancer development in the gastric stump after partial gastrectomy for ulcer. *Ann. Surg.*, **143**, 173–179 (1956).
6.  Hirohata, T. Mortality from gastric cancer and other causes after medical or surgical treatment for gastric ulcer. *J. Natl. Cancer Inst.*, **41**, 895–908 (1968).
7.  Inokuchi, K., Tokudome, S., Ikeda, M., Kuratsune, M., Ichimiya, H., Kaibara, N., Ikejiri, T., and Oka, N. Mortality from carcinoma after partial gastrectomy. *Gann*, **75**, 588–594 (1984).
8.  Krause, U. Late prognosis after partial gastrectomy for ulcer. *Acta Chir. Scand.*, **114**, 341–354 (1958).
9.  Kumashiro, R. and Inokuchi, K. Is the remnant stomach after partial gastretomy more prone to cancer? *In* "A Prospect of Studies on Cancer of the Digestive Tract" (in Japanese), ed. K. Inokuchi and H. Sugano, pp. 255–261 (1984). Gann to Kagakuryoho Sha, Tokyo.
10. Liavaag, K. Cancer development in gastric stump after partial gastrectomy for peptic ulcer. *Ann. Surg.*, **155**, 103–106 (1962).
11. Logan, W.P.D. Social class variations in mortality. *Publ. Health Rep.*, **69**, 1217–1223 (1954).
12. Ross, A.H.M., Smith, M. A., Anderson, J. R., and Small, W. P. Late mortality after surgery for peptic ulcer. *New Engl. J. Med.* **307**, 519–522 (1982).
13. Schafer, L. W., Larson, D. E., Melton, L. J., III, Higgins, J. A., and Ilstrup, D. M. The risk of gastric carcinoma after surgical treatment for benign ulcer disease. A population-based study in Olmsted county, Minnesota. *New Engl. J. Med.*, **309**, 1210–1213 (1983).

14. Stalsberg, H. and Taksdal, S. Stomach cancer following gastric surgery for benign conditions. *Lancet*, **ii**, 1175–1177 (1971).
15. Tokudome, S., Kono, S., Ikeda, M., Kuratsune, M., Sano, C., Inokuchi, K., Kodama, Y., Ichimiya, H., Nakayama, F., Kaibara, N., Koga, S., Yamada, H., Ikejiri, T., Oka, N., and Tsurumaru, H. A prospective study on primary gastric stump cancer following partial gastrectomy for benign gastroduodenal diseases. *Cancer Res.*, **44**, 2208–2212 (1984).
16. Yoshikawa, K. Study on high risk groups for gastric cancer. *In* "Reports of Studies Supported by Grants for Cancer Research from the Ministry of Health and Welfare" (in Japanese), pp. 443–445 (1978). National Cancer Center, Tokyo.

# INTESTINAL BACTERIA AND THE INITIATION
# OF CANCER

B. S. Drasar and P.G.S. Cook

*Department of Medical Microbiology, London School
of Hygiene and Tropical Medicine\**

Colonisation of the gastrointestinal tract by bacteria seems to render those areas colonised liable to develop cancer. Colonisation of the intestine stimulates the normal growth of mucosal cells. Turnover of intestinal cells is faster in conventional than germ free animals, thus more cells are exposed to any mutagenic/carcinogenic agent and there is a greater chance of transformation occurring. Diet, the intestinal flora, and other aspects of the chemical environment have all been implicated; though particular factors have been enthusiastically canvassed no general agreement has been reached. The magnitude of the bacterial contribution to the initiation of cancers cannot at present be quantified, in part because of the technical problems of investigating intestinal bacteria. The possibility remains, however, that bacterial action is a major cause of cancer.

Cancers of the gastrointestinal tract are among the more numerous malignant conditions. Gastrointestinal tumours are an important cause of morbidity and mortality throughout the world. The location of tumours within the gut is different in different societies. Indeed a low incidence of stomach cancer together with a high incidence of colonic and rectal cancers may be regarded as characteristic of a consumer orientated society. Cancer of the stomach seems to occur more frequently in traditional societies while small intestinal lymphoma with a chain disease has some links with poverty and environmental contamination. The cause of gastrointestinal tumours remains obscure though various theories have been put forward.

Diet, the intestinal flora, and other aspects of the chemical environment have all been implicated; though particular factors have been enthusiastically canvased no general agreement has been reached. Among dietary factors fibre and fat have proved very popular.

Intestinal tumours usually occur in those parts of intestine that are normally or have become colonised with bacteria. Environmental chemicals, food additives and endogenous substrates may all be sources of carcinogens (Table I).

In this paper the role of the intestinal flora in the causation of cancer of the stomach, small intestinal lymphoma with a chain disease, and large bowel cancer is discussed. The role of the intestinal bacteria has been most extensively investigated for cancers of the colon and rectum, but it may be that these studies provide insights applicable to other tumours. The basic hypothesis is that the intestinal bacteria are able to produce carcinogens and that this process may be modified by the influence of diet on the flora (1).

---

\* Keppel Street (Gower Street), London WC1E 7HT, U.K.

TABLE I.    Some Potential Sources of Intestinal Mutagens and Carcinogens
Whose Action May Be Mediated by Bacteria in the Intestine

| Source | Substrate | Mutagen/carcinogen | Reference |
|---|---|---|---|
| Endogenous | Tyrosine | Phenol | 24 |
| | Trypotophan | Indole | |
| | Methionine | Ethionine | |
| | Biochonin A | Gentistein | |
| | Furmentonetin | Claidzein | |
| | Bile acids | Aromatic hydrocarbons | 16, 17 |
| | Cholesterol | Cholesterol epoxide | |
| | Biliary conjugates | Retoxified products | 18 |
| Natural products | Cereals | Alklaoid breakdown products | 24 |
| | Pyrrolizidine | Methylazoxymethonel | |
| | Ether alkaloid | | |
| | Cycasin | Methylazoxymethanol | |
| | Amygdalin | Mandelonitrile, cyanide | |
| Drugs | Penathian | Amines | |
| | Chloramphenicol | Arylamines | |
| | Methotrexate | 4-amino-4-deoxy-$N^{10}$-methyl pterocryl gluteric acid | |
| Food additives | Cyclamate | Cyclohexylomine | 9 |
| | Food drugs: | | |
| | Amaranth | a) Naphthionic acid ondamine R acid | 11–13 |
| | Brown FK | b) Amines | 12 |
| | Tartrazine | c) Naphthylamine sulphomate reduction products | |
| | Food dyes | d) Synthetic coal tar dye reduction products | 4, 14, 20, 25, |
| | Food preservatives: nitrite, secondary amines, lecithin | Nitrosamines | 21 |
| Environmental chemicals | Liver metabolites and conjugates, *e.g.* diethylstilbestrol, $\beta$-D-glucaride | Retoxification products Diethylstilbestrol | |
| | $N$-hydroxy N2 fluorenyl acetamide $\beta$ glucuranide | N2 fluorenylactamide | |
| | Benzopyrenol $\beta$ glucuronide | Benzo($a$)pyrene | |
| *Bacteroides thetiotao-micron* and other intestinal bacteroides | Unknown | Faecapentaenes | 27 |

## The Intestinal Bacteria

The intestinal flora has been extensively reviewed (5–7, 15). Most studies have been of people in Europe and North America though there have been sufficient studies in other parts of the world to allow us to delineate some general principles.

The majority of bacteria in the intestine are non-sporing anaerobes; some 200–300 species are thought to be usually present. There is some doubt if all the types of bacteria present have yet been cultured. Gram positive cocci can often be seen in stained preparations of small intestinal contents but few are grown.

Bacteria are seldom cultured from acid stomach contents. Colonisation of the stomach can be demonstrated in people with gastric achlorhydria whether occurring naturally or

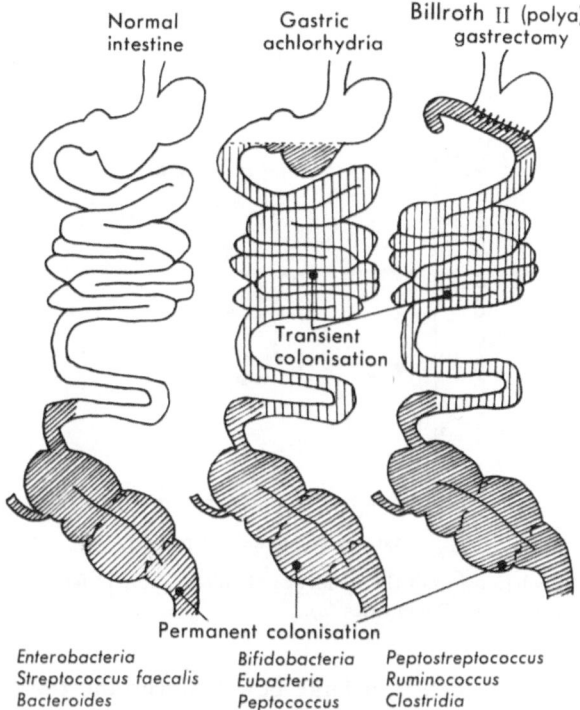

Normal          Gastric          Billroth II (polya)
intestine       achlorhydria     gastrectomy

Transient
colonisation

Permanent colonisation

| Enterobacteria | Bifidobacteria | Peptostreptococcus |
| Streptococcus faecalis | Eubacteria | Ruminococcus |
| Bacteroides | Peptococcus | Clostridia |

FIG. 1.   The distribution of bacteria in the gastrointestinal tract of people with normal gastric acidity, achlorhydria, and a surgical blind loop.

as a result of gastric surgery and in persons with drug induced depression of acid secretion.

The small intestine in Europeans and North Americans contains very few cultivable bacteria though a permanent flora is thought to be present in the lower ileum. More bacteria can be isolated when the stomach is colonised. A transient flora may be present after a meal even when acid secretion is normal. The small intestine in people in developing countries contains a diverse mixture of cultivable bacteria. Gram negative bacteria particularly Enterobacteriaceae and Bacteroides are usually present.

The large intestine harbours a diverse and complex flora. Some 99% of the bacteria are non-sporing anaerobes Bacteroides, Bifidobacteria Eubacteria, Rumino-cocci, and other groups usually present. Enterobacteriaceae, usually *Escherichia coli* and faecal streptococci are also constant components of the flora. Studies on the large intestinal and faecal flora have been associated with major advances in the techniques of the growth of anaerobes and in our understanding of their taxonomy (*e.g.*, Ref. *22*). Figure 1 summarizes the different types of intestinal flora.

### Intestinal Bacteria and Cancer

Cancer of the large intestine is primarily a disease of developed countries. In international comparisons there is a very strong correlation between the incidence of colon cancer and the fat consumption (Fig. 2). It has been suggested that there is a negative

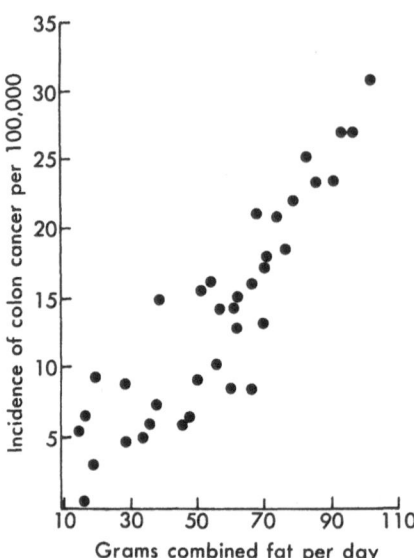

F IG . 2.  The relationship of the incidence of colon cancer to fat intake in an international comparison of 37 countries (8).

correlation between the incidence of large bowel cancer and the intake of fibre in the diet (3). However, because of the problems associated with the measurements of fibre intake this relationship remains speculative.

In view of the high incidence of large bowel tumours in Europe and North America and the association with diet, attention has been focused on food additives as carcinogens directly when ingested, as metabolic substrates for intestinal flora or as carcinogens after bacterial metabolism. Bacteria can convert food additives into various products, e.g., the food dyes tartrazine, Brown FK, amaranth are cleaved by bacterial azoreductase. Hazardous conversions can occur when food contains nitrate and nitrite as preservatives; such compounds are activated by bacterial metabolism in the gut perhaps to produce nitrosamines.

Numerous conversions occur mediated by the intestinal bacteria, but only a few produce carcinogenic products. *In vitro* experiments using *Streptococcus faecalis* and *Proteus vulgaris* revealed that a flavin system mediated azo-food-dye reductions, producing amines. Reduction rates of azo-dyes are altered by dietary carbohydrate, bile acids, and other food additives (*e.g.*, sucrose polyester, dioctylsodium sulphosuccinate) when investigated in *in vitro* incubation experiments. Colonic bacteria alter their metabolic pattern depending upon the intestinal luminal contents, *i.e.*, dietary components. Nitrofuradantin, sucrose polyester, and lecithin mixtures can result in altered bacterial metabolism. The sucrose polyester alters the gut anaerobes' ability to metabolise bile acids. This food additive has the characteristics of other widely used food emulsifiers and resembles dietary fats. The potential of such food emulsifiers to act as modifiers of bacterial metabolic systems may be of particular importance.

A further potential problem with food emulsifiers is that the macromolecular types, the starches, gums, carragenin, alginates may cause malfunction of the macrophage-phagocyte system (MPS). The MPS is the site of gut mucosal antigen processing, interference here was proposed as an effect resulting from persorption of these macro-

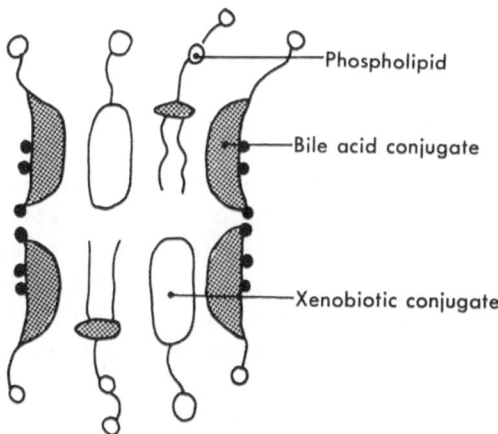

FIG. 3. The insertion of a biliary conjugate, *e.g.*, a glucuronide in a mixed micelle.

molecular additives, which are relatively undegraded in the colon. The proposal was that gut epithelia are penetrated by such compounds causing interference with MPS resulting in abnormal functioning of the immune response. Increased epithelial susceptibility to carcinogens might be a consequence. Nevertheless, evidence of the involvement of food additives in the aetiology of gastrointestinal cancer is not convincing. Denmark has a high incidence of colon cancer although the range of food additives allowed is comparatively restricted. Further countries in which a major part of the diet is industrially produced or processed usually have a low incidence of stomach cancer.

The role of the intestinal flora in the aetiology of large bowel cancer has been extensively investigated by groups of workers in Europe and North America with the help of other investigators in Japan, India, and parts of Africa. Results of many of these studies were reviewed in 1980 (2). A range of candidate carcinogens have been identified (Table I) but no definite conclusions have been reached.

Bile acids are thought to be of particular importance; they may be the substrate from which the gut bacteria can produce carcinogens; they may act as cocarcinogens and they may be important in the transport of biliary conjugates in mixed micelles (Fig. 3). The importance of bile acids is underlined by studies demonstrating that faecal levels of bile acids are dependent on dietary intakes of fat.

The basic theory is that large bowel cancer is caused by carcinogens produced or activated by the gut bacteria under the influence of diet. Fundamental to this theory is the belief that diet controls the gut flora. Unfortunately, the complexity of the flora renders definitive proof of this contention difficult to obtain by classical bacteriological techniques. An alternative approach is to examine the metabolic function of the flora with respect to chosen substrates. In this model the large bowel flora is considered as an organ analogous to the liver.

The role of bacteria in gastric cancer is more speculative. It has been suggested that colonisation of the stomach can result in the development of gastric cancer. The bacteria that colonise natural or surgically produced blind loops belong to the same groups as those in the large intestine. These same bacterial genera are found in the stomach of achlorhydrics. The suggestion is that if bacteria can produce carcinogens in the colon similar reactions could occur in the stomach. If such reactions occur there would be greater opportunity for some reactions to occur in the stomach than in other parts of the gut. Thus, for example, formation of nitrosamines would be more likely in that nitrate and nitrite are rapidly absorbed and are unavailable for reactions in the colon. There is some evidence to suggest that in patients treated with cimetidine gastric colonisation is associated with nitrosamine production (26). This hypothesis requires further investigation.

The role of bacteria in the aetiology is seen mainly in terms of the production of carcinogens and cocarcinogens, however, this is not the sole possibility.

Primary lymphoma of the upper small intestine occurs most frequently in young adults from the Middle East. Cases have been reported from Africa, the Middle East, the Far East, South America, and Southern Europe, and it has been suggested that this disease is characteristic of intermediate populations (10), that is, those populations which are becoming industrialised.

Patients suffer from malabsorption and diarrhoea as a result of the infiltration of the gut by plasma cells. This plasma cell infiltration may develop to form a frankly malignant condition involving the mesenteric lymph nodes. Incomplete immunoglobulin A heavy chains, synthesized by the plasma cells, have been found in the sera of the majority of these patients. While the lesion in the intestine remains confined to the lamina propria, a complete remission of the disease can result from treatment with antibiotics.

The use of antibiotics in the treatment of this disease suggests that it is caused by bacteria. Intestinal infections are common in developing countries. Studies have shown the small intestinal flora of normal people in developing countries to be different from that of normal people in North America and Western Europe. The bacteria present in the small intestine of these people include large numbers of the bacterial species present in the colon. In some way the flora is analogous to that occurring in the blind loop syndrome. It is unclear if this small intestinal contamination is the result of gastric achlorhydria or represents a difference in the ability of the small intestinal mucosa to control the bacteria.

Detailed descriptions of this disease have been published by various authorities (23). The purpose of this brief summary is to draw attention to the possible role of the intestinal flora.

The ability to synthesize incomplete heavy chains is probably genetically determined but although such defective clones may occur in many individuals, this genetic potential is only seldom expressed. The production of immunoglobulins results from the stimulation of the immune system by antigen. B lymphocytes are stimulated to divide and to produce antibodies. Under normal circumstances the continued multiplication of a clone of B lymphocytes and production of antibody would be controlled by a feedback mechanism mediated by the antibody produced. The affinity of an antibody for the antigen stimulating its production depends upon the dose of the antigen. Thus, a small amount of antigen will stimulate production of antibodies of very high affinity while a larger dose of antigen will give more antibody but with a lower average affinity. The incomplete $\alpha$ heavy chains found in this disease may be regarded as antibodies of very low affinity and may act as cell surface antibody receptors. This would mean that B cells committed to the production of such $\alpha$ heavy chains could be stimulated by a massive dose of antigen, such as persistent infection of the small intestine. Recent studies have shown the presence of bacterial overgrowth in the jejunum of patients with this lymphoma.

The induction of the disease could result from an attack of acute diarrhoea involving a colonisation of the jejunal mucosa by enterobacteria. During the attack, the local immune system in the intestine would be exposed to a massive dose of antigen. The abnormal B lymphocytes could be stimulated to grow and produce $\alpha$ heavy chains. If the colonisation of the jejunum was not cleared this antigenic stimulation might continue. The success of antibiotics in treating the initial stages of the disease may be explained in terms of the removal of this antigenic stimulus. With the removal of this stimulus the $\alpha$ chain producing clone would cease to grow and the tumour would regress as a result of the normal processes of cell death.

This hypothesis explains the distribution and cause of the disease. The existence of cells able to produce only incomplete chains is consistent with the clonal selection theory of antibody production. The idea that such cells can be induced to form a lymphoma by massive doses of antigen should be amenable to experimental examination.

In conclusion, it must be said that the magnitude of the bacterial contribution to the initiation of cancers cannot at present be quantified, in part because of the technical problems of investigating intestinal bacteria. The possibility remains, however, that bacterial action is a major cause of cancer.

Colonisation of the intestine stimulates the normal growth of mucosal cells. Turnover of intestinal cells is faster in conventional than germ free animals, thus more cells are exposed to any mutagenic/carcinogenic agent and there is a greater chance of transformation occurring.

Colonisation of the gastrointestinal tract by bacteria seems to render those areas colonised liable to develop cancer.

## REFERENCES

1. Aries, V., Crowther, J. S., Drasar, B. S., Hill, M. J., and Williams, R.E.O. Bacteria and the aetiology of cancer of the large bowel. *Gut*, **10**, 334–335 (1969).
2. Banbury Report No. 7, Gastrointestinal Cancer, Endogenous Factors. (1981). Cold Spring Harbor Laboratory, New York.
3. Burkitt, D. P. Epidemiology of cancer of the colon and rectum. *Cancer*, **28**, 3 (1971).
4. Chung, K. T., Fulk, G. E., and Andrews, A. W. The mutagenicity of methyl orange and metabolites produced by intestinal anaerobes. *Mut. Res.*, **58**, 375–379 (1978).
5. Clarke, R.T.J. and Bauchop, T. "Microbial Ecology of the Gut" (1977). Academic Press, London.
6. Drasar, B. S. and Barrow, P. A. "Intestinal Microbiology" (1984). Van Nostrand Reinhold, U.K.
7. Drasar, B. S. and Hill, M. J. "Human Intestinal Flora" (1974). Academic Press, London.
8. Drasar, B. S. and Irving, D. Environmental factors and cancer of the colon and breast. *Br. J. Cancer*, **27**, 167–172 (1973).
9. Drasar, B. S., Renwick, A. G., and Williams, R. T. The role of the gut flora in the metabolism of cyclamate. *Biochem. J.*, **129**, 881–890 (1972).
10. Dutz, W. Immune modulation and disease patterns in population groups. *Medical Hypotheses*, **1**, 197–203 (1975).
11. Ershoff, B. H. and Thurston, E. W. The effect of diet upon amaranth (F.D.+C. Red No. 2) Toxicity in the rat. *J. Nutr.*, **104**, 937–942 (1974).
12. Fore, H., Walker, R., and Golberg, L. Studies on Brown FK II degradative changes undergone *in vitro* and *in vivo*. *Food Cosmet. Toxicol.*, **5**, 459–473 (1967).
13. Haveland-Smith, R. B. and Combes, R. D. Amaranth studies about toxicity. *Food Cosmet. Toxicol.*, **18**, 215–221 (1979).

14. Hartman, C. A., Andrews, A. W., and Chung, K. T. Production of a mutagen from Ponceau 3R by a human intestinal microbe. *Infect. Immun.*, **23**, 686–689 (1979).

15. Hentges, D. J. (ed). "Human Intestinal Microflora in Health and Disease" (1983). Academic Press, London-New York.

16. Hill, M. J. "Gut Bacteria, Steroids of the Large Bowel in Some Implications of Steroid Hormones in Cancer," ed. D. C. Williams and M. H. Briggs, p. 94 (1971), London.

17. Hill, M. J. Steroid nuclear dehydrogenation and colon cancer. *Am. J. Clin. Nutr.*, **27**, 1475–1480 (1974).

18. Hill, M. J., Drasar, B. S., Aries, V., Crowther, J. S., Hawksworth, G., and Williams, R.E.O. Bacteria and aetiology of cancer of the large bowel. *Lancet*, **i**, 95 (1971).

19. Khera, K. S. and Manra, I. C. A review of the specifications and toxicity of synthetic food colours permitted in Canada. *CRC Crit. Rev. Toxicol.*, **6**, 81–133 (1979).

20. Kirby, A.H.M. and Peacock, P. R. Liver tumours in mice infected with commercial food dyes. *Glasgow Med. J.*, **30**, 364 (1949).

21. Khubes, P. and Jondorf, W. R. Dimethylnitrosamine formation from sodium nitrite and dimethylamine by bacterial flora of rat intestine. *Res. Commun. Chem. Pathol. Pharmacol.*, **2**, 24 (1971).

22. Mitsuoka, T. "A Colour Atlas of Anaerobic Bacteria" (1980) (in Japanese) Sobunsha, Tokyo.

23. Rambaud, J. C. and Seligman, M. Alpha-chain disease. *Clin. Gastroenterol.*, **5**, 341–358 (1976).

24. Scheline, R. R. Metabolism of foreign compounds by gastrointestinal microorganisms. *Pharmac. Rev.*, **25** (4), 451–523 (1973).

25. Shubik, P. Potential carcinogenicity of food additives and contaminants. *Cancer Res.*, **25** (11-12), 3475 (1975).

26. Stockbrugger, R. W., Cotton, P. B., Eugenides, N., Bartholomew, B., Hill, M. J., and Walters, C. L. Intragastric nitrites, nitrosamines and bacterial overgrowth during cimetidine treatment. *Gut*, **23**, 1048–1054 (1982).

27. Wilkins, T. D. Relationships of faecal mutagens to colonic cancer. *Natl. Large Bowel Cancer Proj. Newsl.*, **11**, 52–53 (1984).

# BILE ACID AS A CAUSATIVE FACTOR OF CARCINOMA

Nobuaki Kaibara and Shigemasa Koga

*Department of Surgery I, Tottori University School of Medicine**

We examined the relationship between the operative procedure and the incidence of remnant stomach carcinoma in rats orally treated with $N$-methyl-$N'$-nitro-$N$-nitrosoguanidine (MNNG). The incidence of gastric carcinoma was 39% in rats that had received Billroth II reconstruction resulting in a greater extent of duodenogastric reflux, 25% in those receiving short Roux-en Y procedure resulting in moderate reflux, and 7% in those receiving long Roux-en Y reconstruction resulting in a lesser extent of reflux. This indicates a higher incidence of gastric carcinoma in rats with a greater amount of reflux of duodenal juice including bile. In the *in vitro* test system using a C3H 10T1/2 clone 8 cell line, cultures exposed to bile acids after MNNG treatment exhibited an increased number of transformed cell foci as compared with the group treated with MNNG alone. The number of transformed foci in cultures treated first with bile acids and then with MNNG did not differ appreciably from the counts in cultures treated with MNNG alone, indicating that bile acids act as promoters of cellular transformation. Based on the above, we suggest that the duodenogastric reflux, especially that of bile acids, is implicated in the development of remnant stomach carcinoma.

Although a controversy exists as to whether gastric resection for benign ulcers enhances the potential for the subsequent development of gastric carcinoma, there are a number of studies relating the risk for carcinoma development in the resected stomach (3, 5, 8, 10, 12). The tumor site in the resected stomach tends to be in the gastroenteric anastomotic region; tumor development is reportedly more frequent after Billroth II procedure than after Billroth I reconstruction (12). Thus the extent of duodenogastric reflux may be related to the development of remnant stomach carcinoma.

## Remnant Stomach Carcinoma in Rats

Male Wistar rats were divided into 5 groups: Group 1 underwent gastrectomy removing half of the glandular stomach and received Billroth II reconstruction; Group 2 underwent gastrectomy, alimentary continuity was reconstructed by the Roux-en Y procedure, and the distance between the gastroenterostomia and entero-enterostomia was 10 cm (short Roux-en Y group); Group 3 was subjected to gastrectomy and received Roux-en Y reconstruction, the distance between the gastroenterostomia and entero-enterostomia was 30 cm (long Roux-en Y group); Group 4 received gastrotomy alone; Group 5 served as a non-operated control. Starting with the first postoperative month and for the next 6 months, rats received MNNG (120 $\mu$g/ml) in their drinking water.

---

* Nishi-machi 86, Yonago, Tottori 683, Japan (貝原信明, 古賀成昌).

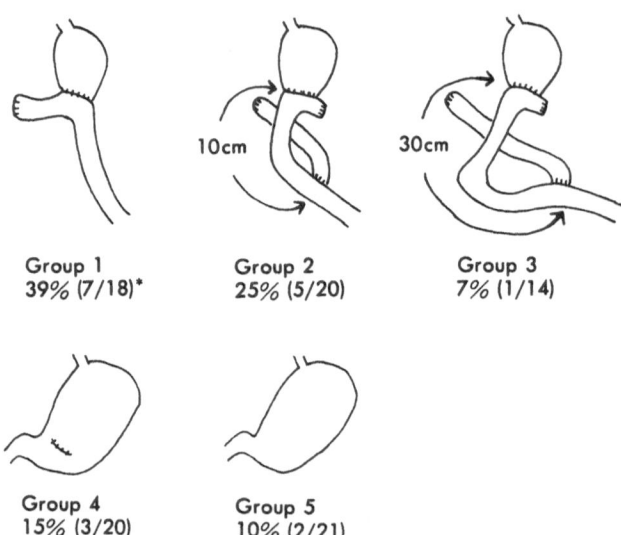

Group 1
39% (7/18)*

Group 2
25% (5/20)

Group 3
7% (1/14)

Group 4
15% (3/20)

Group 5
10% (2/21)

FIG. 1. Incidence of MNNG-induced carcinoma in rats subjected to gastric surgery.
* $p < 0.05$, compared with Groups 3 and 5.

They were sacrificed 9 months after surgery to examine the development of remnant stomach carcinoma.

Carcinoma developed in the gastrotomy group and in the non-operated control group at an incidence of 15 and 10%, respectively (Fig. 1). The incidence of gastric remnant carcinoma was 39% in rats that had received Billroth II reconstruction resulting in a greater extent of duodenogastric reflux, 25% in those receiving short Roux-en Y reconstruction with moderate reflux, and 7% in those receiving long Roux-en Y reconstruction with lesser extent of reflux. This points to a higher incidence of gastric carcinoma in rats with a greater amount of reflux of duodenal juice including bile.

*Effect of Bile Acids on Cell Growth in Vitro*

In order to examine the effect of bile acids on cell growth *in vitro*, C3H 10T1/2 clone 8 cells (*13*) ($1 \times 10^2$ cells per petri dish) were cultivated for 6 hr and then graded concentrations of bile acids were added. After 10-day incubation, cell colonies were counted.

The bile acids produced no appreciable cytotoxic effect at concentrations between 1–100 $\mu$M in the cultures. However, at higher concentrations, lithocholic acid (LCA) and deoxycholic acid (DCA) ($>100$ $\mu$M), chenodeoxycholic acid (CDCA, $>150$ $\mu$M), and cholic acid (CA, $>500$ $\mu$M) were remarkably cytotoxic. Interestingly, cell colonies formed in the presence of 50–100 $\mu$M of LCA, 100 $\mu$M of DCA or CDCA, and 500 $\mu$M of CA were noticeably larger than in the control group. The incidence of colonies measuring $\geqq 5$ mm in diameter was significantly high in cells treated with CDCA and in those exposed to LCA (Fig. 2). A similar tendency was observed in cells treated with CA and DCA. These findings indicate that at the concentrations used, the bile acids promoted cell proliferation.

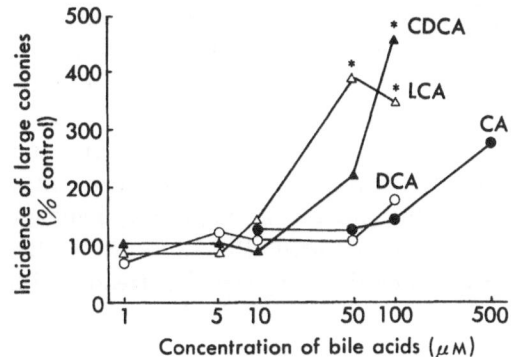

FIG. 2. Increase in the size of C3H 10T1/2 cell colonies formed *in vitro* in the presence of bile acids.

The incidence of colonies measuring $\geq 5$ mm in diameter is expressed as a percent of the control (mean incidence in the controls, 11.2%). Quintuplicate cultures were set up for each group. * $p < 0.01$, compared with the control group.

### Effect of Bile Acids on Cellular Transformation in Vitro

Cultures ($1 \times 10^4$ cells per petri dish) were incubated for 24 hr; MNNG (13.6 $\mu$M) was present in the medium for the next 24 hr, then the cells were incubated for 48 hr in fresh, MNNG-free medium. Thereafter, the cultures were incubated for 3 weeks in the presence of bile acids and subsequently were maintained for 17 days with fresh, bile acid-free medium. After 6-week incubation, the number of transformed cell foci in each culture was counted. As a result, cultures treated with bile acids alone showed no foci of transformed cells. The mean number of transformed cell foci per petri dish was 0.5 in the group treated with MNNG alone. All cultures exposed to bile acids after MNNG treatment exhibited an increased mean number of transformed foci as compared with the group treated with MNNG alone.

TABLE I. Effect of Bile Acids on the MNNG-Induced Transformation of C3H 10T1/2 Cells *in Vitro*

| Groups | | No. of transformed foci per petri dish (No. of dishes with transformed foci / No. of dishes used) |
|---|---|---|
| No treatment | | 0 (0/15) |
| CA | (500 $\mu$M) | 0 (0/10) |
| CDCA | (100 $\mu$M) | 0 (0/10) |
| DCA | (100 $\mu$M) | 0 (0/10) |
| LCA | ( 50 $\mu$M) | 0 (0/10) |
| MNNG | | 0.5 (7/15) |
| MNNG + | CA | 1.3 (12/15)* |
| | CDCA | 1.6 (12/15)* |
| | DCA | 1.5 (12/15)* |
| | LCA | 1.7 (13/15)* |
| CA | | 0.5 (7/15) |
| CDCA | + MNNG | 0.5 (7/15) |
| DCA | | 0.5 (7/15) |
| LCA | | 0.4 (6/15) |

* $p < 0.05$, compared with MNNG alone.

In another set of experiments designed to examine the effect of pretreatment with bile acids, cells were incubated for 3 weeks in medium containing graded concentrations of the acids. Subsequently, $1 \times 10^4$ cells per petri dish were subcultured in the presence of MNNG as described above; transformed foci were counted as in the preceding experiment. The mean number of transformed foci in cultures treated with bile acids and MNNG did not differ appreciably from the mean counts in cultures treated with MNNG alone. These results indicate that the bile acids produced enhancement of *in vitro* transformation of cells when they were added after exposure to the carcinogenic agent. No such enhancement occurred when the cells were first treated with the bile acids and then exposed to MNNG.

## COMMENT

There are many reports presenting experimental and clinical data which suggest that bile acids may promote the development of gastrointestinal malignancies (*2, 9, 11, 14*). Currently available data from *in vivo* studies indicate that only the secondary bile acids act as promoters in the carcinogenic process.

We found that cultures of C3H 10T1/2 cells treated with MNNG for initiation of transformation and then maintained with medium containing bile acids showed an increased incidence of transformed cell foci as compared to cultures treated with MNNG alone. This shows that bile acids act as promoters of cellular transformation. Although the relative magnitude of their effect as promoters of C3H 10T1/2 cell transformation remains unclear, it is of profound interest that even the primary bile acids exerted promoting action in the *in vitro* test system.

Treatment of C3H 10T1/2 cells with the bile acids alone did not lead to formation of transformed cell foci in our study, thus indicating that these bile acids are devoid of activity in initiating transformation of the cells. Kelsey and Pienta (*7*) described that colonies of transformed cells occurred in cultures of Syrian hamster embryo cells treated with DCA or LCA alone. The cells used in their study are known to have a high liability to malignant transformation and, accordingly, there remains the possibility that bile acids may initiate a carcinogenic process in some types of cells.

The mechanism(s) whereby bile acids exert their effects as promoters of cell transformation remains unknown. There have been reports demonstrating an enhanced DNA synthesis in the epithelium of large intestine of rats after administration of CA (*2*), and an increase in the number of epithelial cells constituting lacunae of the large intestine of rats receiving DCA or LCA enemas (*4*). Furthermore, the increased $^3$H-thymidine uptake by liver cells and bile duct epithelium of mice dosed with DCA or LCA (*1*), and the growth promotion of cultured rat liver cells in the presence of LCA (*6*) have also been reported. Our study has demonstrated that the bile acids act to promote the proliferation of C3H 10T1/2 cells *in vitro* when added to culture medium at certain concentrations. These findings indicate that bile acids act to accelerate cellular turnover, which might constitute their action mechanism as promoters of cell transformation.

Our study has also shown that promoter activity is demonstrable not only with the secondary bile acids as has generally been recognized, but with the primary bile acids as well. This represents an important finding which suggests possible participation of bile acids in the pathogenesis of carcinoma of the remant stomach.

## REFERENCES

1. Bagheri, S. A., Solt, M. G., Boyer, J. L., and Palmer, R. H. Stimulation of thymidine incorporation in mouse liver and biliary tract epithelium by lithocholate and deoxycholate. *Gastroenterology*, **74**, 188–192 (1978).
2. Cohen, B. I., Raicht, R. F., Deschner, E. E., Takahashi, M., Sarwal, A. N., and Fazzini, E. Effect of cholic acid feeding on $N$-methyl-$N$-nitrosourea-induced colon tumors and cell kinetics in rats. *J. Natl. Cancer Inst.*, **64**, 573–578 (1980).
3. De Jode, L. R. Gastric carcinoma following gastro-enterostomy and partial gastrectomy. *Br. J. Surg.*, **48**, 512–514 (1961).
4. Glauert, H. P. and Bennink, M. R. Influence of diet or intrarectal bile acid injections on colon epithelial cell proliferation in rats previously injected with 1, 2-dimethylhydrazine. *J. Nutr.*, **113**, 475–482 (1983).
5. Helsingen, N. and Hillestad, L. Cancer development in the gastric stump after partial gastrectomy for ulcer. *Ann. Surg.*, **143**, 173–179 (1956).
6. Jeannin, J. F., Chessebuf, M., Martin, M. S., Lagneau, A., and Martin, F. Proliferative effect of lithocholic acid on rat liver cells in culture. *Biomedicine*, **31**, 207–209 (1979).
7. Kelsey, M. I. and Pienta, R. J. Transformation of hamster embryo cells by neutral sterols and bile acids. *Toxicol. Lett.*, **9**, 177–182 (1981).
8. Morgenstern, L., Yamakawa, T., and Seltzer, D. Carcinoma of the gastric stump. *Am. J. Surg.*, **125**, 29–38 (1973).
9. Narisawa, T., Magadia, N. E., Weisburger, J. H., and Wynder, E. L. Promoting effect of bile acids on colon carcinogenesis after intrarectal instillation of $N$-methyl-$N'$-nitro-$N$-nitrosoguanidine in rats. *J. Natl. Cancer Inst.*, **53**, 1093–1097 (1974).
10. Nishidoi, H., Koga, S., and Kaibara, N. Possible role of duodenogastric reflux on the development of remnant stomach carcinoma induced by $N$-methyl-$N'$-nitro-$N$-nitrosoguanidine in rats. *J. Natl. Cancer Inst.*, **72**, 1431–1435 (1984).
11. Peitsch, W. and Burkhardt, K. Zur Pathogenese und Klinik des Magenstumpfcarcinoms. *Langenbecks Arch. Chir.*, **341**, 195–203 (1976).
12. Peters, H., Schubert, H. J., and Reifferscheid, M. Das carcinom im Restmagen nach Resektion wegen gutartiger Befunde. *Langenbecks Arch. Chir.*, **336**, 219–233 (1974).
13. Rezinikoff, C. A., Brankow, D. W., and Heidelberger, C. Establishment and characterization of a cloned line of C3H mouse embryo cells sensitive to postconfluence inhibition of division. *Cancer Res.*, **33**, 3231–3238 (1973).
14. Weisburger, J. H., Wynder, E. L., and Horn, C. L. Nutritional factors and etiologic mechanisms in the causation of gastrointestinal cancers. *Cancer*, **50**, 2541–2549 (1982).

# INFLUENCE OF GASTRO-JEJUNAL ANASTOMOSIS ON GASTRIC CARCINOGENESIS IN RATS

Ken Kondo,[*1] Harumi Suzuki,[*2] and Takeo Nagayo[*3]

*Yokoyama Gastrointestinal Hospital,[*1] Shizuoka General Hospital,[*2] and Laboratory of Pathology, Aichi Cancer Center Research Institute[*3]*

The effect of reflux of the duodenal contents into the remnant stomach on development of a stump carcinoma was studied using male rats. Under our specifically designed surgical procedures, most adenocarcinomas were developed in the gastric mucosa close to the gastro-jejunal anastomosis, at which the proximal jejunal segment was drained. Furthermore, it is important to note that we found adenocarcinomas not only in carcinogen-exposed rats but also in non-exposed rats. These findings strongly suggest an intimate correlation between the exposure of mucosa at the site of the anastomosis to the duodenal contents and the development of adenocarcinoma.

In our previous study of human gastric stump carcinomas we experienced 29 lesions (*1*). When we compared the incidence of carcinoma by development site, 13 lesions (44.8%) were found in the resected stomachs close to the anastomosis and in nine of the 13 lesions the anastomoses were made by Billroth II resection without Braun's anastomosis.

Billroth II resection without Braun's anastomosis must lead to a chronic duodenogastric reflux into the gastric remnant. In order to clarify the relation between duodenogastric reflux and the development of the gastric stump carcinoma we carried out an animal experiment, applying the technique of diverting the flow of bile and pancreatic juice into the resected stomach.

## Experimental Design and Operative Procedures

The operative technique for diversion of duodenal contents is shown in Fig. 1. Partial resection of the glandular stomach including antrum and pylorus is performed and the cut end of the duodenum is oversewn. The jejunum approximately 20 cm distal from the duodenal onset is then cut out. The proximal cut end of the jejunum is connected with the greater curvature of the glandular stomach by end-to-side anastomosis (hereafter referred to as anastomosis A), then the distal cut end is anastomosed end-to-end with the gastric stump (hereafter referred to as anastomosis B).

The Roux-en Y resection, thought to be the technique eliciting the minimal duodenogastric reflux is also performed. The efferent jejunal loop is anastomosed to the greater curvature of the glandular stomach. The anastomotic site of the stomach (hereafter referred to as anastomosis A') is the same position as in anastomosis A.

---

[*1] Chiyoda 3-11-20, Naka-ku, Nagoya, 460, Japan (近藤　建).

[*2] Kitaando 4-27-1, Shizuoka 420, Japan (鈴木春見).

[*3] Kanokoden 81-1159, Tashiro-cho, Chikusa-ku, Nagoya 464, Japan (長与健夫).

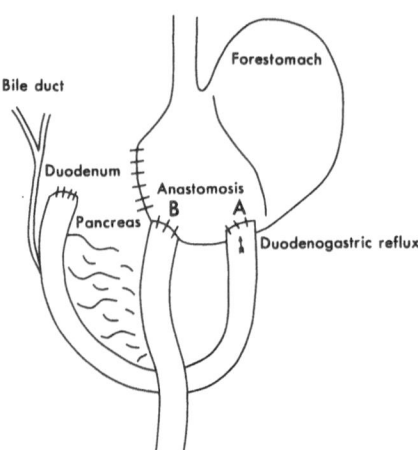

FIG. 1.   Gastrectomy with diversion of duodenal contents.

A total of 80 male Wistar rats, 6 weeks old and weighing 180–200 g, were treated as follows.

Group I (MNNG+operation): one week after single oral administration of $N$-methyl-$N'$-nitro-$N$-nitrosoguanidine (MNNG), the rats were operated by the surgical technique for diversion of duodenal contents.

Group II (MNNG+Roux-en Y operation): one week after MNNG administration by the same method the rats were operated by Roux-en Y resection.

Group III (MNNG): the rats were administered MNNG by the same method, without operation.

Group IV (Operation): the rats were operated by surgical technique for diversion of duodenal contents without MNNG administration.

Group V: non-treated rats.

All surviving rats were sacrificed after the 40th week of the experiment. The average body weight at the end of the experiment was almost the same among the 5 groups.

In order to clarify chronological changes of carcinogenesis, we performed the same operation for diversion of duodenal contents in rats. Two rats were killed at 5 weeks, 6 rats were killed at 10 weeks, 14 rats were killed at 20 weeks, 9 rats were killed at 40 weeks, and 11 rats were killed more than 50 weeks after the operation.

Atypical hyperplasia of the gastric mucosa seen on the anastomotic site of the experimental animals were classified into two grades (low and high) according to the intensity of cellular and structural abnormalities. In low-grade atypical hyperplasia, a few proliferated and dilated glands lined with hyperplastic epithelia were displaced into the tunica submucosa. On the superficial layer of these elevated lesions, erosions or pseudopyloric glandular metaplasia were also often observed. In high-grade atypical hyperplasia, markedly proliferated glands with cyst formation invaded the tunica submucosa, the tunica muscularis propria, or scarred tissue and sometimes caused a bulging of the anastomosed mucosa to form polypoid elevations.

*Frequencies and Characteristics of Cancer Developed in the Remnant Stomachs*

### 1. Incidence of tumors

Adenocarcinoma developed in six out of the 15 rats (40%) in group I and in three of the 13 rats (23%) in group IV, but none developed in groups II, III, or V. Thus, adenocarcinomas were observed in the remnant stomachs of rats with and without MNNG administration (Table I). There was no significant difference in the incidence of adenocarcinoma between the two groups. Macroscopically, the advanced adenocarcinomas showed an elevated mass with central erosion, 1–2 cm in diameter. Microscopically, they were composed of tubular or cystic glands with structural abnormality and cellular atypia, diagnosed as mucoid adenocarcinoma. In group II, one adenoma was found at the jejuno-jejunostomy. The rats of groups I, II, and III also had multiple tumors in the forestomach. All the tumors of the forestomach were histologically squamous cell papilloma with basal cell proliferation or keratotic squamous cell carcinoma. There was significant difference in the incidence between groups I and III.

The incidence of mucosal changes of the glandular stomach in carcinogen-exposed rats are shown in Table II. All the adenocarcinomas arose from anastomosis A. The incidences of low-grade atypical hyperplasia were almost the same among anastomosis A, anastomosis B, and anastomosis A', but the incidence of high-grade atypical hyperplasia was significantly higher in anastomosis A than in the other two. Ulcer, foveolar hyperplasia, and mucosal atrophy were also found usually close to anastomosis A.

TABLE I. Incidence of Tumors of Stomach and Jejunum

| Group | Effective No. of rats | Glandular stomach | | Forestomach | | | Jejunum | |
| | | Adeno-carcinoma | Sarcoma | Papilloma | Squamous cell carcinoma | Sarcoma | Adenoma | Adeno-carcinoma |
| --- | --- | --- | --- | --- | --- | --- | --- | --- |
| I (MNNG-operation) | 15 | 6 (40%) | 1 (7%) | 2 (13%) | 8 (53%) | 0 | 0 | 0 |
| II (MNNG-operation) | 10 | 0 | 0 | 3 (30%) | 2 (20%) | 0 | 1 (10%) | 0 |
| III (MNNG) | 13 | 0 | 0 | 5 (38%) | 2 (15%) | 0 | 0 | 0 |
| IV (Operation) | 13 | 3 (23%) | 0 | 0 | 0 | 0 | 0 | 0 |
| V (Control) | 6 | 0 | 0 | 0 | 0 | 0 | 0 | 0 |

Operation: gastrectomy with diversion of duodenal contents (Groups I, IV); gastrectomy with Roux-en Y gastrojejunal anastomosis (Group II).

TABLE II. Histological Findings in the Resected Stomach of Carcinogen-Exposed Rats (Groups I, II)

| Site | Effective No. of rats | Ulcer | Foveolar hyperplasia | Atrophy | Intestinal metaplasia | Atypical hyperplasia | | Adeno-carcinoma |
| | | | | | | Low | High | |
| --- | --- | --- | --- | --- | --- | --- | --- | --- |
| Anastomosis A | 15 | 4 (27%) | 14 (93%) | 13 (87%) | 6 (40%) | 4 (27%) | 11 (73%) | 6 (40%) |
| Anastomosis B | 15 | 1 (7%) | 2 (13%) | 1 (7%) | 0 | 3 (20%) | 1 (7%) | 0 |
| Anastomosis A' | 10 | 0 | 1 (10%) | 1 (10%) | 0 | 4 (40%) | 0 | 0 |

TABLE III.   Histological Findings in the Resected Stomach of
Carcinogen-Nonexposed Rats (Group IV)

| Site | Effective No. of rats | Ulcer | Foveolar hyperplasia | Atrophy | metaplasia Intestinal | Atypical hyperplasia | | Adeno-carcinoma |
|------|------|------|------|------|------|------|------|------|
| | | | | | | Low | High | |
| Anastomosis A | 13 | 3 (23%) | 11 (85%) | 11 (85%) | 3 (23%) | 7 (54%) | 5 (38%) | 3 (23%) |
| Anastomosis B | 13 | 0 | 1 (8%) | 2 (15%) | 0 | 2 (15%) | 0 | 0 |

In carcinogen-nonexposed rats, the result was almost the same as in the carcinogen-exposed group. That is, adenocarcinomas and atypical hyperplasias were found predominantly in the mucosa close to anastomosis A (Table III).

## 2.   Chronological study in carcinogen-nonexposed rats
*Anastomosis A*

The first adenocarcinoma was found 20 weeks after operation. The incidence of adenocarcinoma was 3/14 (21%) at 20 weeks, 3/9 (33%) at 40 weeks, and 4/11 (36%) at more than 50 weeks, so the incidence was apt to rise in parallel with passing of the weeks. Mucosal changes found at 5–10 weeks were mainly low grade atypical hyperplasia and atrophy of the fundic gland. The highest incidence of intestinal metaplasia and high grade atypical hyperplasia were found in the more than 50 weeks follow up group.
*Anastomosis B*

The incidence of carcinoma development was 2/14 (14%) at 20 weeks, 0% at 40 weeks, and 2/11 (18%) at more than 50 weeks. The incidence and grade of several mucosal changes including adenocarcinoma was much lower than in anastomosis A.

## Comments on the Experiment

We carried out the surgical operation for diversion of duodenal contents in 61 rats with and without carcinogen administration. In comparing the overall incidence of adenocarcinoma development with the location, the difference between anastomosis A and B is evident; 16/61 (26%) in anastomosis A and 4/61 (6.6%) in anastomosis B. It is obvious that adenocarcinoma especially developed close to anastomosis A with intensified exposure of the gastric mucosa to duodenal contents. No adenocarcinomas developed in rats of group II (Roux-en Y operation). These results suggest that duodenogastric reflux is the major causative factor for carcinoma development of gastric stump.

We were unable to demonstrate in our experiment what element of duodenal contents is most essential for the development of carcinoma, even though reflux of bile acid is the most suspect. Mucosal atrophy and atypical regenerative hyperplasia following repeated erosion in the early stage seem to be the initial changes of the carcinoma. Further experiments are needed to clarify the nature of the carcinogenic effect of duodenogastric reflux in the anastomotic area.

## REFERENCE

1.   Kondo, K., Suzuki, H., and Nagoya, T. Pathology of gastric stump carcinoma. *Jpn. J. Cancer Clin.*, **28**, 1615–1623 (1982).

# MULTIDISCIPLINARY APPROACH
# TO CANCER PREVENTION

# INTRODUCTORY REMARKS ON MULTIDISCIPLINARY APPROACH TO CANCER PREVENTION

Gerald P. MURPHY

*Roswell Park Memorial Institute**

Prevention and detection of cancer is as important as treatment and cure. It is estimated that up to 90% of all cancers may be the result of environmental and lifestyle exposures that may be avoided. It has been estimated that as much as 65% of all cancer deaths may be attributable to the effects of tobacco and diet. Human genetics, epidemiology of infectious diseases, and molecular biology are brought to bear on the study of the role of viruses in cancer. Improving accuracy in the detection of cancer and lowering the cost of cancer screening through sensitive and targeted approaches may significantly alter the cost effectiveness ratio and make early cancer detection available to larger numbers of persons at risk.

The preceding session on long-term survival and cancer cure provides appropriate background to the presentations that follow. While the progress being made in the fields of medical, surgical, and radiation oncology is impressive, it remains true that it is better to prevent than to cure. In the United States, there are several cancers which have shown substantial improvement in 5-year relative survival rates for the long-term follow-up of patients diagnosed in the early 1970s (*1*) (Table I). This progress has continued and studies are showing even further advances for patients being diagnosed more recently. On the other hand, there are a number of tumors for which the progress in the overall improvement in treatment results has been relatively modest (Table II). Unfortunately, many of these tumors are very frequent in their occurrence and collectively represent the majority of cancer deaths in the United States.

Thus, it is imperative that the objectives of cancer control be explored through prevention and detection as well as through treatment and cure. Various experts have

TABLE I.   Cancers Showing Gains of 9% or More in Relative 5-Year Survival

| Site | 1960–1963 (%) | 1970–1973 (%) | Points increase |
|---|---|---|---|
| Larynx | 53 | 62 | 9 |
| Kidney | 37 | 46 | 9 |
| Lymphomas (non-Hodgkin's) | 31 | 41 | 10 |
| Prostate | 50 | 63 | 13 |
| Leukemia (chronic lymphocytic) | 35 | 63 | 16 |
| Leukemia (acute lymphocytic) | 4 | 28 | 24 |
| Hodgkin's disease | 40 | 67 | 27 |

From Ref. *1*.

* 666 Elm Street, Buffalo, New York 14263, U.S.A.

TABLE II.  Cancer Showing Gains of 8% or Less in Relative 5-Year Survival

| Site | 1960–1963 (%) | 1970–1973 (%) | Points increase |
|------|---------------|---------------|-----------------|
| Lung/bronchus | 8 | 10 | 2 |
| Stomach | 11 | 13 | 2 |
| Ovary | 32 | 36 | 4 |
| Breast | 63 | 68 | 5 |
| Uterine cervix | 58 | 64 | 6 |
| Colon/rectum | 41 | 48 | 7 |
| Bladder | 53 | 61 | 8 |
| Uterine corpus | 73 | 81 | 8 |

From Ref. *1*.

TABLE III.  Age-Adjusted Death Rates for Cancer (1976–1977)

| Male | Per 100,000 | Female | Per 100,000 |
|------|-------------|--------|-------------|
| Netherlands | 262 | Denmark | 171 |
| France | 256 | England / Wales | 156 |
| England / Wales | 232 | Chile | 154 |
| Denmark | 232 | Netherlands | 143 |
| U.S.A. | 214 | U.S.A. | 136 |
| Poland | 213 | Poland | 126 |
| Chile | 198 | France | 125 |
| Japan | 187 | Japan | 109 |
| Philippines | 62 | Philippines | 55 |
| Thailand | 37 | Thailand | 25 |

From Ref. *5*.

TABLE IV.  Male Variations in Cancer Incidence

| Site | High incidence | Low incidence | Ratio |
|------|----------------|---------------|-------|
| Esophagus | Iran (N.E.) | Nigeria | 300 : 1 |
| Skin | Australia (Queensland) | India (Bombay) | >200 : 1 |
| Liver | Mozambique | England | 100 : 1 |
| Prostate | U.S. Blacks | Japan | 40 : 1 |
| Lung and bronchus | England | Nigeria | 35 : 1 |
| Stomach | Japan | Uganda | 25 : 1 |

From Ref. *2*.

estimated that as much as 90% of all cancers may be the result of environmental and lifestyle exposures that may be avoided. Evidence in support of this is the great variability in cancer incidence and mortality that can be observed on an international scale. Data derived from the careful statistical analyses of cancer mortality carried out by Segi for so many years and now continued by the Segi Institute (*5*) show the variability in the overall importance of cancer as a cause of mortality in different nations (Table III). In light of several migrant studies that show that the populations moving from one region to another tend to adopt the cancer risk of their host nation, these differences probably relate to different patterns of lifestyle, culture, and environmental exposure that are found in the different countries.

If one examines, as have Doll and Peto and others (*2*), variations in cancer incidence by tumor type, we observe that there are tremendous ranges of incidence associated with different tumors (Table IV). For example, the incidence of esophageal cancer is estimated to be 300 times greater in the littoral of Iran compared to Nigeria. Primary liver cancer is 100 times more common in Mozambique than in England. Prostate cancer is 40 times more common in U.S. Blacks than in men in Japan. And, stomach cancer is 25 times more common in Japan than in Uganda. For women, we see large differences in the relative risk of uterine cancer, cervical cancer, breast cancer, and ovarian cancer (Table V).

In an attempt to quantify the relative importance of different kinds of environmental and lifestyle exposure, Doll and Peto (2) have a summary of their estimates (Table VI). Their best estimate suggests that as much as 65% of all cancer deaths may be attributable to the effects of tobacco and diet. Far lesser proportions of cancer mortality are attributed to other categories such as pollution, occupational exposure, geophysical factors such as radiation and sunlight but, for all of these factors, Doll and Peto acknowledge that there is uncertainty as to their true significance.

All of these data point to the great importance of cancer prevention, and the diversity of tumor types, the variations in regional distribution, and the number of types of risk factors involved all suggest that cancer prevention research requires a multidisciplinary and international perspective. In fact, it is very difficult to think of any major research topic in the field of cancer prevention that does not have a multidisciplinary component. In the field of diet and cancer, there is the integration of the work of nutritionists, biochemists, epidemiologists, experts in carcinogenesis and mutagenesis, and bacteriologists, just to name a few. The models for experimentation include not only *in vivo* and *in vitro* laboratory systems. Now we are observing the emergence of clinical trials in human populations designed to assess the prophylactic value of dietary interventions and other chemopreventive interventions.

TABLE V.  Female Variations in Cancer Incidence

| Site | High incidence | Low incidence | Ratio |
|---|---|---|---|
| Uterine corpus | U.S.A. (Calif.) | Japan | 30:1 |
| Uterine cervix | Columbia | Israel (Jewish) | 15:1 |
| Breast | Canada (B.C.) | Israel (Non-Jewish) | 7:1 |
| Ovary | Denmark | Japan | 6:1 |

From Ref. 2.

TABLE VI.  Estimated Proportion of Cancer Deaths Attributable to Different Source of Risk

| Factor | Best estimate | Acceptable estimates |
|---|---|---|
| Tobacco | 30 | 25–40 |
| Diet | 35 | 10–70 |
| Infection | 10? | 1–? |
| Reproductive and sexual history | 7 | 1–13 |
| Occupation | 4 | 2–8 |
| Geophysical | 3 | 2–4 |
| Alcohol | 3 | 2–4 |
| Pollution | 2 | 1–5 |
| Medicine/medical procedures | 1 | 0.5–2 |
| Industrial products | 1 | 1–2 |

From Ref. 2.

TABLE VII.   American Cancer Society Recommendations on Nutrition and Cancer

1. Avoid obesity.
2. Cut down total fat intake.
3. Eat more high fiber foods.
4. Include foods rich in vitamins A and C in the daily diet.
5. Include cruciferous vegetables in the diet.
6. Be moderate in consumption of alcohol.
7. Be moderate in consumption of salt-cured, smoked, and nitrite-cured foods.

TABLE VIII.   Estimated Costs of Each Added Person-Year of Life
Expectancy Achieved by Different Interventions

| | |
|---|---|
| Triennial pap smear   (>20) | $500 |
| Annual fecal occult blood test   (>50) | $500 |
| Annual fecal occult blood test and sigmoidoscope   (>50) | $1,000 |
| Annual breast exam. and biennial mammography   (>50) | $4,500 |
| Hypertension detection and follow-up | $10,000 |

From Refs. *3* and *6*.

Although our knowledge of the true nature and extent of the relationship between diet and cancer remains to be fully explored, the American Cancer Society has made some recommendations on the basis of available evidence concerning dietary practices that may prevent cancer (*4*). Table VII summarizes the seven recommendations of the American Cancer Society which, as a precondition to their consideration, required multidisciplinary data.

Students of the role of viruses in cancer etiology are finding that it is now necessary to incorporate the perspectives of human genetics, of infectious disease epidemiology, and of molecular biology to understand the importance of such factors as the human T-cell leukemia viruses, acquired immune deficiency syndrome, and the associated Kaposi's sarcomas. In the case of primary liver cancer, we have seen the integration of perspectives of researchers working within such diverse settings and with such different models as African, Chinese, Taiwanese, and Korean populations as well as with the animal model of the North American woodchuck.

In the field of cancer detection we know that the problems require the attention of not only the pathologist and radiologist but also the health economist, the behavioral scientist, and the epidemiologist who all may contribute to the assessment of cost and effectiveness of different screening procedures. Some costs in U.S. dollars adapted from work reported by Dr. Eddy (*3, 6*) in his assessments of the costs and effectiveness of different disease detection procedures are shown in Table VIII. It suggests a wide range of costbenefit ratios that we need to consider and also indicates the possible benefit of cancer screening that may be achieved compared with what the costs and benefits are in other fields such as hypertension detection. Improving the detection accuracy and lowering the cost of screening through sensitive and targeted approaches may significantly alter the cost effectiveness ratio and bring early cancer detection to larger numbers of persons at risk.

Our program illustrates further the contribution that the multidisciplinary approach has made to the topic of cancer prevention. I hope that my brief introductory remarks here document the potential range and importance of a multidisciplinary approach which is the essence of so much of our effort in the UICC and the cancer centers represented in this program.

## REFERENCES

1. "Cancer Patient Survival Experience," NIH Publication No. 80-2148 (1980).
2. Doll, R. and Peto, R. The causes of cancer: quantitative estimates of avoidable risks of cancer in the United States today. *J. Natl. Cancer Inst.*, **66**, 1191–1308 (1981).
3. Eddy, D. M. Cost-effectiveness of colorectal cancer screening. Paper presented at the International Symposium on Colorectal Cancer (1983).
4. Nutrition and cancer: cause and prevention. *Ca-A Cancer J. Clin.*, **34**, 121–126 (1984).
5. Segi Institute of Cancer Epidemiology. "Age-Adjusted Death Rates for Cancer for Selected Sites in 43 Countries in 1977" (1982).
6. The value of mammography for women over fifty. Report of the Subcommittee on Mammography to the American Cancer Society National Committee on Cancer Detection (1984).

# PREVENTION OF LIVER CANCER BY HEPATITIS B VACCINES

Arie J. Zuckerman

*Department of Medical Microbiology and WHO Collaborating Centre for Reference and Research on Viral Hepatitis, London School of Hygiene and Tropical Medicine (University of London)\**

Unique opportunities exist for the first time to prevent a frequent cancer by immunisation. Epidemiological data based on cohort or prospective studies have shown high relative risks for hepatocellular carcinoma among carriers of hepatitis B surface antigen and that the carrier state frequently precedes transformation of cells by many years. Infection by hepatitis B virus during early life may well be a critical factor.

The evidence of the association between the carrier state of hepatitis B and hepatocellular carcinoma in the majority of patients is such that active immunisation with hepatitis B vaccines is being evaluated in field trials in several countries as a means of preventing infection and the long-term risk of developing primary liver cancer. The evidence demonstrates that the scientific knowledge accumulated to date in the case of hepatitis B and hepatocellular carcinoma now allows such measures to be taken by active immunisation using the currently licensed plasma-derived hepatitis B vaccines. Rapid progress is also being made with subunit polypeptide vaccines prepared by recombinant DNA techniques and with chemically synthesized vaccines.

Viral hepatitis is a major public health problem in all parts of the world. The term human viral hepatitis refers to infections caused by four or more different viruses or groups of viruses, hepatitis A, hepatitis B, the more recently identified forms of hepatitis, non-A, non-B hepatitis which are caused by more than two viruses and probably by several different viruses, epidemic non-A hepatitis (previously referred to as epidemic non-A, non-B hepatitis) and the $\delta$ virus. Hepatitis A and hepatitis B can be differentiated by sensitive laboratory tests for specific antigens and antibodies and the viruses have been characterised. Specific laboratory tests are available for the $\delta$ agent, a defective virus, which replicates in individuals infected with hepatitis B virus.

## The Biology of Hepatitis B Virus

### 1. Structural and antigenic analysis of the virus

Examination by electron microscopy of plasma containing hepatitis B surface antigen reveals the presence of small spherical particles measuring on average 22 nm in diameter, tubular forms of varying length but with a diameter close to 22 nm, and large double-shelled or solid particles approximately 42 nm in diameter. The 42 nm particle is the

---

\* London WC1E 7HT, U.K.

complete virion and contains a core or nucleocapsid about 27 nm in diameter surrounded by an envelope approximately 14 nm in thickness. The core contains a double-stranded circular DNA with a molecular weight of about $2.3 \times 10^6$. The DNA is approximately 3,200 nucleotides in length, with a single-stranded gap varying from 600–2,100 nucleotides. The core particle also contains a DNA dependent DNA polymerase, which is closely associated with the DNA template, and protein kinase which phosphorylates the major viral specified core polypeptides. Another antigen, hepatitis B e antigen is closely associated with the core and its antigenic reactivity. The core antigen can be converted into e antigen by proteolytic degradation under dissociating conditions. The small spherical 22 nm particles and the tubular forms found in the plasma are non-infectious surplus virus coat protein, which also contain a variable amount of lipid and carbohydrate.

There is evidence which suggests the presence of specific structural receptors for polyalbumin on the complete virion and on purified hepatitis B surface antigen particles and polypeptides particularly if derived from e antigen-positive plasma. Polyalbumin receptors are also present on the surface of hepatocytes with polymerised serum albumin acting as a linker molecule between the surface antigen and the cell. The virion polyalbumin receptors are species and ligand specific and they react only with polymerised serum albumin, whereas the hepatocyte associated polyalbumin receptors are not ligand specific and they react with polymeric and monomeric albumins from different species. The polyalbumin receptors are probably encoded by the genome of the hepatitis B virus.

After the virus attaches to the surface of the hepatocyte, penetration of the virus into the cell may occur by two mechanisms: endocytosis of intact virions with subsequent release from endosomes or fusion between the viral envelope and the liver cell plasma membrane with penetration of the nucleocapsid into the cytoplasm. Replication of the virus in liver cells results in the production of viral proteins and the assembly of the complete virion. Hepatitis B surface antigen and core antigen are expressed on the plasma membrane of infected cells, and subsequently large amounts of the surface antigen and virus are released into the circulation.

The results of studies using monoclonal antibodies suggest that there are distinct determinants which reside on a domain common to all subtypes, but that there are also quantitative and qualitative differences in epitope density among the various subsets, implying that the surface antigen particles are much more heterogeneous than described hitherto. It is therefore now possible to "finger-print" hepatitis B virus, which will permit fine analysis of the evolution of the virus and its epidemiology in different parts of the world.

## 2.  Immune response to acute infection with hepatitis B virus

Infection leads to the appearance in the plasma during the incubation period of hepatitis B surface antigen about 2–8 weeks before biochemical evidence of liver dysfunction or the onset of jaundice. This antigen persists during the acute illness and is usually cleared from the circulation during convalescence. Next to appear in the circulation is the viral DNA polymerase associated with the core of the virus and at about the same time another antigen, the e antigen, becomes detectable, again preceding serum aminotransferase elevations. The e antigen is a distinct soluble antigen which correlates closely with the number of virus particles and relative infectivity. Antibody to the hepatitis core antigen is found in the serum 2–4 weeks after the appearance of the surface antigen, and it is always detectable during the early acute phase of the illness. Core antibody of the immunoglobulin M class becomes undetectable within some months of the onset of uncomplicated acute infection, but IgG core antibody persists after recovery for many years and possibly for life. The next antibody to appear in the circulation is directed against the e antigen, and there is evidence that, in general terms, anti-e indicates relatively low infectivity of serum, although a better measure of infectivity is the presence of hepatitis B virus DNA in serum. Antibody to the surface antigen component, hepatitis B surface antibody is the last marker to appear late during convalescence. Precipitating antibodies reacting with antigen determinants on the complete virus particle have also been described and these antibodies may be relevant to the clearance of circulating hepatitis B virions.

Evidence obtained more recently indicates that at the time of replication of hepatitis B virus, the surface antigen and core antigen are expressed on the plasma membrane of infected liver cells and both cellular and immune responses are initiated. The release of a large amount of surface antigen into the circulation which follows may induce high tolerance and rapid disappearance of the immune response to this antigen. Virions carrying polyalbumin receptors also stimulate the formation of neutralising polymerised human serum albumin antibodies, which prevent attachment and penetration of the virus into uninfected liver cells by reacting with the core antigen on the surface of liver cells. Elimination of the virus thus depends on a combined cellular and humoral response with both receptor neutralising polymerised human serum albumin antibodies and effective cytotoxic T cells. Failure of either of these mechanisms would lead to chronic liver damage and viral persistence. The extent of liver damage then depends on a number of factors which include autoimmune reactions directed at native hepatocyte membrane antigens and modulation of lysis by T cells of infected hepatocytes expressing core antigen on the surface of the cells. This would result eventually in termination of active viral replication with seroconversion to e antibody, with clinical and histological remission. On the other hand, cells with integrated viral genome do not have core antigen expressed on their surface and are protected from T cell lysis. The destruction of hepatocytes containing integrated hepatitis B virus DNA may be dependent on an immune response to hepatitis B surface antigen, and failure of this process of elimination results in persistence of clones of cells with the potential for transformation.

## 3. Hepatitis B virus and hepatocellular carcinoma

Hepatocellular carcinoma is one of the ten most common cancers in the world and one of the most prevalent cancers in developing countries with over 250,000 new cases of liver cancer each year. The actual age-adjusted incidence of hepatocellular carcinoma is over 30 new cases per 100,000 population each year in some parts of Asia and Africa, whereas it is less than 5 new cases per 100,000 per year in most countries in Europe, North America and in Australia. Nevertheless, there appears to be an upward time trend in the majority of the low incidence countries. This form of cancer is more common in males than among females, and it is well established that the incidence of liver cancer increases with age, but in high risk populations the disease occurs in younger age groups. There is a marked increase in incidence in certain ethnic groups (18).

## 4. Epidemiological correlation between hepatitis B infection and hepatocellular carcinoma

Many studies in different parts of the world, particularly in Africa and Asia show a highly significant excess of surface antigen, core antibody, and surface antibody in patients with hepatocellular carcinoma (for review see Refs. *2, 13, 18, 22*). An important factor in the aetiological association between hepatitis B and liver cell carcinoma may lie in an early age of infection. In areas of the world where the prevalence of macronodular cirrhosis and hepatocellular carcinoma is high, infection with hepatitis B virus and development of the persistent carrier state occur most frequently in infants and children.

## 5. *Production of hepatitis B surface antigen by continuous cell lines derived from human hepatocellular carcinoma*

The establishment of continuous cell lines from hepatocellular carcinoma which produce hepatitis B surface antigen provided a laboratory model for the study of various aspects of the biology of hepatitis B. The first of these cell lines, the PLC/PRF/5 cell line produces hepatitis B surface antigen similar in size, morphology, and polypeptide composition to the form which occurs in the serum of naturally infected individuals. The second hepatitis B surface antigen-producing cell line, Hep 3B, differs in some ways from the PLC/PRF/5 cells. A third hepatocellular carcinoma cell line, DELSH-5, releases hepatitis B surface antigen into the medium from the 13th passage onwards and, like the Hep 3B cells, the cells synthesized albumin and $\alpha$-fetoprotein. Other similar cell lines have been derived in other laboratories.

## 6. *Mode of replication of hepatitis B virus*

The inability to cultivate hepatitis B virus *in vitro*, the difficulties of obtaining suitable liver tissue, and, until recently, the lack of suitable experimental systems and techniques, hindered the investigation of the mode of replication of this virus. Summers and Mason (*15*) proposed, on the basis of studies of the duck hepatitis B virus, that the replication cycle of hepatitis B-like viruses is strikingly different from other DNA viruses in that RNA-directed DNA synthesis plays an essential role in the life cycle of these viruses, suggesting a close similarity to the RNA retroviruses. The principal unusual feature is the use of an RNA copy of the genome as an intermediate in the replication of the DNA genome. Infecting DNA genomes are converted to the double-stranded form, which serves as a template for transcription of RNA. Multiple RNA transcripts are synthesized from each infecting genome, and these transcripts have either messenger function or DNA replicative function. The term pre-genomes has been used for the transcripts with DNA replicative function since these are precursors of the progeny DNA genomes; they are assembled into nucleocapsid cores and reverse-transcribed before coating and release from the cell. Each mature virus particle contains, therefore, a DNA copy of the RNA pre-genome and a DNA polymerase.

The pre-genome appears to be a single polyadenylated viral specific plus strand RNA of approximately one genome in length (3Kb). The first DNA to be synthesized is a minus strand, and it is initiated at a unique site on the viral genome. Very small nascent DNA minus strands, as short as 30 nucleotides in length, are covalently attached at the 5′ end of the minus strand to a protein, and the protein probably serves as a primer for the synthesis of the minus strand DNA. Growth of the minus strand is accompanied by degradation of the pre-genome so that a full length single stranded DNA is produced (although hybrid DNA-RNA molecules have also been reported more recently). Plus strand DNA synthesis has been found after completion of the minus strand, and it is initiated at a unique site a few hundred nucleotides from the 5′ end of the minus strand. However, complete elongation of the plus strand is not required for coating and release of the nucleocapsid cores, so that most extracellular virions contain incomplete plus strand, and a single-stranded gap in the genome.

Based on this mode of replication, the ability of an infected cell to produce virus will depend on the continuous presence of a transcriptionally active form of viral DNA or "proviral" DNA. The "proviral" DNA must be present continuously since each pregenomic RNA molecule can give rise to only one virus particle.

Weiser *et al.* (*17*) characterised the major forms of intracellular virus-specific DNA in the livers of experimentally infected ground squirrels. A variety of DNA structures were found, covalently closed circular molecules, relaxed circular molecules, and a heterogeneous collection of molecules associated with protein and containing minus strands in 8- to 10-fold mass excess of plus strands. These results are in agreement with the analysis of intracellular forms of the duck hepatitis B virus and the mode of replication of hepatitis B virus proposed by Summers and Mason (*15*).

Fowler *et al.* (*9*) characterised the DNA replicative intermediates of hepatitis B virus present in the liver of a human and a chimpanzee carrier. The viral DNA forms consisted of a full length 3.2 Kb double-stranded hepatitis B viral DNA in both linear and relaxed circles, partially double-stranded DNA species of heterogeneous length and with mobility in the range of 2.8–2.0 Kb, and single-stranded DNA of heterogeneous length with mobilities relative to double-stranded DNA of 1.6 Kb and less, exclusively in the form of minus strand DNA. The 3.2 Kb double-stranded and single-stranded DNA species are considered to be replicative intermediates since, unlike the partially double-stranded species, they are not found in hepatitis B DNA obtained from plasma. This pattern of single-stranded replicative intermediates exclusively in the form of DNA minus strands is inconsistent with a semiconservative mechanism of DNA replication and is more like the mechanism of asymmetric replication using reverse transcription of an RNA pre-genome, as described above.

Distinct hybrid DNA-RNA molecules have been found in virus particles obtained from the plasma and liver of persistently infected patients and the liver of infected ducks. Examination of the hybrid molecules revealed the presence of viral minus strand DNA hydrogen bonded to plus strand RNA (*17*). Localisation of hepatitis B viral DNA predominantly in the cytoplasm of liver cells by an *in situ* hybridisation technique by Burrell *et al.* (*7*), and the presence in the liver of a patient with chronic active hepatitis B of mainly minus stranded viral DNA in the cytoplasm of hepatocytes using *in situ* hybridisation and by Southern blot analysis are in agreement with the view of replication of the human hepatitis B virus through an RNA intermediate. Thus the mode of replication of three of the Hepadna viruses reported to date is remarkably similar and differs from that known for all other DNA viruses.

## 7.   *Integration of hepatitis B viral DNA in the PLC/PRF/5 cell line*

The PLC/PRF/5 cells contain approximately four copies of viral DNA per haploid, mammalian cell DNA equivalent. Evidence was obtained that DNA from all regions of the viral genome is present in these cells, suggesting that the cells contain most, and possibly all, of the viral genome. Furthermore, the results indicated that the viral DNA is integrated in high molecular weight DNA at three different sites in the cells and that there is no viral DNA in an episomal form. Cellular RNA radiolabelled with [32]P was found to hybridise with all restriction fragments of hepatitis B virus DNA, which suggests that most and possibly all of the viral DNA in these cells is transcribed.

Evidence is also available for integration of the DNA of hepatitis B virus into the host genome of the PLC/PRF/5 cells and for expression of three RNA molecules containing specific sequences of hepatitis B virus. Integration of viral DNA in the cellular genome of human hepatocellular carcinoma tissue and in the PLC/PRF/5 cell line has also been demonstrated. The results suggest the existence of a limited number of integration sites in the cellular DNA, which is consistent either with the development of the liver tumour from one clone with several integration sites or with its development from a few clones each having particular integration sites. Other observations suggest the presence of two or more viral genomes inserted in tandem head-to-tail.

## 8.   Heterotransplantability of the PLC/PRF/5 cells

Desmyter et al. (8) induced tumours in 80% or more of nude mice (Pfd: NMRI/ nu-nu) injected subcutaneously with $5–10\times10^6$ cells. The tumours usually became detectable after 2 weeks and grew up to 15–30% of the body weight of the mice. Metastases were not found. When the cells were inoculated intraperitoneally, multiple tumours developed in various abdominal organs. The histology of the tumours was that of a well differentiated human hepatocellular carcinoma. Hepatitis B surface antigen was demonstrated by immunofluorescence in 0.1–10% of the tumour cells. Hepatitis B surface antigen, but no other serological marker of the virus, was found in the serum of the tumour-bearing mice. Newborn and weanling nude mice were equally susceptible.

The tumours were serially transplantable 3 to 5 times, but the take rates decreased with each passage, although there were no obvious differences between first-passage and later-passage tumours. The take rates were better when pieces of tumour were transplanted rather than trypsinised tumour cells. It was also possible to clone cells from the tumours, and their progeny induced tumours. Similar tumours were obtained in nude, athymic rats (Rowett Pfd: WIST-rnu-rnu), although the rats were less susceptible than nude mice.

## 9.   Integration of hepatitis B virus DNA into the genome of liver cells

Hepatitis B virus DNA has also been found in hepatocellular carcinoma tissue. However, there is no simple correlation between serum markers of hepatitis B and viral DNA in the tumour. Furthermore, in some specimens of liver tissue adjacent to tumours, extra-chromosomal and integrated viral DNA were present. The presence of integrated DNA in non-tumour tissue from patients with hepatocellular carcinoma suggests that integration precedes the development of gross neoplasia.

In carriers of hepatitis B virus with or without histological evidence of chronic liver disease integrated DNA has not been found in most of the carriers with relatively recent history of liver disease. However, in several patients who were long-term carriers, there was diffuse hybridisation in the high molecular weight regions of the gel. Free viral DNA was not identified. In these cases, it is possible that viral DNA is integrated diffusely throughout the host genome. Such integration might precede a stage in persistent infection with hepatitis B virus during which a specific subpopulation of hepatocytes undergoes cellular division into a clonal focus containing integrated viral DNA in one of a few specific sites. Additional factors may then be involved in the development of neoplasia from such a clonal focus.

Brechot et al. (5) used the Southern blot transfer-hybridisation technique to examine tissue extracted DNA immobilized on nitrocellulose paper by hybridisation with cloned hepatitis B virus DNA as a probe labelled with $^{32}$P by the nick translation procedure. Viral DNA was found to be integrated into cellular DNA in both liver tumour and non-tumour tissue in patients with hepatocellular carcinoma as demonstrated by hybridisation of high molecular weight DNA after digestion with *Hind* III and *Eco* RI endonucleases. Integrated viral DNA was also found in patients with cirrhosis with or without chronic active hepatitis. Free hepatitis B virus DNA was found in the liver in two patients with chronic persistent hepatitis and one patient with chronic active hepatitis. Restriction endonuclease patterns in two patients with acute hepatitis B strongly suggested viral DNA integration. If these findings are confirmed by the examination of a large number of patients with acute hepatitis B, then viral integration seems to occur early in the course of infection.

### 10. *Hepatitis B-like viruses in animals: the Hepadna viruses*

A number of human hepatitis B-like viruses in lower animals (other than the great apes) have been identified recently.

Snyder (*14*) reported the presence of liver cancer in 22 out of 76 eastern woodchucks (*Marmota monax*) which lived longer than 4 years in an established colony. In addition, the lesions of chronic active hepatitis and sometimes cirrhosis were usually found in the non-tumour tissue. Examination by electron microscopy of sera collected from the captive woodchucks revealed virus particles which resemble closely human hepatitis B virus (*16*). Human hepatitis B virus and the woodchuck hepatitis virus share the following characteristics. Infection with either virus results in the accumulation in blood of large amounts of excess virus coat protein in the form of spherical and tubular particles measuring 20–25 nm in diameter. Both are 40–45 nm double-shelled or solid particles with a nucleocapsid containing double-stranded circular DNA with a gap and both contain a viral DNA polymerase. Each virus is associated with chronic hepatitis and hepatocellular carcinoma. Antigenic cross-reactivity has been reported between the cores of the two viruses but only minor common antigenic determinants were identified on the virus surface protein. A small region of 100–150 base pairs of nucleic acid homology, measured by liquid hybridisation, was found in the genomes of the two viruses. It seems likely that this 3–5% of nucleic acid homology represents one or two regions of nearly identical nucleotide sequence. The DNA of human hepatitis B virus and the DNA of woodchuck hepatitis virus has been cloned in the vector lambda/gtWES. This was then subcloned into the kanamycin resistant plasmid pA01. Comparison of the recombinant DNAs with authentic virus DNAs by specific hybridisation, size, and restriction enzyme analysis showed that the recombinants contained the complete genome of each virus. The nucleic acid homology between the two viral DNAs was confirmed with the cloned DNAs. Thus the woodchuck hepatitis virus and the human hepatitis virus are phylogenetically related.

Another virus which is related to human hepatitis B has been described in Beechey ground squirrels (*Spermophilus beecheyi*) in northern California. Common features with the human hepatitis B virus include virus morphology, size, and structure of the viral DNA, a virion DNA polymerase which repairs a single-stranded region in the double-stranded circular genome, cross-reacting surface viral antigens, antigen-antibody systems similar to hepatitis B *e* antigen and the core antigen, and persistent infection with viral antigen present continuously in the blood. The antigenic and structural relationships between the surface antigens of the human hepatitis B virus, the ground squirrel hepatitis B virus and the woodchuck hepatitis virus have been described in detail.

The differences in pathogenicity of these three viruses are notable. While persistent infection in infected ground squirrels is common in endemic areas and the titre of the virus, as measured by viral DNA polymerase activity is high, there is little or no evidence of hepatitis in infected ground squirrels. In persistently infected squirrels followed-up in the laboratory for over 2 years, only the mildest form of inflammation of the liver was found in some animals, and none of 25 ground squirrels developed cirrhosis or liver cancer. The complete DNA sequence of the ground squirrel hepatitis virus has not been published at the time of writing, but cross-hybridisation studies show a significant degree of homology between the DNA of human hepatitis B virus and the ground squirrel hepatitis virus. The results to date indicate that the coding sequence for the major surface antigen polypeptide and the major core polypeptide coding sequence of the three mammalian hepatitis viruses have homologous regions with similar locations in relation to the unique physical features of the DNA of the virions.

The fourth member of this group of viruses was discovered in some domesticated ducks (*Anas domesticus*) in the People's Republic of China following the observation of frequent liver cancer in Pekin ducks. Approximately 10% of Pekin ducks in some commercial flocks in the United States carry a hepatitis B-like virus, named duck hepatitis B virus. This species of duck was originally imported from China in the 19th Century. The duck hepatitis B virus is similar morphologically to the three mammalian viruses, although the spherical particles are larger and more pleomorphic and tubular forms have not been found. The viral genome is circular and partially single-stranded and an endogenous DNA polymerase can convert the DNA genome to a complete double-stranded circular form with a size of approximately 3,000 base pairs. Examination for viral DNA in the organs of infected birds revealed preferential localisation in the liver. The virus is transmitted vertically and infected ducklings may develop persistent viraemia. Studies on antigenic analysis and nucleotide sequence are in progress.

In summary, therefore, various studies, including comparative pathology and comparative virology of infected eastern woodchucks and Pekin ducks and the mode of replication of the Hepadna viruses, have established that there is a strong and specific association between persistent hepatitis B infection and hepatocellular carcinoma, and it is likely that this association is causal in up to 80% of such cancers (*18*). However, factors other than hepatitis B virus may be implicated. It is possible that hepatocellular carcinoma is the cumulative result of several cofactors or hepatocarcinogens including genetic, immunological, nutritional, and hormonal factors, mycotoxins, particularly aflatoxin, chemical carcinogens and other environmental influences including alcohol, and that hepatitis B virus acts either as a carcinogen or as a cocarcinogen in persistently infected hepatocytes (for reviews see Refs. *20, 22*, and others).

However, the evidence of the association between the carrier state of hepatitis B and hepatocellular carcinoma in the majority of patients is such that active immunisation with hepatitis B vaccines is being evaluated in field trials in several countries as a means of preventing infection and long-term risk of developing primary liver cancer. Development of "preventive measures specific to cancers that are preventable in the countries concerned, leading to a significant reduction in the incidence of these cancers" is one of the three main targets of the WHO Cancer Control Programme. The evidence outlined above demonstrates that the scientific knowledge accumulated to date in the case of hepatitis B and hepatocellular carcinoma now allows such measures to be taken by active immunisation using the currently licensed plasma-derived hepatitis B vaccines. Rapid progress is also being made with the subunit polypeptide vaccines, vaccines prepared by recombinant DNA techniques and with chemically synthesized vaccines.

### Prevention of the Carrier State of Hepatitis B Virus and of Liver Cancer by Immunisation

#### 1. Passive immunisation

Passive immunisation against hepatitis B by the administration of hepatitis B immunoglobulin has been available for about a decade, and it has been used with substantial effectiveness for post-exposure prophylaxis after a single acute accidental inoculation and for interrupting maternal-to-infant transmission. The results of small non-randomised studies, and more recently controlled studies, have shown that it is possible to prevent perinatal transmission of hepatitis B virus from surface antigen and *e* antigen carrier mothers in 70–80% of infants by the administration of hepatitis B immunoglobulin at birth and at varying intervals thereafter. However, infection still occurs in many instances (range 20–40%). The importance of administering the first dose of immunoglobulin within a few hours of birth should be noted (3).

#### 2. Active immunisation

The development of hepatitis B vaccines from the excess surface antigen protein coat of the virus collected from the plasma of asymptomatic carriers is an ingenious, though highly unusual, solution to the repeated failure to grow the virus in tissue culture. The surface antigen is purified by several physical and biological procedures and inactivated. The currently licensed plasma-derived vaccines which meet WHO requirements have been shown to be safe and effective, and have not been associated with a risk of transmission of AIDS or other infectious agent. Vaccines produced by recombinant DNA techniques in eukaryotic cells, particularly yeast, are at a stage of clinical evaluation (14), progress is being made with the development of chemically synthesized hepatitis B peptide vaccines (see Ref. 6), and live recombinant vaccinia virus vaccines are promising (12).

Although the priorities for immunisation against hepatitis B are not the same for each country or geographical region, since the needs are dictated by differing epidemiological patterns, cultural and sexual practices, socioeconomic factors and the environment, it is evident that the prevention of perinatal transmission has the highest priority for children born to mothers in "high-risk" groups and for susceptible women of childbearing age and their newborn infants in endemic areas. This was clearly demonstrated by the pioneer studies carried out in Senegal by Maupas *et al.* (10) and in Taiwan by Beasley *et al.* (4). The plasma-derived vaccines were highly immunogenic and there was no interference by circulating maternal antibodies. Nevertheless, the protection afforded by the vaccine alone was about 70%, a rate which is similar to the efficacy of passive protection using multiple injections of hepatitis B immunoglobulin.

#### 3. Passive-active immunisation

Various temporal combinations of hepatitis B immunoglobulin and hepatitis B vaccine have now been extensively evaluated in Taiwan (4) and in Hong Kong (19), and smaller studies were conducted in Japan, in Holland and elsewhere. A number of trials are still in progress. Analysis of the results of the trials in Taiwan and Hong Kong, which are high endemic areas, has shown that combined passive-active prophylaxis improved the protective efficacy in infants born to hepatitis B *e* antigen carrier mothers to over 90%, whereas in the untreated group development of the carrier state ranged from 73–88%.

Although it is difficult to recommend precise immunisation schedules at present, since an international standard preparation of the vaccine is not yet available to permit direct comparisons between different vaccines, it is clear that combined prophylaxis is the method of choice for protection of infants born to *e* antigen-positive mothers, and this should be extended to babies born to surface antigen carrier mothers who are *e* antibody-negative. Ideally, it has been suggested that infants born to all surface antigen-positive mothers including those with anti-*e* should be immunised, although it is recognised that the risk of perinatal infection in the latter group is very small. It should be noted, however, that unless these children are actively immunised they are at a continuing risk of infection by horizontal transmission later in life.

However, the relative scarcity of hepatitis B immunoglobulin and its cost and the current high cost of the licensed hepatitis B vaccines preclude large scale prophylaxis at present. Nevertheless, the fact that multiple doses of immunoglobulin as compared with a single dose at birth did not offer significant advantage when combined with a course of vaccine is encouraging. Second, the vaccine is highly immunogenic in infants and the dose could be reduced substantially. Third, vaccines produced by recombinant DNA techniques should prove to be equally effective and substantially cheaper; and there is also the longer term prospect of cheap chemically synthesized vaccines.

Given sufficient resources, protection by combined immunisation against hepatitis B of all newborn infants at risk is within reach. The principal health benefits will include dramatic reduction of the persistent carrier rate, reduction in morbidity and mortality from chronic liver disease and prevention of a substantial proportion of hepatocellular carcinomas (for review see Ref. *21*).

*Acknowledgments*

The hepatitis research programme at the London School of Hygiene and Tropical Medicine is supported by generous grants from the Medical Research Council, the Department of Health and Social Security, the Wellcome Trust, the World Health Organisation and Organon B.V.

The hepatitis B vaccine development project at the London School of Hygiene and Tropical Medicine is generously supported by the British Technology Group (formerly the National Research Development Corporation), the Department of Health and Social Security, the Wellcome Trust and the Commission of the European Economic Community.

## REFERENCES

1.  Arthur, M.J.P., Hall, A. J., and Wright, R. Hepatitis B, hepatocellular carcinoma and strategies for prevention. *Lancet*, **i**, 607–610 (1984).
2.  Beasley, R. P. and Hwang, L.-Y. Hepatocellular carcinoma and hepatitis B virus. *Semin. Liver Dis.*, **4**, 113–121 (1984).
3.  Beasley, R. P., Hwang, L.-Y., Lin, C.-C., Stevens, C. E., Wang, K.-Y., Sun, T.-S., Hsieh, F.-J., and Szmuness, W. Hepatitis B immune globulin (HBIG) efficacy in the interruption of perinatal transmission of hepatitis B carrier state. *Lancet*, **ii**, 388–393 (1981).
4.  Beasley, R. P., Hwang, L.-Y., Lee, G. C.-Y., Lan, C.-C., Roan, C.-H., Huang, F.-Y., and

Chen, C.-L. Prevention of perinatally transmitted hepatitis B virus infections with hepatitis B immune globulin and hepatitis B vaccine. *Lancet*, **ii**, 1099–1102 (1983).

5. Brechot, C., Hadchouel, M., Scotto, J., Fonck, M., Potet, F., Vyas, G. N., and Tiollais, P. State of hepatitis B virus DNA in hepatocytes of patients with hepatitis B surface antigen-positive and -negative liver diseases. *Proc. Natl. Acad. Sci. U.S.*, **78**, 3906–3910 (1981).

6. Brown, S. E., Howard, C. R., Zuckerman, A. J., and Steward, M. W. Affinity of antibody responses in man to hepatitis B vaccine determined with synthetic peptides. *Lancet*, **ii**, 184–187 (1984).

7. Burrell, C. J., Gowans, E. J., Jilbert, A. R., Lake, J. R., and Marmion, B. P. Hepatitis B virus DNA detection by *in situ* cytohybridization: implications for viral replication strategy and pathogenesis of chronic hepatitis. *Hepatology*, **2**, Suppl., 85–91 (1982).

8. Desmyter, J., de Groote, J., Ray, M. B., Bradburne, A. F., Desmet, V., De Somer, P., and Alexander, J. HBsAg-producing human hepatoma cell line: tumours in nude mice and interferon properties. *In* "Virus and the Liver," ed. L. Bianchi, W. Gerok, K. Sinkinger, and G. A. Stalder, pp. 217–221 (1980). MTP Press, Lancaster.

9. Fowler, M.J.F., Monjardino, J., Tsiquaye, K. N., Zuckerman, A. J., and Thomas, H. C. The mechanism of replication of hepatitis B virus: evidence of asymmetric replication of the DNA strands. *J. Med. Virol.*, **13**, 83–91 (1984).

10. Maupas, P., Chiron, J.-P., Barim, F., Coursaget, P., Goudeau, A., Perrin, J., Denir, P., and Diop Mar, I. Efficacy of hepatitis B vaccine in prevention of HBsAg carrier state in children. Controlled trial in an endemic area (Senegal). *Lancet*, **i**, 289–292 (1981).

11. Miller, R. H., Tran, C.-T., Marion, P. L., and Robinson, W. S. Replication of hepatitis B virus DNA. *In* "Viral Hepatitis: Proceedings of the 1984 International Symposium" (1984), in press.

12. Moss, B., Smith, G. L., Gerin, J. L., and Purcell, R. H. Live recombinant vaccinia virus protects chimpanzees against hepatitis B. *Nature*, **311**, 67–69 (1984).

13. Sherman, M. and Shafritz, D. A. Hepatitis B virus and hepatocellular carcinoma: molecular biology and mechanistic considerations. *Semin. Liver Dis.*, **4**, 98–112 (1984).

14. Snyder, R. L. Hepatomas of captive woodchucks. *Am. J. Pathol.*, **52**, 32 (1968).

15. Summers, J. and Mason, W. S. Replication of the genome of a hepatitis B-like virus by reverse transcription of an RNA intermediate. *Cell*, **29**, 403–415 (1982).

16. Summers, J., Smolec, M. J., and Snyder, R. L. A virus similar to human hepatitis B virus associated with hepatitis and hepatoma in woodchucks. *Proc. Natl. Acad. Sci. U.S.*, **75**, 4533–4537 (1978).

17. Weiser, B., Gane, D., Seeger, C., and Varmus, H. E. Closed circular viral DNA and asymmetrical heterogeneous forms in livers from animals infected with ground squirrel hepatitis virus. *J. Virol.*, **48**, 1–9 (1983).

18. World Health Organisation. Prevention of primary liver cancer. Report of a WHO meeting. World Health Organisation Technical Report Series, No. 691 (1983). WHO, Geneva.

19. Wong, V.C.W., Ip, H.M.H., Reesink, H. W., Lelie, P. N., Reerlink-Brongers, E. E., Yeung, C. Y., and Ma, H. K. Prevention of the HBsAg carrier state in newborn infants of mothers who are chronic carriers of HBsAg and HBeAg by administration of hepatitis B vaccine and hepatitis B immunoglobulin. *Lancet*, **i**, 921–926 (1984).

20. Zuckerman, A. J. Primary hepatocellular carcinoma and hepatitis B virus. *Trans. R. Soc. Trop. Med. Hyg.*, **76**, 711–718 (1982).

21. Zuckerman, A. J. Perinatal transmission of hepatitis B. *Arch. Dis. Child.* (1984), in press.

22. Zuckerman, A. J., Sun, T.-T., Linsell, A., and Stjernsward, J. Prevention of primary liver cancer. *Lancet*, **i**, 463–465 (1983).

# SIGNIFICANCE OR INSIGNIFICANCE OF MASS SCREEN-ING PROGRAM FOR STOMACH CANCER

Shigeru HISAMICHI,[*1] Akira FUKAO,[*1] Tooru YANBE,[*2] and Nobuyuki SUGAWARA[*2]

*Department of Public Health, Tohoku University School of Medicine[*1] and Cancer Detection Center of Miyagi Cancer Society[*2]*

A mass screening program for stomach cancer has been systematical-ly performed since 1960 in Japan and the number of examinees now amounts to over 4,000,000 a year. The age-adjusted death rate for this disease has been on a downward trend during the past two decades in Ja-pan. During the same period, gastric mass surveys have been conducted regularly throughout the country as a secondary prevention for cancer, thus attempting to reduce the mortality from stomach cancer by its early detection.

Long-term follow-up studies clearly suggest that the gastric mass sur-veys have contributed toward reducing deaths from stomach cancer. A significant reduction was observed in a group screened compared to one unscreened in Miyagi Prefecture. It is said, however, that several biases are possible in evaluating the trend of reduced death rate by mass screening for cancer, such as incidence bias and lead time bias. The 10-year survival rate of patients with stomach cancer detected by the mass survey was higher than the rate of those detected by outpatient clinics, even if a lead time bias was considered. Furthermore, the percent decrease in death rate for stomach cancer from 1960 to 1980 in this prefecture was observed to be larger than the percent decrease of incidence rate during the same period, one of the most important beneficial effects of gastric mass survey being to eliminate incidence bias.

We also indicated the "insignificance," the problems of false negative screening accuracy and possible or potential radiation hazard due to re-peated mass radiography.

*History of Gastric Mass Survey*

The 1948 photofluorography conducted on 10,000 persons by Roach *et al.* (*13*) is con-sidered to be the first full-scale type of gastric mass survey. The first survey in Japan was carried out by Irie and Kadota (1953) (*8*). However, the first such systematic survey by governmental supports using an X-ray car was conducted in Miyagi Prefecture in 1960 (*4*).

**Gastric mass surveys thus originally started in the U.S.** but then completely dis-appeared. However, since 1960 they have been disseminated nationwide in Japan, along with some improvements in the diagnostic technique. The number of examinees has been increasing annually since 1968 and amounted to over 4 million in 1981.

---

*1 Seiryo-machi 2-1, Sendai 980, Japan (久道 茂, 深尾 彰).
*2 Kamisugi 5-7-10, Sendai 980, Japan (山家 泰, 菅原伸之).

The following background lies behind such dissemination in Japan: mortality from stomach cancer was the highest among malignant diseases; a gastric cancer, if treated in its early stage, is clinically curable; and the mass survey using X-ray cars was easily adapted to public health communities and the health control systems which had already been created for mass screening programs for pulmonary tuberculosis. In addition to the primary prevention, early detection and early treatment is considered to be most effective for persons who have already accumulated cancer risk factors.

### Natural History of Cancer and Role of Gastric Mass Survey

Miller (10) proposed the following three hypotheses as assumptions in conducting mass screening for cervical cancer: 1) the histological abnormalities identified in an asymptomatic stage or an early stage, if left untreated, in an early stage will progress in the majority of cases to symptomatic invasive cancer and a proportion of these will result in death; 2) all invasive cancers arise in this way; and 3) providing a sufficient number of women are screened, the morbidity and eventually the mortality of the disease will be reduced. These three hypotheses are also applicable to a gastric mass survey. The natural history model formed for cervical cancer shows that the progress of the disease, from cancer onset *in situ* to micro invasive cancer, occult invasive cancer, clinical invasive cancer, and finally to death, progresses according to age. This phenomenon is very useful in understanding Dr. Miller's hypotheses and is also very convincing (10).

Figure 1 shows the natural history of gastric cancer compiled on the basis of our own data. The number of patients with stomach cancer detected by the mass survey was 2,295. The average age at the time of diagnosis was first recorded, and average age at the time of death was also obtained for those who died later. The average age of gastric

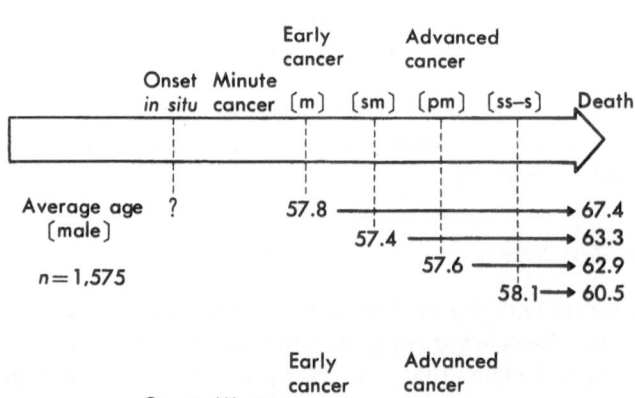

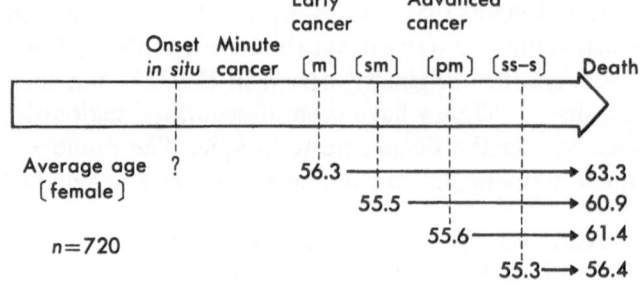

FIG. 1.   Model of natural history of stomach cancer; from cases (n=2,295) detected by gastric mass survey in Miyagi Prefecture, 1970–1982.

cancer patients who were detected by the mass survey is around 57 in males and 55 in females, showing no correlation with the progressive degree at each stage. The natural history of gastric cancer is, therefore, not so simple as that of cervical cancer. The findings which attracted our attention were that the shallower the depth of cancer infiltration at the time of detection, the older the patient's age was at the time of death. The primary prevention, which means measures against the causes, is fundamentally important. However, the relationship of the risk factors which induce gastric cancer and degree of these factors contributing to the mortality from stomach cancer is not as clear as that of smoking causing pulmonary carcinoma. This is the reason the mass survey method as a . secondary prevention is regarded as the most important in Japan.

Incidentally, the case in which surgical removal of precancerous lesions such as severe dysplasia of the uterine cervix and atypical epithelium of the stomach can reduce carcinogenesis is called by the authors "the primary-and-a-half prevention for cancer." Such an idea is also presented in the concept "CANSCREEN" advocated by Sutnick et al. (17).

## Conditions of the Mass Survey for Cancer

In conducting a mass survey for cancer, there are several conditions in addition to those of a gastric mass survey. These are: 1) cancer with high morbidity and mortality should be targeted, 2) a screening test adaptable for a mass population should be used, 3) a high degree of diagnostic accuracy should be possible, 4) the effect of early treatment should be expected by early detection, 5) the cost-benefit ratio should be well balanced, 6) the survey method should be efficient and effective, 7) the screening test should be safe and without any side effects, and 8) globally, the merits should outweigh demerits. A mass survey for cancer of any specific organ is valuable if these conditions are all satisfied. The gastric mass survey being made in Japan completely satisfies conditions 1), 2), and 4). However, its evaluation on the other conditions is controversial. This is perhaps not surprising since an evaluation is always affected by the difference in importance given to a gastric cancer survey, the value of human life, levels of other diagnostic techniques, economic situations, and sometimes, religious or philosophical concepts which differ to a considerable extent from country to country.

## Evaluation of the Gastric Mass Survey and Its Problems

In view of the conditions cited above, the gastric mass survey can be assessed by: 1) an epidemiological evaluation, 2) an evaluation for diagnostic accuracy, 3) an economic evaluation by a cost-benefit analysis, 4) a political or administrative evaluation, and 5) a social and ethical evaluation. The most important of all these is the epidemiological evaluation.

Evaluation is actually made by 1) monitoring, 2) case study, 3) survey research, 4) trend analysis, and 5) experimental design (9). There is, however, a dispute over the methods of evaluation between clinical doctors and epidemiologists. The point of their argument is "Is the mass survey for cancer really effective and useful as a secondary prevention?" No agreement has yet been reached concerning this. Sackett (14) an epidemiologist, claimed that the only acceptable method of evaluating a mass survey is a randomized controlled trial. However, only two kinds of studies have been made using this randomized controlled method. These were a breast cancer screening (HIP Study) (16) and a mass screening for lung cancer (Mayo Lung Project) (3). The former study was evaluated as effective while the latter was not. Cole and Morrison (2), on the other hand, said that the evaluation of a survey can only be made as a non-experimental study. They stressed the difficulty in conducting randomized controlled trials on humans. In fact, the American Cancer Society (ACS) (1) evaluated highly the effectiveness of mass survey for cervical cancer recommending models with concrete ages and test intervals to be used, although such a survey has not yet been evaluated by a randomized controlled trial.

A gastric mass survey has not been made using the randomized controlled method in Japan. Due to the Law of Health and Medical Service for the Aged, which became effective February 1983, gastric mass surveys which are needed by community residents are now one of the administration policies of the Government. Therefore, adoption of the randomized controlled trial is now all the more difficult. What is important in the evaluation is how well the biases, such as length, lead time, self-selection, and incidence biases which are all caused when randomized controlled trial is not applicable, are removed. The UICC International Workshop (18), referring to the evaluation of the mass survey for cancer, pointed out that a "second best" method of measuring effectiveness might be possible by comparing cancer incidence and mortality in a defined population before and after the introduction of a screening program and comparing intensively screened areas with non-screened areas. Effectively preventing cancer death by early detection and early treatment should also be stressed using the critical point hypothesis.

Many published studies have proved the effectiveness of gastric mass survey in the prevention of deaths from stomach cancer (5–7, 11, 12, 19). Various studies were published in which a comparison was made between the long-term survival rate of patients with stomach cancer detected by mass survey and that of those diagnosed at general outpatient departments. In contrast, a study by Sakka et al. (15) was carried out on one of the demerits of the gastric mass survey, i.e., the relationship between leukemia and low-level radiation caused by gastric photoradiography. No excess incidence of leukemia in a screened group compared with an unscreened group was reported.

The problem of defining the false negative rate still remains unsolved in relation to the accuracy in the screening test of the gastric mass survey. Yamagata et al. (19) clarified the false negative rate, its cause, and a method for its improvement. Many studies are also available on the cost-benefit analysis.

CONCLUSION

A small difference is found in the policies on cancer, namely, the administration and key policies in each country. However, the policy of WHO seems to be fundamentally unchangeable. It places importance on primary as well as secondary prevention, aftercare including rehabilitation, education and training regarding cancer, information collection and dissemination. The gastric mass survey will be further disseminated in Japan. It will take an important role in the prevention of cancer in such countries where morbidity as well as mortality by gastric cancer are rather high. For that purpose, the significance and purpose of the mass survey program should be recognized.

Furthermore, in order that the gastric mass survey program should not be evaluated as "high efforts, low effects," a much more detailed study as well as a more careful approach to the survey should be taken.

# REFERENCES

1. ACS Report on the Cancer-Related Health Checkup. Approved by Board of Directors on February 8, 1980, pp. 1–39 (1980). American Cancer Society, Inc., U.S.A.
2. Cole, P. and Morrison, A. S. Basic issues in population screening for cancer. *J. Natl. Cancer Inst.*, **64**, 1263–1272 (1980).
3. Fontana, R. S., Sanderson, D. R., Wooler, L. B., Miller, W. E., Bernatz, P. E., Payne, W. S., and Taylor, W. F. The Mayo lung project for early detection and localization of bronchogenic carcinoma: a status report. *Chest*, **67**, 511–522 (1975).
4. Hisamichi, S. "Principles and Practice in Gastric Mass Examination," (in Japanese) pp. 4–6 (1978). Kanahara-Shuppan, Tokyo.
5. Hisamichi, S. Public health and gastric mass survey (in Japanese). *J. Gastroenterol. Mass Surv.*, **64**, 23–28 (1984).
6. Hisamichi, S., Sasaki, R., Sugawara, N., Yanabe, T., and Yamagata, S. Stomach cancer in various age groups (Japan) as detected by gastric mass survey. *J. Am. Geriatr. Soc.*, **27**, 439–443 (1979).
7. Hisamichi, S. and Sugawara, N. Mass screening for gastric cancer by X-ray examination. *Japan. J. Clin. Oncol.*, **14**, 211–223 (1984).
8. Irie, H. and Kadota, H. Early detection of stomach cancer by mass photofluorography (in Japanese). *Nihonijishinpou*, **1513**, 1589–1591 (1953).
9. Kaluzny, A. D. and Veney, J. E. Evaluating health care programs and services. *In* "Introduction to Health Services," ed. S. J. Williams and P. R. Torrens, pp. 433–457 (1984). John Wiley & Sons, New York.
10. Miller, A. B. Evaluation of mass screening programmes for carcinoma of the cervix. *In* "Cancer Campaigns, Detection Rehabilitation, Clinical Classification," Proc. Vol. 4, pp. 204–218 (1974), XI Int. Cancer Congr., Florence.
11. Oshima, A. and Fujimoto, I. Cancer of the stomach. *In* "The Epidemiology of Cancer," ed. G. J. Bourke, pp. 116–130 (1983). Croom Helm, London-Sydney / The Charless Press, Publishers, Philadelphia.
12. Oshima, A., Hanai, A., and Fujimoto, I. Evaluation of a mass screening program of stomach cancer. *In* "Second Symposium on Epidemiology and Cancer Registries in the Pacific Basin," Natl. Cancer Inst. Monogr. 53, NIH Publication No. 79-1864, pp. 181–186 (1979). NIH. NCI, Bethesda, Maryland.
13. Roach, J. F., Sloan, R. D., and Morgan, R. H. The detection of gastric carcinoma by photofluorographic methods. Part I. Introduction. *Am. J. Roentgenol.*, **61**, 183–187 (1949).
14. Sackett, D. Periodic examination of patients at risk. *In* "Cancer Epidemiology and Prevention," ed. C. Schottenfeld, pp. 437–456 (1975). Charles C. Thomas, Springfield.
15. Sakka, M., Hisamichi, S., Takano, A., Hashizume, T., Sasano, N., and Uzuka, Y. Mass survey of gastric cancer and leukemia in Miyagi Prefecture, Japan. *Tohoku J. Exp. Med.*, **138**, 239–243 (1982).
16. Shapiro, S., Strax, P., and Venet, L. Periodic breast cancer screening in reducing mortality from breast cancer. *J. Am. Med. Assoc.*, **215**, 1777–1785 (1971).
17. Sutnick, A. I., Miller, D. G., Samson, B., Dean, D. H., Kudowski, K. M., Haopern, L., Jefferys, C., and Bahn, A. D. Population cancer screening. *Cancer*, **38**, 1367–1372 (1976).
18. UICC Technical Report Series, Vol. 40, "Screening in Cancer," ed. A. B. Miller, pp. 334–338 (1978). UICC, Geneva.
19. Yamagata, S., Hisamichi, S., and Sugawara, N. Mass screening for cancer in Japan, present and future. *In* "Recent Advances in Cancer Control," ed. S. Yamagata, T. Hirayama, and S. Hisamichi, pp. 33–45 (1983). Excerpta Medica, Amsterdam-Oxford-Princeton.

# NUTRITION AND CANCER PREVENTION: GASTROINTESTINAL CANCER

J. H. Weisburger

*Naylor Dana Institute for Disease Prevention,
American Health Foundation**

The complex process of carcinogenesis involves a series of steps that include initiation, development, and progression. Initiation stems from specific changes caused by genotoxic carcinogens. For cancers of the colon, breast, prostate, and perhaps even pancreas, these may be the mutagens-carcinogens seen in fried or broiled meat or fish. Gastric cancer has distinct associated factors, namely, pickled or salted fish or beans, or geochemical or agricultural sources of nitrate. The genotoxic carcinogen is postulated as an alkylnitrosamide or diazonium type of chemical, and the formation of such compounds is inhibited by vitamin C, vitamin E, and certain anti-oxidants. Vitamin A and carotene may play a role in delaying later stages in gastric cancer development.

Promoting agents play a major role in the development of colon cancer. Human and animal model studies show that the amounts of dietary fat and fiber are critical. Dietary fat controls bile acid biosynthesis, and since bile acids are promoters of colon tumors, fat promotes colon tumor development. Cereal bran fibers increase intestinal bulk and reduce the concentration of promoters. Calcium salts lower the toxicity of fatty and bile acids. The action of promoters is dose and time dependent, and a reduction in dose leads to a lower risk. Even colon cancer patients may benefit from dietary intervention as an effective adjuvant therapy.

In many parts of the world, lifestyle is the main factor associated with the locally prevailing types of neoplastic diseases. Cancers in the respiratory tract, kidney, bladder, and in part, pancreas are associated with the habit of smoking. Oral cavity and esophageal cancers are related to chewing of tobacco-containing products, or smoking combined with excessive drinking, anywhere in the world where these habits are practiced. In the Western World, traditional nutritional customs involving the consumption of 40–45% of total calories as dietary fat with relatively little cereal fiber, and frequent use of fried meats are mainly associated with the occurrence of cancer of the colon, breast, prostate, endometrium, and also in part, pancreas. Such dietary practices also relate to atherosclerosis, coronary heart disease, and diabetes. On the other hand, in the Orient and in part, in Nordic, Eastern European, and Latin American countries, the dietary traditions involving intake of salted, pickled, or smoked fish, or similarly processed vegetables, or meat are associated with cancer of the glandular stomach; in some areas with cancer of the nasopharynx and esophagus, and through other mechanisms, with hypertension and thence cerebrovascular accidents.

---

* Valhalla, New York, 10595-1599, U.S.A.

In this paper, we will review briefly the procedures used to define risk factors and discuss the evidence obtained from studies in human subjects, in animal models, and in cell culture systems in the light of the current understanding of the mechanisms of cancer causation.

### Procedures for the Delineation of Risk Factors

The causative and modifying factors for any specific disease can be detected by considering a set of essential data (Table I).

1.   Comparative incidence and mortality data from different geographic areas are most useful in leading to classification of the populations as high- or low-risk groups. Disease incidence also can be determined in certain populations within an area whose lifestyles are related to religious or ethnic traditions.

2.   Changes in disease incidence in migrants from low to higher risk regions or *vice versa* is considered.

3.   Long-term observations of incidence or mortality, recorded by established, reliable cancer registries in different parts of the world, provide information on changes over time.

4.   Studies in human subjects by the techniques of metabolic epidemiology, in animal models, and by other suitable techniques delineate the effect of suspected risk factors from 1, 2, and 3 and acquire information on the underlying mechanisms of action.

TABLE I.   Factors in the Etiology of Human Cancers

---

  I.  Epidemiology
      A.  Geographic pathology
      B.  Special populations
      C.  Time trends
 II.  Laboratory Studies
      A.  Metabolic and biochemical epidemiology-population studies
      B.  Model studies in animals
      C.  Model studies in cell and organ cultures
      D.  Definition of mechanisms
III.  Development of Hypotheses
      A.  Established risk factors and their mode of action
          1.  Genotoxic carcinogens (chemical, virus, radiation)
          2.  Nongenotoxic promoting or enhancing stimulus (chemical, viral)
          3.  Data on amount and duration of exposure to each kind of agent
          4.  Possible inhibition of action of agents
      B.  Suspected risk factors and their possible role

---

### Mechanisms of Carcinogenesis

Cancer causation and development requires a series of sequential steps. An early event in neoplasia is a somatic mutation, an alteration of the genetic material (*18, 41, 43*). One type of alteration is direct attack on DNA by radiation, viruses, or chemicals. Chemical carcinogens, classified into nine classes, belong, in turn, to two main groups: 1) genotoxic carcinogens, 2) agents operating by nongenotoxic or epigenetic pathways such as promotion (*33*). This classification is important in delineating the role of each agent —genotoxic carcinogen, cocarcinogen, or promoter—in the overall carcinogenic process for each kind of cancer. This key early set of events has been reviewed elsewhere (see Refs. *18*, *32*, *33*, *41*, *43*).

### Cancer of the Upper Gastrointestinal Tract

#### 1. Nitrosamines—possible carcinogens for head and neck cancer

Appreciable levels of certain nitrosamines such as nitrosonornicotine are present in tobacco (*11*). These carcinogens may be responsible for tobacco-associated cancers (lung, pancreas, kidney, urinary bladder) or in the presence of heavy alcohol intake, for cancers of the oral cavity and esophagus.

A geographic belt of high incidence of esophageal cancer is evident in eastern Iran, southern Soviet Union, and central China, where this disease occurs in people who do not smoke and drink. The key risk factors remain to be discovered, but in China (*20*), nitrosamines appear to be present in some foods. Nutritional intake of the antidotes to nitrite, vitamins C and E, contained in green and yellow vegetables, fruits, and other foods is low (*2*), and thus, through this association, the endogenous formation of nitrosamines cannot be excluded.

#### 2. Nitrosamides or diazo compounds—possible carcinogens for gastric cancer

Cancer of the glandular stomach has a high incidence in Japan, Iceland, the mountainous interior regions of Central and Western Latin America, and some Eastern European countries. Over the last 40 years, the gastric cancer rate in the United States has steadily declined from 30 to 9.0/100,000 for men and 22 to 3.7/100,000 for women (*31*). Dietary risk factors are a high intake of dried, salted fish; pickled vegetables; smoked fish, and also a low fruit and vegetable intake, particularly on a seasonal basis (*3*, *8*, *12*, *17*, *19*). A higher intake of uncooked vegetables such as celery, lettuce, tomatoes, and fresh fruit juices by Japanese migrants to Hawaii correlated with a lower risk of gastric cancer compared to indigenous Japanese and first generation Japanese migrants to Hawaii.

Alkylnitrosoureido compounds such as $N$-methyl-$N'$-nitro-$N$-nitrosoguanidine (MNNG) are the specific carcinogens used to induce glandular stomach cancer in animal models (*17*). Such carcinogens are formed through the reaction of nitrite and suitably substituted secondary amines or amides. Mirvish (*19*) discovered that ascorbic acid had an inhibitory effect on the nitrosation of methylurea and alkylamines.

An isolate from soy sauce, 1-methyl-1,2,3,4-tetrahydro-$\beta$-carboline-3-carboxylic acid, treated with nitrite under acidic conditions akin to stomach acidity, led to direct-acting mutagenic activity (*23*). Another promutagen identified in soy sauce, tyramine, upon nitrosation, led to a new type of direct-acting mutagen 4-(2-aminoethyl)-6-diazo-2,4-cyclohexadienone (*23*). Agaritine, $\beta$-$N$-[$\gamma$-L(+)-glutamyl]-4-hydroxymethylphenylhydrazine, from the mushroom *Agaricus bisporus* yields 4-(hydroxymethyl)phenylhydrazine upon hydrolysis, and the corresponding diazonium compound induced glandular stomach cancer in mice (*38*). **Reaction of nitrite with fava beans** yielded direct-acting mutagenic activity in the form of chloroindoles (*25*, *44a*).

Alkylating activity was discovered in several kinds of fish treated with nitrite (*45*). Our laboratory has tested fish species *sanma* and *aji*, frequently eaten in high-risk regions for stomach cancer; beans consumed in Latin America, and borscht in Eastern Europe. Direct-acting mutagenic activity was found upon reaction with nitrite at pH 3, a reaction blocked by vitamin C. A mutagenic extract induced adenocarcinomas of the glandular stomach in Wistar rats (42).

Thus, human consumption of salted, picked, and smoked foods may result in gastric cancer through the action of an active agent (or agents) formed from nitrite and undefined substrates. The formation of such carcinogens may be blocked by vitamin C or by vitamin E. Reduced use of salted and pickled foods and better nutrition accounts for the sharp decline of gastric cancer in the United States, a decline also beginning in other areas of the world (12, 42). Joossens and Geboers (12) document a parallelism in international trends between gastric cancer and stroke. Kono et al. (13) found a strong association between salt use and stroke in Japan but not with gastric cancer. This result is consistent with salt as a potentiator or cocarcinogen in human gastric cancer, rather than the initial causative stimulus. This, in turn, suggests that the carcinogen is already preformed in pickled and smoked foods, with salt acting mainly as an enhancing element.

Under these conditions, the protection afforded by yellow-green vegetables and fruits may suggest that the vitamin A or $\beta$-carotene content also deserves consideration in inhibiting the development of neoplasia (34, 35).

### 3. Comments and recommendations for prevention

One key element is avoidance of pickled, salted, or smoked foods. In addition, regular daily intake of fresh fruits, vegetables, or salads as sources of vitamins C, E, and A is important from early childhood onward to lower the risk for cancer of the glandular stomach and also of the esophagus.

### Carcinogens in Large Bowel Cancer

The specific carcinogens causing large bowel cancer and its anatomic subsegments, ascending, transverse, descending colon, and rectal cancer, are not known. For cancer of the rectum, associations with beer, stout, or ale drinking have been made (1, 26, 30). For colon cancer, several leads have appeared. The stools of individuals in high-risk populations contain mutagenic activity, and one mutagen is identified as (S)-3-(1,3,5,7,9-dodecapentienyloxy)-1,2-propanediol (7, 9). Vegetarian populations showed no fecal mutagenic activity. The mutagenic activity can be lowered by cereal fiber or increased amounts of vitamin C or E (7). Individuals with familial polyposis had its consistent neoplastic change moderated by vitamin C, a finding under further study (4).

Sugimura and associates (36) discovered that charcoal broiled fish or meat contained powerful mutagenic activity. These mutagens form during pan frying and broiling but not during cooking in water or in a microwave oven. These mutagens belong to a new class of heterocyclic amines: 2-amino-3-methylimidazo[4,5-$f$]quinoline (IQ), 2-amino-3,4-dimethylimidazo[4,5-$f$]quinoline (MeIQ), 2-amino-3,8-dimethylimidazo[4,5-$f$]quinoxaline (MeIQ$_x$), and the 3,7,8-trimethyl analog (Me$_2$IQ$_x$). Their structures resemble that of 3,2'-dimethyl-4-aminobiphenyl, which causes colon, breast, and prostate cancer in rats. These mutagens are highly active in the DNA repair test in liver cells (42) and have induced cancer of intestine, liver, ear duct, kidney, mammary gland in rats and mice (24, 37, 37a). Whether the mutagenicity found in human stools contains metabolites of these mutagens is not yet known.

Mutagen formation depends on the temperature, length of frying, and the fat content of the meat (42). Addition of soy protein, antioxidants, or ethylene diamine tetraacetic acid (EDTA) inhibits mutagen formation, whereas iron salts increase it (42).

### 1. Geographic pathology, migrant studies, special populations

Descending colon cancer exhibits a high incidence in the United States, in Western and Northern Europe, and other Anglo-Saxon countries (27). Finland is an exception with a rate as low as Japan. Vegetarian and Mormon populations frequently show a lower incidence of colon cancer (see Phillips et al. and Lyon et al. in Ref. 44). Migrants from any low-incidence region in the world to areas with a higher risk show a rapid increase in incidence (29).

### 2. Time trends

The incidence of colon cancer in the United States during the last 50 years shows a small increasing trend in males and a slight decrease in females, but in the last few decades, virtually no change in age-corrected incidence per 100,000 is noted. Mortality has also been stable or has been decreasing, more so in females (31). However, in other areas of the world, such as Scandinavia and Japan where 50 years ago the incidence was lower than in the United States, an increasing trend has appeared. These trends parallel those for coronary heart disease, postmenopausal breast cancer, and prostate cancer (10).

### 3. Definition of risk factors
#### a) Promoting effect of fat, inhibiting effect of cereal fibers

In countries with a high incidence of colon cancer, populations consume 40–45% of the daily caloric intake in total fat, saturated plus unsaturated, or about 130–150 g fat per day. In contrast, the traditional dietary fat intake in Japan accounted for 10–15% of calories with more of the fat unsaturated as fish oils. Another element is cereal fiber. People in rural Finland (Kuopio) have a traditional high intake of cereal fiber, yielding in turn a considerable stool bulk and, in part, increasing stool frequency (27). In addition, Domellöf et al. (5) and Graham (6) describe populations in northern Sweden and in the United States who, despite a sizable fat intake had a lower risk of colon cancer, intermediate between that of the population in New York and that of Japan or Finland. The lower-risk population consume more cereal fiber in northern Sweden, or in the U.S., more yellow-green vegetables. Mormons in Utah have a basically American dietary pattern, but their customary nutrition includes cereal products and bread made from stone ground grains with a higher fiber content than that of the control American population who consumed baked goods made from refined flours.

#### b) Evidence from animals

Rats on a diet containing 20% total fat (saturated and unsaturated, 40% of calories) have a higher incidence of chemically-induced colon cancer than when the fat content is 10% of calories. These animal studies, without exception, reproduce the observations made in population groups at high and low risk. Experiments with cereal fiber gave results that are not as clear-cut but usually showed that cereal fiber such as wheat bran inhibited colon carcinogenesis. Studies where a protective effect could not be demonstrated or, in a few cases where an increased incidence was found, can be explained mainly by the large dose of colon carcinogen used, or by excessive amounts of cereal bran, which have an irritating effect on the colon mucosa (14, 39). Pectin with different chemical properties inhibited the effect of carcinogens requiring biochemical activation, such as azoxymethane, but not that of direct-acting carcinogens such as $N$-nitrosomethylurea (27). Few laboratory studies have been done to account for the effect of yellow-green vegetables, especially cabbage. Wattenberg (40) noted that a laboratory chow yielded higher levels of benzo-(a)pyrene hydroxylase in rat intestines than a purified diet. Brussel sprouts or cauliflower contain indole derivatives that act as enzyme inducers and as inhibitors of the carcinogenic process (40). Butylated hydroxyanisole also inhibited colon carcinogenesis (28). Calcium salts have been suggested for reducing colon cancer risk (22).

### c) Mechanism of dietary fat and cereal fiber

Humans and animals on a 40% fat calorie diet uniformly excrete more bile acids, 12 mg/g of stool compared to 4 mg/g in groups on a low-fat (10% of calories) diet. Importantly, the population in Kuopio, Finland also had a concentration of bile acids of about 4 mg/g because of the diluting effects of larger stool bulk compared to that of the corresponding New York or Copenhagen populations (27). Bile acids do not have the properties of genotoxic carcinogens but act as promoting agents. As currently noted, the effect of promoters is highly dependent on dose and on chronicity of exposure. A comparison of the concentration of bile acids in a typical New York population with that in Japan or Finland, the difference between high- and low-risk groups, is 12:4 or only 3. Since the effect of promoters is reversible, the risk of colon cancer development can be reduced by lowering the concentration of bile acids by either a lower fat intake or a higher cereal fiber intake, or by a combination of both actions.

In familial polyposis coli and hereditary colon cancer, the fecal excretion of undegraded cholesterol is high, but that of the microbial metabolites of cholesterol is low compared with the control population (15). While the reason for this unique biochemical difference in fecal constituents is unknown, the cholesterol may stem from cells shed into the lumen. The higher fecal cholesterol level would signify a higher cell turnover and shedding rate (14, 16, 21). The chemical analysis of stools might be useful for screening.

### 4.  Comment

Fairly conclusive information on risk and protective factors bearing on the etiology of large bowel cancer has been acquired.

a.   Separate etiologic factors apply to cancer in the ascending and transverse colon than in the descending colon to the recto-sigmoid junction, or to rectal cancer.

b.   For cancer in the descending colon, the total level of dietary fat intake is a major element. A Western level of 40% fat calories represents a high-risk situation and an Asian diet of 10–15% of fat calories a low-risk situation. The underlying mechanism is control of the endogenous production of bile acids. Calcium salts may decrease the effect of bile and fatty acids as promoters.

c.   Cereal fiber or bran in adequate amounts increases stool bulk, diluting the effectors (bile acids) in colon carcinogenesis.

d.   Intake of yellow-green vegetables seems to protect, but more data are needed on the mechanisms.

e.   The genotoxic carcinogens for colon cancer are not yet fully known. High-risk individuals have bacterially-produced fecal mutagens. Also relevant are certain mutagens/carcinogens in fried foods such as aminoimidazoquinolines or quinoxalines.

f.   On the basis of currently *established* facts, lower risk for colon cancer may be secured by recommending a total fat intake of about 20% of calories, an increased consumption of bran type fibers titrated to yield a daily stool of about 200 g, and a good supply of calcium ions as found in low-fat dairy products.

## Overall Recommendations for Prevention

The causative and modifying factors for head and neck, and gastric cancers are clearly quite different from those elements related to the other nutritionally-linked cancers as cancer of the colon, breast, prostate, and endometrium that are seen more frequently in the Western World. It is desirable to distinguish between causative factors that are classified as genotoxic carcinogens and others that act by promoting mechanisms. Exposure to genotoxic elements need not last a lifetime, especially if such exposure occurred early in life. The effect of dietary fat mechanistically relates to promoting effects, which are reversible and highly dose-dependent. A lower intake can be practiced in any population at any age. It is likely to be effective in lowering the risk of recurrence in individuals who have had colon or breast cancer. Increasing intake of bran-containing cereal fiber to increase stool bulk is desirable to effect a lower risk for cancer of the colon and possibly other intestinal diseases.

Another dietary change follows almost automatically, namely, an increased intake of fruits, vegetables, and salads (without high-fat dressings) since this will be necessary to balance the daily caloric requirements. Useful calcium and magnesium are obtained from an adequate intake of skim milk or other nonfat dairy products such as yoghurt or low-fat cheese.

The last recommendation is to lower the intake of heavily fried or broiled fish or meats and to lower the formation of mutagens and carcinogens by antioxidants or chelating agents. Soy protein can be mixed with ground meat before frying to decrease mutagen/carcinogen content.

Anywhere in the world, the occurrence of nutritionally-linked cancers can be lowered by avoiding the use of highly salted, pickled, or smoked foods, or foods containing mycotoxins; by eating no more than 20% of calories in total fat; by consuming an adequate amount of cereal fiber to ensure proper stool bulk, and by eating a sizable part of the daily caloric needs as complex carbohydrates found in whole grains, cereal products, fruits, and vegetables. Such a new dietary tradition would most likely also lower the risk for hypertension and stroke, hypercholesterolemia, atherosclerosis, and coronary heart disease.

## Acknowledgments

These investigations were supported by United States Public Health Service grants through the National Cancer Institute grants CA-29602 and CA-24217. Mrs. Clara Horn has provided excellent editorial services.

## REFERENCES

1. Anonymous. Beer drinking and the risk of rectal cancer. *Nutr. Rev.*, **42**, 244–247 (1984).
2. Bright-see, E. Vitamins C and E (or fruits and vegetables) and the prevention of human cancer. *In* "Nutrition Factors in the Induction and Maintenance of Malignancy," ed. C. E. Butterworth, Jr. and M. L. Hutchinson, pp. 217–223 (1983). Academic Press, New York.

3.  Correa, P., Cuello, C., Fajardo, L. F., Haenszel, W., Bolanos, O., and de Ramirez, B. Diet and gastric cancer: Nutrition survey in a high-risk area. *J. Natl. Cancer Inst.*, **70**, 673–678 (1983).

4.  DeCosse, J. J. Potential for chemoprevention. *Cancer*, **50**, 2550–2553 (1982).

5.  Domellöf, L., Darby, L., Hanson, D., Mathews, L., Simi, B., and Reddy, B. S. Fecal sterols and bacterial β-glucuronidase activity: a preliminary metabolic epidemiology study of healthy volunteers from Umea, Sweden, and Metropolitan New York. *Nutr. Cancer*, **4**, 120–127 (1982).

6.  Graham, S. Results of case-control studies of diet and cancer in Buffalo, New York. *Cancer Res.*, **43**, 2409–2413 (1983).

7.  Gupta, I., Baptista, J., Bruce, W. R., Che, C. T., Furrer, R., Gingerich, J. S., Grey, A. A., Marai, L., Yates, P., and Krepinsky, J. J. Structures of fecapentaenes, the mutagens of bacterial origin isolated from human feces. *Biochemistry*, **22**, 241–245 (1983).

8.  Hill, M. J. Environmental and genetic factors in gastrointestinal cancer. *In* "Precancerous Lesions of the Gastrointestinal Tract," ed. P. Sherlock, B. C. Morson, L. Barbara, and U. Veronesi, pp. 1–22 (1983). Raven Press, New York.

9.  Hirai, N., Kingston, D.G.I., Van Tassell, R. L., and Wilkins, T. D. Structure elucidation of a potent mutagen from human feces. *J. Am. Chem. Soc.*, **104**, 6149–6150 (1982).

10. Hirayama, T. Diet and cancer. *Nutr. Cancer*, **1**, 67–80 (1979).

11. Hoffmann, D. and Adams, J. D. Carcinogenic tobacco specific N-nitrosamines in snuff and in the saliva of snuff dippers. *Cancer Res.*, **41**, 4305–4308 (1981).

12. Joossens, J. V. and Geboers, J. Epidemiology of gastric cancer. *In* "Precancerous Lesions of the Gastro-intestinal Tract," ed. P. Sherlock, B. C. Morson, L. Barbara, U., and Veronesi U., pp. 97–114 (1983). Raven Press, New York.

13. Kono, S., Ideda, M., and Ogata, M. Salt and geographical mortality of gastric cancer and stroke in Japan. *J. Epidemiol. Community Health*, **37**, 43–46 (1983).

14. Lipkin, M., Blattner, W. A., Gardner, E. J., Burt, R. W., Lynch, H., Deschner, E., Winawer, S., and Fraumeni, J. F., Jr. Classification and risk assessment of individuals with familial polyposis, Gardner's syndrome, and familial non-polyposis colon cancer from [³H]thymidine labeling patterns in colonic epithelial cells. *Cancer Res.*, **44**, 4201–4207, (1984).

15. Lipkin, M., Reddy, B. S., Weisburger, J. H., and Schecter, L. Nondegradation of fecal cholesterol in subjects at high risk for cancer of the large intestine. *J. Clin. Invest.*, **67**, 304–307 (1981).

16. Luk, G. D. and Baylin, S. B. Ornithine decarboxylase as a biologic marker in familial colonic polyposis. *New Engl. J. Med.*, **311**, 80–83 (1984).

17. Magee, P. N. (ed.) Banbury Report 12, "Nitrosamines and Human Cancer" (1982). Cold Spring Harbor Lab., Cold Spring Harbor, New York.

18. Miller, E. C. and Miller, J. A. Mechanisms of chemical carcinogenesis. *Cancer*, **47**, 1055–1064 (1981).

19. Mirvish, S. S. The etiology of gastric cancer. *J. Natl. Cancer Inst.*, **71**, 631–647 (1983).

20. Muñoz, N., Crespi, M., Grassi, A., Qing, W. G., Qiong, S., and Cai, L. Z. Precursor lesions of oesophageal cancer in high-risk populations in Iran and China. *Lancet*, **i**, 876–879 (1982).

21. Narisawa, T., Sato, M., Sano, M., and Takahashi, T. Inhibition of development of methylnitrosourea-induced rat colonic tumors by peroral administration of indomethacin. *Gann*, **73**, 377–381 (1982).

22. Newmark, H. L., Wargovich, M. J., and Bruce, W. R. Colon cancer and dietary fat, phosphate, and calcium: a hypothesis. *J. Natl. Cancer Inst.*, **72**, 1323–1326 (1984).

23. Ochiai, M., Wakabayashi, K., Nagao, M., and Sugimura, T. Tyramine is a major mutagen precursor in soy sauce, being convertible to a mutagen by nitrite. *Gann*, **75**, 1–3 (1984).

24. Ohgaki, H., Kusama, K., Matsukura, N., Morino, K., Hasegawa, H., Sato, S., Takayama, S., and Sugimura, T. Carcinogenicity in mice of a mutagenic compound, 2-amino-3-methyl-imidazo[4, 5-*f*]quinoline, from broiled sardine, cooked beef and beef extract. *Carcinogenesis*, **5**, 921–924 (1984).

25. Piacek-Llanes, B. G. and Tannenbaum, S. R. Formation of an activated *N*-nitroso compound in nitrite-treated fava beans (*Vicia faba*). *Carcinogenesis*, **3**, 1379–1384 (1982).

26. Pollack, E. S., Nomura, A.M.Y., Heilbrun, L. K., Stemmermann, G. N., and Green, S. B. Prospective study of alcohol consumption and cancer. *New Engl. J. Med.*, **310**, 617–621 (1984).

27. Reddy, B. S., Cohen, L. A., McCoy, D., Hill, P., Weisburger, J. H., and Wynder, E. L. Nutrition and its relationship to cancer. *Adv. Cancer Res.*, **32**, 237–245 (1980).

28. Reddy, B. S., Maeura, Y., and Weisburger, J. H. Effect of various levels of dietary butylated hydroxyanisole on methylazoxymethanol acetate-induced colon carcinogensis in CF/mice. *J. Natl. Cancer Inst.*, **71**, 1299–1305 (1983).

29. Schottenfeld, D. and Fraumeni, J. F., Jr., (eds.) "Cancer Epidemiology and Prevention" (1982). W. B. Saunders Co., Philadelphia.

30. Seitz, H. K., Czygan, P., Waldherr, R., Veith, S., Raedsch, R., Kässmodel, H., and Kommerell, B. Enhancement of 1, 2-dimethylhydrazine-induced rectal carcinogenesis following chronic ethanol consumption in the rat. *Gastroenterology*, **86**, 886–891 (1984).

31. Silverberg, E. and Lubera, J. A. Cancer statistics. *CA-A Cancer J. Clin.*, **34**, 2–25 (1984).

32. Slaga, T. J. Overview of tumor promotion in animals. *Environ. Health Perspect.*, **50**, 3–14 (1983).

33. Slaga, T. J. and Montesano, R. (eds.) Tumour promotion and human cancer. *Cancer Surv.*, **2**, 519–621 (1983).

34. Sporn, M. B. and Roberts, A. B. Role of retinoids in differentiation and carcinogenesis. *Cancer Res.*, **43**, 3034–3040 (1983).

35. Stähelin, H. B., Buess, E., Rösel, E., Widmer, L. K., and Brubacher, G. Vitamin A, cardiovascular risk factors, and mortality. *Lancet*, **i**, 394–395 (1982).

36. Sugimura, T. and Sato, S. Mutagens-carcinogens in food. *Cancer Res.*, **43**, 2415s–2421s (1983).

37. Takayama, S., Nakatsuru, Y., Masuda, M., Ohgaki, H., Sato, S., and Sugimura, T. Demonstration of carcinogencity in F344 rats of 2-amino-3-methylimidazo[4, 5-*f*]quinoline from broiled sardine, fried beef and beef extract. *Gann*, **75**, 467–470 (1984).

37a. Tanaka, T., Barnes, W. S., Williams, G. M., and Weisburger, J. H. Multipotential carcinogenicity of the fried food mutagen 2-amino-3-methylimidazo [4, 5-f] quinoline in rats. *Jpn. J. Cancer Res.* (*Gann*), **76**, 570–576 (1985).

38. Toth, B., Nagel, D., and Ross, A. Gastric tumorigenesis by a single dose of 4-(hydroxymethyl)benzenediazonium ion of *Agariscus bisporus*. *Br. J. Cancer*, **46**, 417–422 (1982).

39. Vahouny, G. V. and Kritchevsky, D. (eds.) "Dietary Fiber in Health and Disease" (1982). Plenum Press, New York.

40. Wattenberg, L. V. Inhibition of neoplasia by minor dietary constituents. *Cancer Res.*, **43**, 2448s–2453s (1983).

41. Weinberg, R. A. Oncogenes of spontaneous and chemically induced tumors, *Adv. Cancer Res.*, **36**, 149–164 (1983).

42. Weisburger, J. H., Horn, C. L., and Barnes, W. S. Possible genotoxic carcinogens in foods in relation to cancer causation. *Semin. Oncol.*, **10**, 330–341 (1983).

43. Weisburger, J. H. and Williams, G. M. Bioassay of carcinogens: *in vitro* and *in vivo* tests. *In* "Chemical Carcinogens," ed. C. E. Searle, pp. 1323–1373 (1984). American Chemical Society, Washington, D. C.

44. Wynder, E. L., Leveille, G. A., Weisburger, J. H., and Livingston, G. (eds.) "Environmental Aspects of Cancer: the Role of Macro and Micro Components of Foods" (1983). Food and Nutrition Press, Westport, Conn.

44a. Young, D., Tannenbaum, S. R., Büchi, G., and Lee, G. C. M. 4-Chloro-6-methoxyindole
     is the precursor of a potent mutagen (4-chloro-6-methoxy-2-hydroxy-1-nitroso-indoline-
     3-one oxime) that forms during nitrosation of the fava bean (*Vicia faba*). *Carcinogenesis*,
     **5**, 1219–1224 (1984).
45.  Yano, K. Alkylating activity of processed fish products treated with sodium nitrite in
     simulated gastric juice. *Gann*, **72**, 451–454 (1981).

# AUTHOR INDEX

# SUBJECT INDEX

278